Study Guide

to accompany

Wong's Nursing Care of Infants and Children

Seventh Edition

Study Guide

to accompany

Wong's Nursing Care of Infants and Children

Seventh Edition

By

Anne Rath Rentfro, MSN, RN, CS

Associate Professor of Nursing
The University of Texas at Brownsville
in partnership with Texas Southmost College
Brownsville, Texas

Linda Sawyer McCampbell, MSN, APRN, BC

Family Nurse Practitioner
Rural Clinics of South Texas
Port Isabel Health Clinic
Port Isabel, Texas

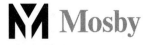

An Affiliate of Elsevier Science
St. Louis   London   Philadelphia   Sydney   Toronto

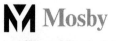 Mosby

An Affiliate of Elsevier Science

11830 Westline Industrial Drive
St. Louis, Missouri 63146

Study Guide to accompany *Wong's Nursing Care of Infants and Children*   ISBN 0-323-01732-0
Seventh Edition
Copyright © 2003,   Mosby, Inc.   All rights reserved.

Notice

Pharmacology is an ever-changing field. Standard safety precautions must be followed, but as new research and clinical experience broaden our knowledge, changes in treatment and drug therapy may become necessary or appropriate. Readers are advised to check the most current product information provided by the manufacturer of each drug to be administered to verify the recommended dose, the method and duration of administration, and contraindications. It is the responsibility of the licensed prescriber, relying on experience and knowledge of the patient, to determine dosages and the best treatment for each individual patient. Neither the publisher nor the editor assumes any liability for any injury and/or damage to persons or property arising from this publication.

The Publisher

Vice President/Publishing Director, Nursing: Sally Schrefer
Executive Editor: Loren S. Wilson
Senior Developmental Editor: Michele D. Hayden
Project Manager: Gayle May Morris
Design Manager: Bill Drone

WB/EB

Printed in the United States of America

Last digit is the print number: 9   8   7   6   5   4   3   2   1

Preface

This Study Guide accompanies the seventh edition of *Wong's Nursing Care of Infants and Children*. Students may use the Study Guide not only to review content but also to enhance their learning through critical thinking. The Study Guide is designed to assist students in mastering the content presented in the text, developing problem-solving skills, and applying their knowledge to nursing practice.

Each chapter in the Study Guide includes questions that will assist students to meet the objectives of each corresponding textbook chapter. Because most students using this Study Guide will also be preparing to pass the nursing examination (NCLEX), we have primarily used a multiple-choice format. A Critical Thinking section is also included for each chapter, with questions designed to help students analyze the chapter's content and address their own attitudes about pediatric nursing practice. Case Studies were used in many of the Critical Thinking sections to give students experience in addressing specific practice issues. All case presentations are fictitious but designed to address situations that are frequently encountered by the nurse in practice. This new edition also includes features to help students learn and retain pediatric terminology used in each chapter.

How to Use the Study Guide

We intend for students to use this Study Guide as they study a chapter in the textbook, processing the material chapter by chapter and section by section. For this reason we chose to present the questions in an order that follows the textbook's content. Students will find the answers to the questions for each chapter at the end of the Study Guide. Page numbers from the textbook have been included to facilitate finding content related to the answers.

It is our hope that this Study Guide will function as both an aid to learning and a means for measuring progress in the mastery of pediatric nursing practice.

Anne Rath Rentfro
Linda Sawyer McCampbell

Contents

CHAPTER 1

Perspectives of Pediatric Nursing

1. The following terms are related to health during childhood. Match each term with its corresponding definition or description. (This exercise is continued on next page.)

a. Health
b. Mortality
c. Morbidity
d. National Health Promotion and Disease Prevention Objectives
e. Vital statistics
f. Mortality statistics
g. National Center of Health Statistics (NCHS)
h. Infant mortality rate
i. Neonatal mortality
j. Postneonatal mortality
k. Birth weight

l. Low birth weight (LBW)
m. Family Medical Leave Act of 1993
n. Perinatal mortality rate
o. Violent deaths
p. Suicide
q. Morbidity statistics
r. Acute illness
s. Disability
t. New morbidity
u. Accident
v. Injury
w. Host
x. Environment

y. Agent
z. Passive strategies
aa. Active strategies
bb. Consumer Product Safety Commission (CPSC)
cc. Financial barriers
dd. System barriers
ee. Knowledge barriers
ff. Prospective payment system
gg. Diagnosis-related groups (DRG)
hh. Health maintenance organization (HMO)

_____ Companies that provide health care within a managed care framework

_____ Symptoms severe enough to limit activity or require medical attention

_____ A form of self-violence; the third leading cause of death among teenagers and young adults 15 to 24 years of age

_____ Commonly defined as the number of fetal deaths (fetuses of 28 weeks or more gestation) and deaths in infants under 7 days of age per 100 live births

_____ Responsible for the collection, analysis, and dissemination of data on the health of Americans

_____ Death

_____ The object that is the direct cause of an injury

_____ A major change in health care delivery that bases payment on pretreatment billing

_____ Describes the incidence or number of individuals who have died over a specific period of time

_____ Illness

_____ Statistical rate expressed as the number of deaths within 28 days of birth

_____ Categories that define prospective billing for almost all U.S. hospitals reimbursed by Medicare

_____ A state of complete physical, mental, and social well-being and not merely the absence of disease

_____ A key factor contributing to the fact that neonatal mortality rates are higher in the United States than in other developed countries

_____ The major determinant of neonatal death in technologically developed countries

_____ A chaotic, random event that is based on luck or chance

_____ The legislation that determines eligibility to take leave from work to care for infants

_____ Measured in days off from school or days confined to bed

_____ The person affected by an injury

_____ An occurrence that has steadily increased recently among young people between the ages of 10 and 25 years, especially blacks and males

_____ The time and place of an injury

_____ Increase the span of healthy life for Americans, reduce health disparities among Americans, and achieve access to preventive services for all Americans

_____ Established by the U.S. government to protect the public against unreasonable risk for injury and death associated with products

_____ The preferred term to use when discussing the leading cause of death in children over age 1 year; connotes a sense of responsibility and control

_____ Examples include a lack of understanding about the need or value of prenatal or child health supervision or an unawareness of the services that are available

_____ Examples include not having insurance, having insurance that does not cover certain services, or being unable to pay for services

_____ Pediatric social illness; behavioral, social, family, and educational problems

_____ Prevention strategies used to persuade individuals to change their behavior for increased self-protection, such as the use of seat belts

_____ The prevalence of a specific illness in the population at a particular time, generally presented as rates per 1000 population

_____ Prevention strategies providing automatic protection by product and environment design, such as air bags

_____ Examples include the need to travel great distance for health care or state-to-state variations in Medicaid benefits

_____ The number of deaths during the first year of life per 1000 live births

_____ The number of deaths that occur from 28 days to 11 months of life

_____ Figures describing rates of occurrence of events such as death in children

2. Match each pediatric nursing term with its definition or description.

a. Definition of nursing
b. Family-centered care
c. Enable
d. Empowerment
e. Parent-professional partnership
f. Atraumatic care
g. Therapeutic care
h. Setting
i. Personnel
j. Interventions
k. Psychologic distress
l. Physical distress

m. Clinical practice guidelines
n. Agency for Health Care Policy and Research (AHCPR)
o. Therapeutic relationship
p. Nontherapeutic
q. Caring
r. Pediatric nurse practitioner (PNP)
s. Clinical nurse specialist (CNS)
t. Advanced nurse practitioner (ANP)

u. Autonomy
v. Nonmaleficence
w. Beneficence
x. Justice
y. Nursing process
z. Community-based health driven system
aa. Standard of practice
bb. Provider of care
cc. Manager of care
dd. Unlicensed assistive personnel
ee. Evidence-based practice

_____ Recognizes the family as the constant in a child's life

_____ A mechanism for enabling and empowering families where parents serve as respected equals with professionals and have the rightful role in deciding what is important for themselves and their family; a relationship in which the professional's role is to support and strengthen the family's ability to nurture and promote its members' development in a way that is both enabling and empowering

_____ The diagnosis and treatment of human responses to actual or potential health problems

_____ The patient's right to be self-governing

_____ Therapeutic care provided through the use of interventions that eliminate or minimize the psychologic and physical distress experienced by children and their families in the health care system

_____ A systematic problem-solving method used routinely by nurses

_____ Creating opportunities and means for all family members to display their present abilities and competencies and to acquire new ones that are necessary to meet the needs of the child and family

_____ Includes anyone directly involved in providing therapeutic care

_____ Describes the interaction of professionals with families in such a way that families maintain or acquire a sense of control over their family lives

_____ Individuals who are trained to function in an assistive role to the registered professional nurse in the provision of care activities as delegated by and under the supervision of the registered professional nurse

_____ May include anxiety, fear, anger, disappointment, sadness, shame, or guilt

_____ Encompasses the prevention, diagnosis, treatment, or palliation of chronic or acute conditions

_____ Reflects the research that has been conducted relative to a specific disease or illness

_____ Refers to the place in which care is given

_____ A meaningful relationship with children and their families that has well-defined boundaries that separate the nurse from the child and family

_____ The level of performance that is expected of a professional

_____ A relationship where boundaries that separate the nurse from the child and family are blurred

_____ A role that combines the responsibilities of clinical nurse specialist and nurse practitioner

_____ A specialized ambulatory or primary care role for pediatric nurses

_____ May range from sleeplessness and immobilization to the experience of disturbing sensory stimuli such as pain, temperature extremes, loud noises, bright lights, or darkness

_____ Expressing compassion and empathy for others

_____ Approaches ranging from psychologic interventions, such as preparing children for procedures, to physical interventions, such as providing space for a parent to room-in with a child

_____ A U.S. federal agency founded in 1989 for the purpose of developing national guidelines and enhancing the quality, appropriateness, and effectiveness of care

_____ A role developed in an attempt to provide expert nursing care; serves as a role model, a researcher, a change agent, and a consultant

_____ The obligation to minimize or prevent harm

_____ The traditional role of the nurse, in the which the focus is promotion, maintenance, and restoration of health

_____ The system of the future, in which the nurse's role will expand to health care planning, particularly on a political or legislative level

_____ The obligation to promote the patient's well-being

_____ The concept of fairness

_____ A role of the nurse that requires a shift in thinking and different skills from those needed for health promotion, health maintenance, and health restoration; a shift from performing tasks to collaborative practice

_____ A system of nursing that involves questioning why something is effective and whether there is a better approach

3. Match each term with its definition or description.

a. Critical thinking
b. Nursing diagnosis
c. Problem statement
d. Risk factors
e. Etiology
f. Signs and symptoms

g. Dependent activities
h. Interdependent activities
i. Independent activities
j. Outcome
k. Standard care plans
l. Individualized care plans

m. Joint Commission on Accreditation of Healthcare Organizations (JCAHO)
n. Continuous quality improvement (CQI)

_____ Issues contributing to a person's or population's susceptibility to a potential health problem

_____ The governing body from which many types of health care providers (including hospitals, nursing homes, ambulatory services, and home health agencies) are required to obtain accreditation status to receive federal funds, such as Medicare or Medicaid.

_____ A clinical judgment about individual, family, or community responses to actual and potential health problems/life processes

_____ Refers to a cluster of cues and/or defining characteristics that are derived from patient assessment and that indicate actual health problems

_____ Purposeful, goal-directed thinking that assists individuals to make judgments based on evidence rather than guesswork

_____ Those areas of nursing practice that hold the nurse accountable for implementing the prescribed treatment

_____ The process of ongoing review of systems, problem identification, and resolution; allows the institution to establish and maintain quality care

_____ The first component of the nursing diagnosis; describes the response to health pattern deficits

_____ Those areas of nursing practice in which nursing responsibility and accountability overlap with other disciplines, such as medicine, and require collaboration between the two disciplines

_____ Plans that are sufficiently broad to account for situations that may develop in patients with particular problems

_____ The second component of the nursing diagnosis; describes the physiologic, situational, and maturational factors that cause the problem or influence its development

_____ Those areas of nursing practice that are the direct responsibility of the nurse

_____ Care plans that are concerned only with those diagnoses that apply to the particular patient situation

_____ The projected change in a patient's health status, clinical condition, or behavior that occurs after nursing interventions have been instituted

4. According to Healthy People 2010, priority areas for the nation include all *except*:
   a. decreasing tobacco use.
   b. increasing innovative treatments.
   c. decreasing substance abuse.
   d. increasing immunization.

5. Which one of the following statements is true about infant mortality in the United States?
   a. There has been a recent dramatic increase in infant mortality in the U.S.
   b. The U.S. currently holds its highest infant mortality rate ever.
   c. Most countries with lower infant morality rates than the U.S. have national insurance programs.
   d. The U.S. has lower infant mortality rates than most other developed countries.

6. The major determinant of neonatal death in technologically developed countries is:
   a. birth weight.
   b. short gestation.
   c. long gestation.
   d. HIV infection.

7. Which one of the following causes of death accounts for the most deaths in infants under 1 year of age?
   a. Pneumonia and influenza
   b. Infections specific to the perinatal period
   c. Accidents and adverse effects
   d. Congenital anomalies

8. Neural tube defects are expected to decrease as much as 50% with the current recommendation by the

   American Academy of Pediatrics for all women of childbearing age to receive _____

   _____ supplementation.

9. Which of the following differences is seen when infant death rates are categorized according to race?
   a. Infant mortality for Native Americans has decreased dramatically in the last two decades.
   b. Infant mortality for Hispanic infants is much higher than for any other group.
   c. Infant mortality for black infants is much higher than for any other group.
   d. Infant mortality for white infants is the same as for other races.

10. After a child reaches the age of 1 year, the leading cause of death is from:
    a. human immunodeficiency virus (HIV).
    b. congenital anomalies.
    c. cancer.
    d. accidents.

11. Causes of violence against children can usually be attributed to:
    a. the presence of firearms in the household.
    b. numerous socioeconomic influences.
    c. depression.
    d. poor safety devices on firearms.

12. The disease that continues to be a leading cause of death in all age groups of children is:
    a. heart disease.
    b. acquired immunodeficiency syndrome (AIDS).
    c. cancer.
    d. infectious disease.

13. Morbidity statistics that depict the prevalence of a specific illness in the population are:
    a. presented as rates per 100 population.
    b. difficult to define.
    c. denoting acute illness only.
    d. denoting chronic disease only.

14. Fifty percent of all acute conditions of childhood can be accounted for by:
    a. injuries and accidents.
    b. bacterial infections.
    c. parasitic disease.
    d. respiratory illness.

15. Identify one major category of disease that children tend to contract in infancy and early childhood.

16. List three factors that contribute to increasing the morbidity of any disorder in children.

17. The degree of disability in children can be measured by:
    a. days of hospitalization.
    b. developmental stages.
    c. days absent from school or confined to bed.
    d. physical growth patterns.

18. Another term for "the new morbidity" is:
    a. pediatric social illness.
    b. pediatric noncompliance.
    c. learning disorder.
    d. dyslexia.

19. Which one of the following statements about injuries in childhood is *false*?
    a. Developmental stage determines the prevalence of injuries at a given age.
    b. Most fatal injuries occur in children under the age of 9 years.
    c. Developmental stage helps to direct preventive measures.
    d. Children ages 5 to 9 years are at greatest risk for bicycle injuries.

20. When evaluating a child's injury and the circumstances under which it occurred, the nurse should:
    a. provide anticipatory guidance.
    b. judge whether this injury could have been prevented.
    c. analyze the specific type of injury in regard to age.
    d. decide whether the cause of injury was intentional.

21. Identify the following strategies as either passive or active prevention measures.

    a. _____ Childproof medicine caps

    b. _____ Airbags

    c. _____ Smoke detectors

    d. _____ Seat belts

    e. _____ Safety restraints

    f. _____ Automatic seat belts

    g. _____ Warning labels

    h. _____ Automatic fire sprinklers

    i. _____ Education about firearms

    j. _____ Anticipatory guidance

    k. _____ Window guards

    l. _____ Mandatory seat belt laws

    m. _____ Bicycle helmet laws

    n. _____ Childproof cigarette lighters

    o. _____ Swimming pool fences

    p. _____ Swimming pool surface alarm

22. Which one of the following statements about injury prevention in children is true?

    a. A teaching strategy that includes only the mother may be the most effective with the Hispanic population.

    b. Research indicates that influential members of the Hispanic child's family should be included in education about child car restraints.

    c. Parents of two or more children are likely to be familiar with all areas of child safety.

    d. Parents are usually aware of their child's developmental progress and capabilities.

23. _____ _____ refers to the teaching and counseling given to parents and others about developmental expectations that serve to alert parents to the issues that are most likely to arise at a given age.

24. Child health care in the United States has evolved from the colonial era, with its many hazards and epidemics, to the advances of the twentieth century, when studies of economic and social factors stimulated the creation of better standards of care for mothers and children.

    Indicate whether each of the following is more characteristic of colonial times or modern (industrial) times.

    a. _____ Nurses need to be aware of economics.

    b. _____ Milk stations are common.

    c. _____ Many parents are illiterate.

    d. _____ Knowledge barriers (e.g., not knowing about available services) are common.

    e. _____ Services include rooming in, sibling visitation, child life (play) programs.

    f. _____ Books are scarce.

    g. _____ This period is the dawn of improved health care.

    h. _____ Maternal and child health services, disabled children's services, and child welfare services are instituted.

    i. _____ Quackery is common.

    j. _____ Lina Rogers becomes the first full-time school nurse.

k. _____ There is a decline in infant mortality.

l. _____ Exposure to new fatal diseases is common.

m. _____ Prevention and health promotion measures are important issues.

n. _____ Lillian Wald founds the Henry Street Settlement.

o. _____ Spitz and Robertson demonstrate the effects of isolation and maternal deprivation.

p. _____ Statistics on childhood mortality are unavailable.

q. _____ Parents are prohibited from visiting sick children.

r. _____ Isolation and maternal deprivation are common.

s. _____ Midwives are untrained; practice is based on past experiences.

t. _____ Lillian Wald founds the field of community nursing.

u. _____ Parent education becomes an important issue.

v. _____ Few physicians have any formal training.

w. _____ Epidemic diseases are common.

x. _____ Cow's milk is the chief source of bovine tuberculosis.

y. _____ Financial issues pose barriers to health care (e.g., lack of health insurance).

z. _____ Smallpox, measles, mumps, chickenpox, and influenza are common.

aa. _____ School health helps to develop pediatric courses.

bb. _____ Diagnosis-related groups (DRGs) are used to measure a facility's delivery of care.

cc. _____ Diphtheria, yellow fever, cholera, and whooping cough are common.

dd. _____ Cow's milk is the chief source of infantile diarrhea.

ee. _____ Nurses are employed to teach parents and children.

ff. _____ Prehospitalization preparation

gg. _____ Dysentery is common.

hh. _____ Abraham Jacobi becomes known as the father of pediatrics.

ii. _____ Measures for controlling diseases are unknown.

jj. _____ Sanitation and pasteurization of cow's milk is practiced.

kk. _____ System barriers, such as state-to-state variations, exist.

ll. _____ American Medical Association opposes the Maternity and Infancy Act.

mm. _____ American Academy of Pediatrics is created.

nn. _____ Medical care is generally limited to the wealthy.

oo. _____ Title V of the Social Security Act is passed.

pp. _____ There is a shortage of physicians.

qq. _____ White House Conference on Children is held.

25. Match each federal program with the impact it has on maternal and child health.

    a. Education of the Handicapped Act Amendments of 1986 (P.L. 99-457)
    b. Social Services Block Grant
    c. Alcohol, Drug Abuse, and Mental Health Block Grants
    d. Education for All Handicapped Children Act (P.L. 94-142)
    e. Medicaid
    f. Family and Medical Leave Act (FMLA)
    g. Aid to Families with Dependent Children (AFDC)
    h. MCH Service Block Grant
    i. Women, Infants, and Children (WIC)
    j. Omnibus Budget Reconciliation Act of 1990

    _____ Created in 1965, the largest maternal-child health program; program under which the Child Health Assessment Program (CHAP) provides services for children and pregnant women, with eligibility varying from state to state

    _____ Created in 1935 as a cash grant to aid needy children without fathers

    _____ Provides services to reduce infant mortality, disease, and disabilities and to increase access to care

    _____ Established in 1981 to fund projects related to substance abuse and treatment of mentally disturbed children

    _____ Provides funds for child protective services, family planning, and foster care

    _____ Started in 1974 to provide nutritious food and education to low-income childbearing women, infants, and children up to age 5 years

    _____ Passed in 1975 to provide free public education to disabled children

    _____ Provides funding for multidisciplinary programs for disabled infants and toddlers

    _____ Allows employees to take unpaid leave (1993)

    _____ Requires states to extend Medicaid coverage to children 6 to 18 years of age with family incomes below 133% of poverty level

26. List three barriers to health care in the United States and give an example of each one.

27. Define the following components of prospective payment.

    Prospective payment system based on diagnosis-related groups:

    Health maintenance organizations:

    Managed health care:

28. Two basic concepts in the philosophy of family-centered pediatric nursing care are:
    a. enabling and empowerment.
    b. empowerment and bias.
    c. enabling and curing.
    d. empowerment and self-control.

29. The role of the nurse in the parent-professional partnership is to:
    a. decide what is most important for the family.
    b. decide what is most important for the child.
    c. strengthen the family's ability to nurture.
    d. manipulate the available resources.

30. An example of atraumatic care would be to:
    a. eliminate all traumatic procedures.
    b. restrict visiting hours to adults only.
    c. perform invasive procedures only in the treatment room.
    d. remove parents from the room during painful procedures.

31. _____ _____ is a health care delivery system that balances quality and cost and that has been shown to improve satisfaction, decrease fragmentation, and measure patient outcomes.

32. As the movement for providing care based on guidelines continues, nurses will be using:
    a. Agency for Health Care Policy and Research (AHCPR) guidelines in place of guidelines developed locally.
    b. guidelines that are based on traditional practice.
    c. timelines that are developed locally.
    d. guidelines that reflect current research but decrease job satisfaction.

33. Match each role of the pediatric nurse with its description.

    a. Family advocacy/caring   f. Restorative care
    b. Disease prevention/health promotion   g. Coordination/collaboration
    c. Health teaching   h. Ethical decision making
    d. Support   i. Research
    e. Counseling   j. Health care planning

    _____ A mutual exchange of ideas and opinions
    _____ Extending to include the community or society as a whole
    _____ Health maintenance strategies
    _____ Working together as a member of the health team
    _____ Providing physical and emotional care (feeding/bathing)
    _____ Systematically recording and analyzing observations
    _____ Attention to emotional needs (listening/physical presence)
    _____ Transmitting information
    _____ Using patient/family/societal values in care
    _____ Acting in the child's best interest

Critical Thinking—Case Study

Marisa Gutierrez arrives with her infant Sara in the well-baby clinic. Sara, who is 14 months old, is the youngest of three children. Her mother has brought her to the clinic for well-child care. Sara's two brothers, who are 7 and 8 years old, have come along. As the nurse interviews the mother, Sara explores the examination room. She reaches for her older brothers' marbles and puts one in her mouth.

34. After organizing the data into similar categories, the nurse makes which one of the following decisions?
    a. No dysfunctional health problems are evident.
    b. High risk for dysfunctional health problems exists.
    c. Actual dysfunctional health problems are evident.
    d. Potential complications are evident.

35. The nurse then identifies a possible human response pattern to further classify the data. Which one of the following functional health patterns would be *best* for the nurse to select?
    a. Role-relationship pattern
    b. Nutritional-metabolic pattern
    c. Coping-stress tolerance pattern
    d. Self-perception/self-concept pattern

36. Based on the data collected, which one of the following nursing diagnoses would be most appropriate?
    a. Altered family process
    b. Altered family coping
    c. Altered individual coping
    d. Altered parenting

37. Which one of the following patient outcomes is individualized for Sara?
    a. Sara will receive her immunizations on time.
    b. Sara will demonstrate adherence to the nurse's recommendations.
    c. Marisa Gutierrez will verbalize the need to keep small objects away from Sara to avoid aspiration.
    d. Sara's brothers will verbalize the need to stop playing with small objects.

38. During the evaluation phase, which one of the following responses by Sara's mother would indicate that the expected outcomes have been met?
    a. "I will have to go through all of the boys' things when we get home to be sure there aren't any other small objects that could hurt Sara."
    b. "I had forgotten how curious babies are. It has been many years since the boys were babies, and they didn't have an older child's toys around."
    c. "I will have to start to discipline Sara now so that she knows not to play with the older children's belongings."
    d. "I am afraid she cannot receive her immunizations. She had a fever after her last one."

39. At Sara's next well-baby visit, what information will be most important to document in the chart?
    a. Written evidence of progress toward outcomes
    b. The standard care plan
    c. Broad-based goals
    d. Interventions applicable to patients like Sara

CHAPTER 2

Social, Cultural, and Religious Influences on Child Health Promotion

1. Match each term with its definition or description.

a. Transcultural nursing orientation

b. Culture

c. Race

d. Socialization

e. Material overt/manifest culture

f. Nonmaterial covert culture

g. Subcultures

h. Roles

i. Primary group

j. Secondary group

k. Ethnic stereotyping

l. Absolute standard of poverty

m. Visible poverty

n. Invisible poverty

o. Relative standard of poverty

p. Episodically poor

q. Chronically poor

r. Parens patriae

s. Homeless individual

_____ Characterized by limited intermittent contact; generally less concern for members' behavior; usually offer little in terms of support or pressure toward conformity except in rigidly limited areas

_____ A division of humankind possessing traits that are transmissible by descent and sufficient to characterize it as distinct human type

_____ An awareness of the nurse's own frame of reference with a conscious effort to recognize and appreciate the views and beliefs of the health care recipients

_____ The process by which children acquire the beliefs, values, and behaviors of a given society in order to function within that group

_____ Individual groups related to the larger culture, each having an identity of its own

_____ Income that falls below the official poverty line from time to time, reflecting short-term fluctuations in household composition or economic circumstances

_____ Refers to those aspects that cannot be observed directly, such as ideas, beliefs, customs, and feelings of a culture

_____ Refers to social and cultural deprivation; for example, limited employment opportunities; inferior educational opportunities; lack of, or inferior, medical services/health care facilities; and absence of public services

_____ Labeling that stems from ethnocentric views

_____ Characterized by intimate, continued, face-to-face contact, mutual support of members, and the ability to order or constrain a considerable proportion of individual members' behavior and role assumption; examples—the family and the peer group

_____ A pattern of assumptions, beliefs, and practices that unconsciously frames or guides the outlook of a group of people

_____ Cultural creations that define patterns of behavior for persons in a variety of social positions

_____ Delineates a basic set of resources needed for adequate existence

_____ Reflects the median standard of living in a society; refers to childhood poverty in the U.S.

_____ Legal principle that says the state has an overriding interest in the health and welfare of its citizens

_____ Refers to a lack of money or material resources; for example, insufficient clothing, poor sanitation, and deteriorating housing

_____ Characterized by incomes below the poverty line year after year

_____ The observable components of a culture such as material objects and actions

_____ Those persons who lack resources and community ties necessary to provide for their own adequate shelter

2. Match each cultural term with its definition or description.

a. Biculturation
b. Cultural diversity
c. African American
d. Asian/Pacific Islander

e. American Indian/ Alaska Native
f. Hispanic
g. Cultural shock
h. Cultural sensitivity

i. Culturally competent care
j. Acculturation
k. Assimilation
l. Cultural pluralism
m. Cultural relativity

_____ A person who has origins in any of the indigenous peoples of the Far East, Southeast Asia, the Indian subcontinent, or the Pacific Islands

_____ The differences that exist as the minority population increases and the majority white population decreases

_____ A person having origins in the indigenous peoples of North America and who maintain cultural identification through tribal affiliations or community recognition

_____ A person whose lineage includes ancestors who originated from any of the black racial groups of Africa

_____ Care that goes beyond the awareness of similarities and differences to implementing care that is sensitive

_____ The process of developing a new cultural identity

_____ A person of Mexican, Puerto Rican, Cuban, Central or South American, or other Spanish culture or origin, regardless of race

_____ An awareness of cultural similarities and differences

_____ The concept that any behavior must be judged first in relation to the context of the culture in which it occurs

_____ Feelings of helplessness, discomfort, and disorientation experienced by an outsider attempting to comprehend or effectively adapt to a different cultural group; caused by differences in cultural practices, values, and beliefs

_____ The attitude that supports the rights of group differences and promotes a mutual respect for the existence of cultural differences

_____ Gradual changes produced in a culture by the influence of another culture, causing one or both cultures to be more similar to the other

_____ The straddling of two cultures; involves the ability to efficiently bridge the gap between an individual culture of origin and the dominant culture

3. The following terms are related to cultural/religious influences on health care. Match each term with its definition and description.

a. Miseries
b. Locked bowels
c. Caida de la molera
d. Susto
e. Dolor/duels/lele
f. La diarrhea

g. Chi
h. Mal ojo
i. Yin/yang
j. Curandero/curandera
k. Acupuncture

l. Acupressure
m. Moxibustion
n. Kahunas
o Ho' oponopono

_____ The term for diarrhea used by some Hispanic people

_____ The term used by some Hispanic people to denote the "evil eye"

_____ The term used by some Hispanic people for a fallen fontanel resulting from dehydration

_____ The term for pain used by some Hispanic people

_____ The term for pain used by some African Americans

_____ Application of pressure to cure maladies

_____ The Chinese term for the innate energy that leaves the body through the mouth, nose, and ears and flows through the body in definite pathways or meridians at specific time and locations

_____ Hawaiian folk healers

_____ The term for fright used by some Hispanic people

_____ Insertion of needles to cure maladies

_____ The practice of healing family imbalances or disputes among Native Hawaiians

_____ The Chinese terms for the forces of hot and cold that are believed to be out of balance when a person is ill

_____ The term used for constipation by some African Americans

_____ Application of heat to cure maladies

_____ The Mexican-American folk healer

4. The following terms are related to folk medicine practices that may be harmful. Match each term with its definition and description.

a. Coining
b. Forced kneeling
c. Female genital mutilation (female circumcision)

d. Topical garlic application
e. Greta/azarcon, paylooah, surma

f. Azogue
g. Lok

_____ Traditional remedies that contain lead

_____ Haitian folk medicine practice used to rid the newborn of meconium; a mixture of castor oil, grated nutmeg, sour orange juice, garlic, unrefined sugar, and water; may result in dehydration

_____ Removal of, or injury to, any part of the female genital organ; practiced in Africa, the Middle East, Latin America, India, the Far East, North America, Australia, and Western Europe

_____ Child discipline measure of some Caribbean groups

_____ A practice of Yemenite Jews; applied to the wrist to treat infectious disease; can result in blisters or burns

_____ Vietnamese practice; may produce weltlike lesions on the child's back

_____ A mercury compound commonly used in Mexico and sometimes sold illegally to low-income Hispanic families in the United States as a remedy for diarrhea; can cause permanent central nervous system damage

5. When considering the impact of culture on the pediatric patient, the nurse recognizes that culture:
   a. is synonymous with race.
   b. affects the development of health beliefs.
   c. refers to a group of people with similar physical characteristics.
   d. refers to the universal manner and sequence of growth and development.

6. Which of the following social groups is an example of a primary group?
   a. Six inseparable teenagers
   b. A second-grade class
   c. The members of a national church
   d. The city garden club

7. The use of guilt and shame by a culture provides:
   a. feelings of comfort about wrongdoing.
   b. an outlet following wrongdoing.
   c. rewards for culturally acceptable social behavior.
   d. internalization of the cultural norms.

8. Match each of the following subcultural influences with its description or its influence on a child's cultural development.

   a. Ethnicity   e. Homelessness   i. School
   b. Ethnocentrism   f. Migrant families   j. Peers
   c. Social class   g. Affluence   k. Biculture
   d. Poverty   h. Religion

   _____ May result in the adult authority being provided by paid surrogates
   _____ Often results in language becoming a major educational controversy
   _____ Occurs when there is a lack of resources for adequate shelter
   _____ After family, the subcultural influence that has the strongest impact on a child's socialization
   _____ Differentiation within a population that is determined by similar distinguishing factors
   _____ Limit of resources needed for adequate existence
   _____ Belief that one's own ethnic group is superior to others
   _____ Lack of continuity in education and health care
   _____ Dictates the code of morality
   _____ Synonymous with socioeconomic status and usually determined by occupation in the United States
   _____ An increasing influence as child moves through school

9. Currently in North America there is less reliance on tradition, families are fragmented, and transmission of customs is limited because of:
   a. a growing proportion of ethnic minorities.
   b. more emphasis on ethnic diversity.
   c. the frontier background of the American culture.
   d. increasing geographic and economic mobility.

10. Which country has more racial, ethnic, and religious minority groups than any other country?
    a. United States
    b. Mexico
    c. Canada
    d. India

11. Which of the following is the largest minority group in the United States?
    a. Spanish/Hispanic
    b. African American
    c. Asian
    d. Latino

12. A child has become acculturated when:
    a. a gradual process of ethnic blending occurs.
    b. the child identifies with traditional heritage.
    c. ethnic and racial pride emerge.
    d. counteraggressive behavior is eliminated.

13. Which of the following strategies is likely to produce the most conflict when considering the concept of cultural shock?
    a. Teaching the family some of the dominant culture's customs
    b. Having an older son or daughter translate a health history
    c. Identifying some of the usual family customs
    d. Learning tolerance of others' values and beliefs

14. When analyzing cultural components of a nursing assessment, the nurse recognizes that beliefs:
    a. may sometimes expedite the plan of care.
    b. can be manipulated more easily if known.
    c. must be in unison with standard health practices.
    d. are very similar from one culture to another.

15. An innate susceptibility is acquired through:
    a. the child's general physical status.
    b. exposure to environmental factors.
    c. long-term proximity to disease.
    d. generations of evolutionary changes.

16. Match each disease or disorder with the racial/ethnic group with which it is associated.

a. Tay-Sachs disease	d. Phenylketonuria	g. Clubfoot
b. Cystic fibrosis	e. Cleft lip/palate	h. Ear anomalies
c. Sickle cell disease	f. β-thalassemia	i. Werdnig-Hoffman disease

    _____ Greek
    _____ Middle Eastern
    _____ Japanese
    _____ Jewish
    _____ Irish
    _____ Polynesian
    _____ Navajo American Indian
    _____ African American
    _____ White American

17. In which of the following ethnic groups is the finding of phenylketonuria considered unusual?
    a. Scandinavian
    b. Scottish/Irish
    c. Mediterranean
    d. Middle Eastern

18. Compared with parents in other socioeconomic classes, parents of children in lower class families are more likely to:
    a. read and encourage educational play.
    b. value concrete over abstract thought processes.
    c. provide role models that support the value of education.
    d. interact with teachers using abstract expressions.

19. Which one of the following statements about mass media is true?
    a. Clear evidence exists that documents a relationship between television viewing and high-risk behaviors in adolescents.
    b. Educational television programming teaches the habits of mind to be a good leader.
    c. Reading ability and intelligence are linked to the number and type of comic books read.
    d. Mass media and increased use of tobacco by adolescents have been linked.

20. When considering social, cultural, and religious factors in a North American child's development, the nurse recognizes that the most overwhelming influence on health is the individual's:
    a. genetic background.
    b. proximity to the disease.
    c. socioeconomic status.
    d. health beliefs and practices.

21. The concept that any behavior must be judged first in relation to the context of the culture in which it occurs is called:
    a. cultural relativity.
    b. cultural stereotyping.
    c. nonverbal communication.
    d. culturally sensitive interaction.

22. Match each custom or belief with the ethnic group with which it is associated.

    a. Japanese   d. Asian
    b. White American (dominant culture)   e. Native American
    c. Hispanic

    _____ Eye contact is considered a sign of hostility.
    _____ Nonverbal communication is a practiced art.
    _____ Focus is on time; the expression "time flies" is commonly used.
    _____ Fish is a staple food.
    _____ Members believe that infants can develop symptoms of the "evil eye."

23. Which of the following strategies is *not* considered culturally sensitive?
    a. Active listening
    b. Slow and careful speaking
    c. Loud and clear speaking
    d. Repetition and clarification

24. Which of the following groups of food is common in many cultures?
    a. Chicken, milk, rice, apples, corn
    b. Pork, milk, broccoli, noodles, bananas
    c. Sausage, milk, carrots, dry cereal, oranges
    d. Beef, milk, green beans, oatmeal, pears

25. Match each ethnic group with the food it is associated with.

    a.   African American   d.   Chinese
    b.   Hispanic   e.   Vietnamese
    c.   Japanese   f.   Eastern Indian

    _____   Curry
    _____   Raw tuna
    _____   Lychee
    _____   Nopales
    _____   Bok choy
    _____   Chitterlings

26. In order to transmit an attitude of respect for a family's ethnic or religious heritage, the nurse should:
    a. have the dietitian explain why the hospital diet must be followed.
    b. maintain good eye contact.
    c. help the patient by interjecting the correct terms during the interview.
    d. acknowledge concern for differences in food preferences.

27. Voodoo is an example of an influence that is considered:
    a. a supernatural force.
    b. a natural force.
    c. an imbalance of the forces.
    d. an imbalance of the four humors.

28. Adopting a multicultural perspective means that the nurse:
    a. explains that biomedical measures are usually more effective.
    b. uses the patient's traditional health cultural beliefs.
    c. realizes that most folk remedies have a scientific basis.
    d. uses aspects of the cultural beliefs to develop a plan.

29. Which of the following terms is *not* used to describe a kind of folk healer?
    a. Azogue
    b. Curandera
    c. Curandero
    d. Kahuna

30. Which of the following health practices may compromise the health and well-being of either mother or fetus?
    a. The mother reaching her arms above her head
    b. The practice of eating clay
    c. The use of asafetida
    d. The practice of ho'oponopono

31. To provide culturally sensitive care to children and their families, the nurse should:
    a. disregard ones own cultural values.
    b. identify behavior that is abnormal.
    c. recognize characteristic behaviors of certain cultures.
    d. rely on one's own feelings and experiences for guidance.

32. In planning and implementing transcultural patient care, nurses need to strive to:
    a. adapt the family's ethnic practices to the health need.
    b. change the family's long-standing beliefs.
    c. use traditional ethnic practices in every patient's care.
    d. teach the family only how to treat the health problem.

33. Awareness of generalizations about cultural groups is important, because this information helps the nurse to:
    a. learn the similarities between all cultures.
    b. learn the unique practices of various groups.
    c. stereotype groups' characteristics.
    d. categorize groups according to their similarities.

Critical Thinking

34. During assessment the patient reveals that her family uses an acupuncturist occasionally. Based on this information, the nurse realizes that another health practice commonly practiced by the same cultural group is:
    a. voodoo.
    b. moxibustion.
    c. santeria.
    d. kampo.

35. Consideration of cultural assessment data is *most* important for which of the following nursing diagnoses?
    a. Decreased cardiac output
    b. Impaired skin integrity
    c. Ineffective airway clearance
    d. Altered nutrition

36. In planning any meal for a patient whose family holds beliefs of Islam, the nurse would exclude which one of the following foods?
    a. Pork
    b. Corn bread
    c. Rice
    d. Collard greens

37. Using a framework to evaluate transcultural nursing care, the nurse identifies which of the following health practices as typical?
    a. A Japanese family cares for a disabled family member in their home.
    b. An African-American family uses amulets as a shield from witchcraft.
    c. A Puerto Rican family seeks help from a curandera.
    d. A Mexican-American family seeks help from santeros.

CHAPTER 3

Family Influences on Child Health Promotion

1. Match each term with its description or characteristics.

a.	Family	g.	Time-out	m.	Household
b.	Structure	h.	Divided, split custody	n.	Family of origin
c.	Consanguineous	i.	Joint custody	o.	Open family
d.	Coping strategies	j.	Function	p.	Closed family
e.	Discipline	k.	Adoption	q.	Behavior modification
f.	Limit-setting	l.	Step-family		

_____ Establishment of the rules or guidelines for behavior

_____ Family interaction

_____ Persons sharing a common dwelling

_____ A group of people, living together or in close contact, who take care of one another and provide guidance for their dependent members

_____ Blood relationships

_____ A system of rules governing conduct

_____ Family situation in which each parent is awarded custody of one or more of the children, thereby separating siblings

_____ Resources for dealing with stress, such as community services, social support, and the adoption of a future orientation

_____ Family unit into which a person is born

_____ Composition of the family

_____ Refinement of the practice of "sending the child to his or her room"; based on the premise of removing the reinforcer and using the strategy of unrelated consequences

_____ Accepting of new ideas, resources, and opportunities

_____ Family situation in which the children reside with one parent, although both parents act as legal guardians and both participate in childrearing

_____ Resists input; views change as threatening and suspicious

_____ Establishment of a legal relationship of parent and child between persons not related by birth

_____ Family situation that includes married adults, one or both of whom have children from a previous marriage residing in the household

_____ Practice based on the belief that behavior, if rewarded, will be repeated and behavior not rewarded will be eliminated

2. Which one of the following is *not* a correct definition of the term *family* as it is viewed today?
   a. The family is what the patient considers it to be.
   b. The family may be related or unrelated.
   c. The family is always related by legal ties or genetic relationships, and members live in the same household.
   d. The family members share a sense of belonging to their own family.

3. Match each family theory with its description. (Some theories may be used more than once.)

   a. Family systems theory
   b. Family stress theory

   c. Developmental theory
   d. Structural-functional theory

   _____ Crisis intervention strategies are used, with the focus on helping members cope with the challenging event.
   _____ Continual interaction occurs between family members and the environment.
   _____ Focus is on the interactions of family members rather than on an individual member. A problem or dysfunction is not viewed as lying in any one family member but rather in the interactions used by the family.
   _____ Concepts of basic attributes, resources, perception, and coping behaviors or strategies are used in assessing family crisis management.
   _____ Changes in the family over time are addressed, based on the predictable changes in the structure, function, and roles of the family, with the age of the oldest child as the marker for stage transition.
   _____ The family and each individual member must achieve developmental tasks as part of each family life cycle stage.
   _____ Socialization of family members into society is considered the major goal of the family.

4. In working with children, nurses include family members in the plan of care. Which of the following statements does the nurse recognize as *false* when planning nursing interventions for the family?
   a. A complete family assessment is needed to discover family dynamics, family strengths, and family weaknesses.
   b. It is not a nurse's responsibility to recognize situations in which a family should be referred to specialized services.
   c. The intervention used with families depends on the nurse's view of the theoretic model of the family.
   d. The level of assistance a family needs depends on the type of crisis, factors affecting family adjustment, and the family's level of functioning.

5. Debbie is 2 years old and lives with her brother Mark, her sister Mary, and her mother. Her father and mother recently divorced, and now her father lives 1 hour away. Debbie sees her father once a month for a day's visit. Her mother retains custody of Debbie. Debbie's grandparents live in a different state, but she visits them each year. Debbie's family represents which one of the following?
   a. Binuclear family
   b. Extended family
   c. Single-parent family
   d. Reconstituted family

6. Identify three major objectives of the family in relation to children.

7. List indicators that identify vulnerable families.

8. Which one of the following is an effective approach for working with vulnerable families?
   a. Identify and emphasize family deficits.
   b. Offer single-purpose services with responses aimed at solving emergencies.
   c. Emphasize and focus on the troubled individual child or family member.
   d. Identify cultural differences, treating families with respect and honoring their traditions.

9. Identify the following statements as true or false.

   _____   Roles are learned through the socialization process.

   _____   Role continuity is defined as role behavior that is expected of children conflicting with desirable adult behavior.

   _____   All families have strengths and vulnerabilities.

   _____   Each family has its own standards for interaction within and outside the family.

   _____   Role definitions are changing as a result of the changing economy and women's liberation movement. Marital roles, however, are still most segregated among the middle classes.

10. _____ is the type of role that is related to fantasy and is important in childhood as a means of adjustment and socialization. In this role, the child uses the environment as a primary resource for learning the conduct that befits position or status.
    a. Ascribed role
    b. Achieved role
    c. Adopted role
    d. Assumed role

11. Children learn role behavior and to perform in an expected way within the family at a very early age. One factor that influences the role each sibling is assigned within the family structure is the

    _____   _____.

12. Parenting practices differ in small and large families. Which one of the following characteristics is *not* found in small families?
    a. Emphasis is placed on the individual development of the child, with constant pressure to measure up to family expectations.
    b. Adolescents identify more strongly with their parents and rely more on their parents for advice.
    c. Emphasis is placed on the group and less on the individual.
    d. Children's development and achievement are measured against those of children in the same neighborhood and social class.

13. Because age differences between siblings affect the childhood environment, the nurse recognizes that there is more affection and less rivalry and hostility between children whose ages are how many years apart?
    a. 4 or more years
    b. 4 or fewer years
    c. 3 or fewer years
    d. 2 or fewer years

14. Johnny has always been viewed by his parents as being less dependent than his brother, Tommy, or his sister, Julie. Johnny is described as affectionate, good-natured, and flexible in his thinking. He identifies with his peer group and is very popular with classmates. His parents tend to place fewer demands on Johnny for household help. From this description, the nurse would expect Johnny to have what birth position within the family?
    a. Firstborn child
    b. Middle child
    c. Youngest child
    d. Any of the above (birth position does not affect personality)

15. Monozygotic twins are:
    a. the result of fertilization of two ova.
    b. the result of fertilization of one ovum that became separated early in development.
    c. different physically and genetically.
    d. of dissimilar behaviors with greater sibling rivalry.

16 The *most* essential component of successful parenting is which one of the following?
    a. Strong religious and cultural ties to the community
    b. Previous experience with childcare, usually during adolescence as an older sibling or babysitter
    c. An understanding of childhood growth and development
    d. One person responsible for providing childcare within the family structure

17. Which one of the following does *not* identify a method to promote separation-individuation among twins?
    a. Parents discipline and praise twins as a unit.
    b. Parents foster feeling of separateness between twins.
    c. Parents avoid using the phrase "the twins."
    d. Parents foster opportunities to build one-to-one relationships with each twin.

18. List the three basic goals of childrearing.

19. The parenting behavior of warmth-hostility is best described by which one of the following?
    a. The degree of autonomy that parents allow their children
    b. The degree of open or frequent parental affection, combined with the degree of affection mixed with feelings of rejection or hostility that is expressed by the parents to their children
    c. The degree of restrictive control parents impose on their children, combined with the degree of active survey of their children's behavior
    d. The degree to which the parents allow their children to openly display feelings of rejection and hostility, combined with the acceptance of this behavior

20. Identify the following as true or false.

_____   A couple who have attended parenting classes before the birth of their infant can expect no disruption in the role transition to parenthood.

_____   The time between the ages of 18 and 35 years is the best childbearing period.

_____   The role of the father has become less significant to the family's health and well-being as the age of the mother has increased.

_____   Parent education classes taken in high school are more effective in relieving parental transitional stress than are classes taken closer to the childbearing period.

21. Match each parenting style with its description.

    a.   Authoritarian/dictatorial
    b.   Permissive/laissez-faire
    c.   Authoritative/democratic

    _____   Allows children to regulate their own activity; sees the parenting role as a resource rather than a role model
    _____   Establishes rules, regulations, and standards of conduct for children that are to be followed without question
    _____   Respects each child's individuality; directs the child's behavior by emphasizing the reason for rules

22. Child misbehavior requires parental implementation of appropriate disciplinary action. Identify which one of the following would *not* be an appropriate guideline for implementing discipline.
    a. Focus on the child and the misbehavior by using "you" messages rather than "I" messages.
    b. Maintain consistency with disciplinary action.
    c. Make sure all caregivers maintain unity of plan by agreeing on the plan and being familiar with details before implementation.
    d. Maintain flexibility by planning disciplinary actions appropriate to the child's age, temperament, and severity of misbehavior.

23. Which one of the following is a correct interpretation in the use of reasoning as a form of discipline?
    a. Used for older children when moral issues are involved
    b. Used for younger children to "see the other side" of an issue
    c. Used only in combination with scolding and criticism
    d. Used to allow children to obtain lengthy explanations and a greater degree of attention from parents

24. Which one of the following is *not* a description of the use of time-out as a discipline?
    a. Allows the reinforcer to be maintained
    b. Involves no physical punishment
    c. Offers both parents and child "cooling off" time
    d. Facilitates the parent's ability to consistently apply the punishment

25. Johnny spills his milk on the living room rug. His mother smacks him on the bottom and says, "You are a messy, bad boy, Johnny." The discipline strategies used are:
    i.   Consequence
    ii. Corporal punishment
    iii. Scolding
    iv. Behavior modification
    v.   Ignoring

    a. i, ii, and iii
    b. ii and iii
    c. iii and v
    d. ii, iii, and iv

26. Areas of concern for parents of adoptive children include:
    a. the initial attachment process.
    b. telling the children that they are adopted.
    c. identity formation of children during adolescence.
    d. all of the above.

27. Which of the following statements about adoption is true?
    a. Adoptive children should be treated no differently than biologic children.
    b. Acknowledging and encouraging discussion of the adopted child's feelings helps foster positive self-image in the child.
    c. An adopted child does not adapt easily in a family if there is open discussion about the child's birth circumstances.
    d. Older children display less behavioral changes following adoption disclosure than do younger children.

28. Identify the following statements about the impact of divorce on children as true or false.

    _____   Research has shown that children of divorce suffer no lasting psychologic and social difficulties.

    _____   One outcome found in children of divorce is a heightened anxiety about forming enduring relationships as young adults.

    _____   Children of divorce cope better with their feelings of abandonment when there is continuing conflict between parents.

    _____   Preschoolers assume themselves to be the cause of the divorce and interpret the separation as punishment.

    _____   School-age children's teachers and school counselors should be informed because these children will often display altered behaviors.

    _____   Adolescents have concerns and heightened anxiety about their own future as a marital partner and the availability of money for future needs.

29. Which one of the following is *not* considered important by parents when telling their children about the decision to divorce?
    a. Initial disclosure should include both parents and siblings.
    b. Time should be allowed for discussion with each child individually.
    c. The initial disclosure should be kept simple and reasons for divorce should not be included.
    d. Parents should physically hold or touch their child to provide feelings of warmth and reassurance.

30. List and describe the two major phases that children go through when adjusting to a divorce.

31. Single parenting, step-parenting, and dual-earner family parenting add stress to the parental role. Match each family type with an expected stressor or concern.

    a. Single parenting
    b. Step-parenting
    c. Dual-earner family parenting

    _____ Shortages of money, time, and energy are major concerns.
    _____ Overload is a common source of stress, and social activities are significantly curtailed, with time demands and scheduling seen as major problems.
    _____ Competition is a major area of concern among adults, with reduction of power conflicts a necessity.

Critical Thinking—Case Study

Ester and Roberto Garcia are the proud new parents of twin boys Timothy and Thomas. Ester and Roberto have been married less than 1 year. Ester is 17 years old and plans to return to finish school next year. Roberto finished high school and works with his father in a local auto repair shop. He is taking a week off from work to help Ester at home with Timothy and Thomas. Neither Ester nor Roberto attended child parenting classes. You are making a home visit to the couple on the day after they have brought Timothy and Thomas home from the hospital. As you arrive at the house, you see that both Timothy and Thomas are crying. Ester is trying to give Timothy his bath while Roberto is busy trying to get Thomas to take his formula. Both new parents appear tired, and Roberto admits they have been up all night with the infants and that either Timothy or Thomas seems to be crying "all the time" and that "something must be terribly wrong with them."

32. As you begin your assessment of the family, you know that the Garcias are in stage II, families with infants, according to Duvall's developmental stages of the family. Which one of the following is a developmental task of this stage?
    a. Reestablishing couple identity
    b. Socializing children
    c. Making decisions regarding parenthood
    d. Accommodating to parenting role

33. Which of the following is a priority nursing diagnosis for this family?
    a. Altered family process related to gain of family members
    b. Altered growth and development related to inadequate caretaking
    c. Fear related to new parental role
    d. High risk for injury related to unsafe environment

34. As the nurse developing the plan for this new family, you choose which of the following as the priority intervention?
    a. Teach the parents about Duvall's developmental stages, explaining that what they are experiencing is normal transition into parenthood.
    b. Reassure the parents that you will examine both infants but that they appear to be healthy and that the parents are doing a good job.
    c. Take over the feeding and bathing of the infants, explaining to the parents the necessity of child parenting classes.
    d. Check the infant supplies and environment to make sure the home has been made safe for children.

35. Both Thomas and Timothy are now sleeping, and you have completed your family assessment with Roberto and Ester. As a nurse you decide to use the family stress theory to promote adaptation to the family's new role. Which of the following is *not* a capability the family can use to manage the crisis?
    a. Basic attributes of the family
    b. Resources within the family
    c. Perception of the family to the situation
    d. Closed boundary within the family system

36. Identify a long-term goal for the Garcia family and discuss nursing interventions that will foster achievement of this long-term goal.

37. Compare and contrast the following types of consequences and give an example of a discipline technique for each type.

    a. Natural:

    b. Logical:

    c. Unrelated:

38. Discuss the use of corporal punishment and the concerns of using this form of discipline to stop or decrease certain behaviors.

CHAPTER 4

Community-Based Nursing Care of the Child and Family

1. The following terms are related to community health concepts. Match each term with its description.

a. Community
b. Population
c. Target population
d. Community care

e. Community health nursing
f. Roles and functions
g. Core functions

_____ Population-wide services that are based on assessment disease surveillance, policy development, and assurance; a list developed by the Institute of Medicine that guides the work of public health professionals and is directed at providing population-wide services, personal services, and home services for people at risk

_____ Subpopulation; a more narrowly defined population (e.g., obese middle-school children) toward whom nurses direct activities in order to improve the health status of individuals in the group

_____ A group of individuals with shared characteristics or interests who interact with one another

_____ A collaboration of individuals and groups within a specific community, including health care providers, advocates, governments, managed care organizations, businesses, children, and families, whose goal is the provision of services that promote health initiatives

_____ A group of people who live in a community (e.g., school-age children)

_____ Examples: caregiver, advocate, case manager, case finder, counselor, educator, epidemiologist, group process leader, health planner, and manager

_____ Focuses on promoting and maintaining the health of individuals, families, and groups in the community setting

2. The following terms are related to community health research and measurement. Match each term with its description or function.

a. Demography
b. Demographic characteristics
c. Risk
d. Epidemiology
e. Morbidity rates
f. Natality/mortality rates

g. Incidence
h. Prevalence
i. Agent
j. Host factors
k. Environmental factors
l. Primary prevention
m. Secondary prevention

n. Tertiary prevention
o. Screening
p. Economics
q. Cost-effectiveness analysis

_____ Factors such as age, gender, race, ethnicity, socioeconomic status, and education

_____ Level of prevention that focuses on screening and early diagnosis of disease

_____ The science of population health applied to the detection of morbidity and mortality in a population

_____ Factor that is responsible for causing a disease (e.g., *Mycobacterium tuberculosis*)

_____ Used to measure disease and injury

_____ The probability of developing a disease, injury, or illness

_____ The most common type of economic evaluation

_____ Measures the occurrence of new events in a population during a period of time

_____ Variables that provide the setting for the disease or condition, including conditions related to climate, home, neighborhood, and school

_____ Measures existing events in a population during a period of time

_____ The level of prevention that focuses on health promotion and prevention of disease or injury

_____ The rate of death in neonates and individuals, respectively

_____ Characteristics of a disease or condition that are specific to an individual or a group

_____ In health, the measure of the amount of resources individuals and communities are willing to pay for health; allocation of health care dollars and methods for estimating cost of health

_____ A secondary prevention activity used to detect and treat disease early

_____ The level of prevention that focuses on optimizing function for individuals with disabilities or chronic diseases

_____ The study of population characteristics

3. The following terms are related to community nursing process. Match each term with its description.

   a. Community needs assessment
   b. Community nursing diagnosis
   c. Community health
   d. Community nursing interventions
   e. Community nursing evaluation
   f. Goals
   g. Health programs

   _____ The development of community-centered interventions

   _____ Outcomes that give direction to interventions and provide a measure of the change the interventions produced

   _____ Collection of subjective and objective information about the target population or community

   _____ Analysis whether community goals were met

   _____ The form that many community interventions take

   _____ Identification of problems based on community needs

   _____ Measures that enable a community to reach its goals

4. A community that is considered healthy would typically:
   a. have quality medical care.
   b. provide a safe place to live.
   c. provide a nurturing place to grow.
   d. have all of the above.

5. Visit the Website at http://www.healthycommunities.org. List the seven characteristics of a health community identified by this site.

6. When community health nursing is successful, it is because:
   a. the nurse provides what the community needs.
   b. the community is empowered.
   c. acute care services are at their best.
   d. the community is the nurse's personal responsibility.

7. Settings for traditional community health include:
   a. pediatric intensive care units.
   b. neonatal intensive care units.
   c. psychiatric intensive care units.
   d. emergency departments.

8. Which of the following are the categories of standards for community health nursing as established by the American Nurses Association?
   a. Data collection, evaluation, and interdisciplinary collaboration
   b. Demography, epidemiology, and data collection
   c. Surveillance, policy development, and assurance
   d. Data collection, policy development, and surveillance

9. According to the Institute of Medicine, a community health nurse must be able to:
   a. provide care to acutely ill patients.
   b. intervene in disputes with insurance companies.
   c. bring about change in organizations.
   d. administer immunizations.

10. There is an increased risk associated with race and ethnicity that is thought to be due to a complicated relationship between:
    a. genetic predisposition and class.
    b. minority status and socioeconomic status.
    c. low level of education and class.
    d. genetic predisposition and socioeconomic status.

11. If asthma is more prevalent in School A than in School B, the nurse should expect that:
    a. there were more new cases of asthma this year than last year in School B.
    b. there were fewer new cases of asthma this year than last year in both schools.
    c. there are currently more cases of asthma in School A than in School B.
    d. there are currently more cases of asthma in School B than in School A.

12. Screening is an excellent tool to use to detect a disease:
    a. as a one-time program.
    b. that is not well understood.
    c. when treatment is too costly.
    d. with a latent symptomatic stage.

13. An understanding of economics is essential, because it enables the nurse to:
    a. trade resources for patients needs.
    b. participate in discussions about the worth of health programs.
    c. develop new methods for estimating cost.
    d. all of the above.

14. A cost-effectiveness analysis contains results expressed as a ratio, with the numerator as the costs and the denominator as the:
    a. health program.
    b. health unit.
    c. risk program.
    d. cost analysis.

15. The end point of a cost-effectiveness analysis is calculated in:
    a. dollars.
    b. units of time.
    c. health units.
    d. cost-benefit terms.

16. In community nursing the focus of the nursing process shifts from:
    a. the community to the individual.
    b. the target population to the individual.
    c. the individual to the family.
    d. the individual to the target population.

17. The community health nurse collaborates with:
    a. other nurses.
    b. politicians.
    c. religious leaders.
    d. all of the above.

18. An example of a method to collect objective information in a community needs assessment is the:
    a. windshield tour.
    b. patient questionnaire.
    c. direct interview of a patient.
    d. telephone survey.

19. List the eight community systems that the nurse should examine as part of the community needs assessment.

20. An example of comparing the rates in a community with a standard population to evaluate a community needs assessment is to compare:
    a. tuberculosis rates with diabetes rates.
    b. county teen pregnancy rates with state rates.
    c. tuberculosis rates from one year with diabetes rates of another year.
    d. county teen pregnancy rates with tuberculosis rates.

21. Match each evaluation component with its focus.

    a. Structure

    b. Process

    c. Outcome

    _____ Focuses on whether program objectives and community goals were met

    _____ Focuses on the qualifications of personnel; the adequacy of building(s), offices, supplies, and equipment; and the characteristics of the target population

    _____ Focuses on the interaction between the patients and provider, using indicators such as the number of people who attend a program

Critical Thinking

22. Match each health program or intervention with the level of prevention it provides. (Levels of prevention may be used more than once.)

    a. Primary prevention
    b. Secondary prevention
    c. Tertiary prevention

    _____ Diabetes self-management clinic
    _____ Hepatitis B immunization program
    _____ Depression risk education
    _____ Diabetes screening
    _____ Support group for stroke victims
    _____ Battered women's hotline
    _____ Cardiac rehabilitation
    _____ Pap smear testing
    _____ Firearms safety program

Use Community Assessment Box 4-3 (textbook p. 108) to answer questions 23 through 26.

23. Which of the following is an example of a standard used for comparison in the Sabine project?
    a. Poverty level
    b. Level of protein in the meals
    c. Immunization rate for children under 2 years of age
    d. Vision and hearing referral rate

24. Using the *outcome* approach described by Donabedian to evaluate the Sabine project after it was implemented, the evaluator would *most* want to know:
    a. when the nurse addressed the parent association.
    b. the percentage of BMIs above the 95th percentile.
    c. the number of injuries related to school bus accidents.
    d. the type of resources used for the program.

25. Using the *process* approach described by Donabedian to evaluate the Sabine project after it was implemented, the evaluator would *most* want to know:
    a. when the nurse addressed the parent association.
    b. the percentage of BMIs above the 95th percentile.
    c. the number of injuries related to school bus accidents.
    d. the type of resources used for the program.

26. Using the *structure* approach described by Donabedian to evaluate the Sabine project after it was implemented, the evaluator would *most* want to know:
    a. when the nurse addressed the parent association.
    b. the percentage of BMIs above the 95th percentile.
    c. the number of injuries related to school bus accidents.
    d. the type of resources used for the program.

CHAPTER 5

Hereditary Influences on Health Promotion of the Child and Family

1. The following terms are related to genetic influences on health. Match each term with its definition or description.

a. Genes
b. Chromosomes
c. Major structural abnormalities
d. Minor anomalies
e. Syndrome
f. Association
g. Congenital anomalies
h. Chromosomal disorders
i. Structural abnormality
j. Ring chromosome
k. –somy
l. Monosomy
m. Trisomy

n. Gamete formation
o. Postzygotic cell division
p. Nondisjunction
q. Sister chromatid
r. Partial chromosomal abnormalities
s. Classic deletion syndromes
t. Contiguous gene syndromes
u. X inactivation
v. Consanguinity
w. Mutation
x. Variable expression

y. Premutation
z. Genetic anticipation
aa. Genomic imprinting
bb. Prader-Willi syndrome
cc. Angelman syndrome
dd. Uniparental disomy
ee. Single-gene disorders
ff. Karyotyping
gg. Fluorescence in situ hybridization
hh. Mapped
ii. Multifactorial disorders
jj. Teratogens

_____ Malformations that may result from genetic and/or prenatal environmental causes, resulting in serious medical, surgical, or quality-of-life consequences

_____ A recognized pattern of malformations due to a single specific cause

_____ The genetic material responsible for programming the body's physiologic process and characteristics

_____ A nonrandom pattern of malformations for which an etiology has not been determined, such as VATER, vertebral defects, imperforate anus, tracheoesophageal fistula, and radial-renal defects

_____ Structures that are organized from genes and visible only during certain stages of cell division

_____ A deviation from that which is normal or typical

_____ Another term for birth defects

_____ Loss, addition, rearrangement, or exchange of some of the genes of a chromosome

_____ Used to designate that the deviation of a chromosome involves the gain or loss of a chromosome

_____ Deviations in the structure or number of chromosomes that result in a readily observed aberration in the individual; cytogenic disorders that are often severe or lethal

_____ A relatively rare structural abnormality and/or alteration in the chromosome, in which a break occurs in the terminal ends of both arms of a chromosome

_____ Failure of the separation of homologous chromosomes during meiosis or of sister chromosomes during meiosis II or mitosis

_____ Involve a missing (deletion) or extra (duplication) segment of a chromosome

_____ Meiosis

33

_____ Selection of a mate based on geographic, ethnic, or religious restrictions

_____ A cell that contains one more than the total number of chromosomes, resulting in the addition of an extra member to a normal pair

_____ Disorders characterized by a microdeletion or microduplication of smaller chromosome segments, which may require special analysis techniques or molecular testing to detect

_____ A cell that contains one less than the total number of chromosomes; loss of one member of a chromosome pair

_____ Mitosis

_____ Refers to the pair of chromosome strands that constitutes a metaphase (a stage of mitosis) chromosome

_____ The concept that describes differences in the extent and/or severity of manifestations of genetic diseases

_____ Can be detected on a routine chromosome analysis and may include cri-du-chat, Wolf-Herschorn, and chromosome 18 deletions

_____ The concept that certain dominantly inherited disorders tend to worsen or have an earlier age of onset with succeeding generations

_____ Lyon hypothesis; explains the milder physical and mental deficiencies of children with sex chromosomal abnormalities compared with children who have autosomal abnormalities

_____ Any heritable change in the DNA sequence of a gene

_____ Contains a large number of DNA nucleotide repeats that are unstable and can undergo amplification

_____ Characterized by central hypotonia, cognitive dysfunction, dysmorphic appearance, behavioral disturbances, hypothalamic hypogonadism, short stature, and obesity, as well as abnormally low body temperature, an increased tolerance to pain, and diminished salivation

_____ Modification in some instances of genetic material, resulting in phenotypic differences based on whether the genes/chromosomes are from the mother or the father

_____ Diseases and defects that show an increased incidence in some families but have no clear-cut affected/unaffected classification and show no specific mode of inheritance; prenatal and environmental factors appear to play an important role; examples are neural tube defects, cleft lip, congenital hip dislocation and pyloric stenosis

_____ Sometimes called "happy puppet syndrome"; includes severe mental retardation, characteristic facies, abnormal gait, and paroxysms of inappropriate laughter

_____ A new technique of chromosome analysis that uses radioactive or fluorescent probes in a variety of ways to identify chromosome and DNA abnormalities

_____ Disorders that are the result of a defect or mutation of a single gene, rather than a partial or whole chromosomal abnormality

_____ Situation in which both copies of a chromosome pair are determined to have come from one parent, instead of one from each

_____ A pictorial representation of chromosomal analysis

_____ The ability to locate a gene on a specific chromosome or segment of a chromosome

_____ Agents that cause birth defects when present in the prenatal environment

2. The following terms are related to the impact of hereditary disorders on the family. Match each term with its definition or description.

a. Presymptomatic testing
b. False positive
c. False negative
d. Screening test
e. Diagnostic test
f. Maternal triple-marker screening test

g. Fetal blood sampling
h. Fetal biopsy (FB)
i. Fetal echocardiography
j. In vitro fertilization
k. Preimplantation genetic diagnosis
l. Genetic counseling

m. Proband
n. Empiric risks
o. Theoretic risks
p. Pedigree chart
q. Burden of a genetic defect
r. Chronic sorrow

_____ Test results that indicate a problem exists when, in fact, it does not

_____ Test that simply indicates a higher risk than expected in the general population

_____ Family tree; genogram

_____ Test that determines with a high degree of accuracy the presence or absence of a birth defect or genetic disorder

_____ Prenatal genetic testing that can be performed after 18 weeks gestation; used for rapid chromosome analysis and to detect fetal hematologic abnormalities, inborn errors of metabolism, and fetal infection

_____ May be performed for further diagnosis when a cardiac defect is noted; ultrasound

_____ Test results that indicate a problem does not exist when, in fact, it does

_____ Refers to the process of screening for disease in high-risk populations who are currently asymptomatic

_____ May indicate the presence of an open neural tube defect, ventral wall defect, or Down syndrome in the fetus

_____ Used to diagnose certain genetic skin disorders and metabolic disorders when DNA studies are unavailable or uninformative

_____ The genetic counseling term for the affected person or index case

_____ The technique used to implant the embryo after it has been tested for the presence of a specific genetic disorder

_____ The total amount of distress (economic and emotional) that is placed on persons, their families, and society by the birth of an affected child

_____ Risks based on Mendelian inheritance patterns

_____ A communication process that deals with the human problems associated with the risk for occurrence of a genetic disorder in a family

_____ In vitro process in which an embryo can be tested at the six- to eight-cell stage for the presence of a genetic disorder prior to implantation

_____ Risks based on observations of recurrence in similar situations

_____ A grieving process, the resolution of which is delayed while a child with a disability is alive

3. Trisomy 21, or Down syndrome, is an example of a:
   a. congenital chromosomal association.
   b. sex chromosomal abnormality.
   c. autoimmune aberration.
   d. autosomal aberration.

4. All of the following chromosomal disorders are considered sex chromosomal abnormalities *except*:
   a. Turner syndrome.
   b. Klinefelter syndrome.
   c. cri-du-chat syndrome.
   d. triple X syndrome.

5. According to the Lyon hypothesis, when compared with children who have autosomal abnormalities, children with sex chromosomal abnormalities:
   a. usually have milder physical and mental deficiencies.
   b. are shorter in stature with poor coordination.
   c. are more easily identified at birth.
   d. usually have more severe handicaps.

6. Match each disorder with its inheritance pattern. (Inheritance patterns may be used more than once.)

   a. Autosomal-dominant

   b. Autosomal-recessive

   c. Sex-linked (dominant or recessive)

   _____ Wilson disease
   _____ Tay Sachs disease
   _____ Osteogenesis imperfecta
   _____ Neurofibromatosis
   _____ Duchenne muscular dystrophy
   _____ Maple syrup urine disease
   _____ Hemophilia A
   _____ Fragile X syndrome
   _____ Ocular albinism
   _____ Achondroplasia
   _____ Cystic fibrosis
   _____ Galactosemia
   _____ Familial hypothyroidism
   _____ Marfan syndrome
   _____ Myotonic dystrophy
   _____ Noonan syndrome
   _____ Phenylketonuria
   _____ Thalassemia

7. A disease or defect encountered frequently in the population without a clear-cut inheritance pattern is classified as:
   a. a mutation.
   b. a mosaicism.
   c. a uniparental disomy.
   d. multifactorial.

8. Which one of the following disorders is clearly teratogenic?
   a. Type 1 diabetes
   b. Rheumatoid arthritis
   c. Fetal alcohol syndrome
   d. Myasthenia gravis

9. Fetal surgery has been used in particular to treat congenital:
   a. urinary tract abnormalities.
   b. heart disease.
   c. facial and limb deformities.
   d. pyloric stenosis.

10. Phenylketonuria is usually treated by:
    a. diet modification.
    b. hormone replacement.
    c. surgical repair.
    d. vitamin supplement.

11. Most genetic centers recommend that genetic testing should be reserved for children:
    a. prior to their adoption.
    b. when clear medical benefits exist.
    c. who have deleterious recessive genes.
    d. who have deleterious dominant genes.

12. Careful counseling is necessary when screening an individual for carrier status of hereditary disorders because:
    a. this type of screening is controversial.
    b. of possible ethical dilemmas.
    c. this type of screening is expensive.
    d. the emotional threat for the child is always devastating.

13. Which one of the following statements is *not* a part of the controversial aspect of mass genetic screening programs?
    a. Health professionals sometimes lack knowledge about the purpose of the testing.
    b. The public cost of testing does not always outweigh the benefits.
    c. Many well-organized programs have been successful in preventing disease.
    d. The psychologic implications of the carrier states may not be handled properly.

14. Match each type of prenatal genetic test with its purpose.

    a. Triple-marker screen

    b. Ultrasonography

    c. Amniocentesis

    d. Chorionic villus sampling (CVS)

    _____ To perform chromosomal and biochemical analysis
    _____ To estimate gestational age and identify structural abnormalities
    _____ To perform chromosomal analysis at the earliest possible point during pregnancy
    _____ To screen for neural tube defects

15. Preimplantation genetic diagnosis has been used for parents at risk for having a child with:
    a. Down syndrome.
    b. a neural tube defect.
    c. a congenital heart defect.
    d. cystic fibrosis.

16. Which of the following actions is *not* considered an appropriate nursing responsibility in genetic counseling?
    a. Choose the best course of action for the family.
    b. Identify families who would benefit from genetic evaluation.
    c. Become familiar with community resources for genetic evaluation.
    d. Learn basic genetic principles.

17. The most efficient genetic counseling service provided by a group of genetic screening specialists may:
    a. predict the outcome of the disease.
    b. take less than 2 hours.
    c. evaluate the affected child only.
    d. be inaccessible to the people who need it most.

18. *Proband* is the term used in genetic counseling to mean the:
    a. affected person.
    b. genetic history.
    c. clinical manifestations.
    d. mode of inheritance.

19. When teaching families about genetic risks and probabilities, the nurse may need to:
    a. make specific recommendations.
    b. use games such as flipping coins and horse racing.
    c. realize that most people have a basic understanding of biology.
    d. recognize that each pregnancy's probabilities build on the previous pregnancy's probabilities.

20. Which one of the following assessment findings should alert the nurse to the need for genetic counseling?
    a. Individuals with a family history of tuberculosis
    b. Parents who had an infant born at 42 weeks gestation
    c. Couples with a history of infertility
    d. Pregnant adolescents

21. Which one of the following assessment findings in an infant should indicate to the nurse that there is a need for genetic referral?
    a. Vernix caseosa
    b. Acrocyanosis
    c. Mongolian spots
    d. Odorous breath

22. In a drawing of a pedigree genogram, which one of the following facts is *least* significant?
    a. The proband's paternal grandmother had two stillbirth pregnancies.
    b. The proband's sibling died as an infant in a motor vehicle accident.
    c. The proband's paternal grandfather was a carrier for sickle cell disease.
    d. The proband's half brother carries the sickle cell trait.

23. In regard to genetic counseling, which one of the following statements is *false*?
    a. Families have a tendency to be more ashamed of a hereditary disorder than other illness.
    b. The nurse's role in genetic counseling involves sympathy and supportive listening.
    c. The nurse ensures that patients have accurate and complete information to make decisions.
    d. Once the family understands the situation intellectually, they will be able to cope.

Critical Thinking—Case Study

Mr. and Mrs. Jones are waiting in the obstetrician's office for a routine prenatal checkup. They are Roman Catholic and do not believe in abortion. The obstetrician has recommended a screening test to rule out neural tube defects. Mrs. Jones does not see any benefit from this testing procedure and does not want to undergo the procedure.

24. Which one of the following factors is the *least* important consideration during the assessment phase of this visit?
    a. The nurse is not Roman Catholic.
    b. The test is a venipuncture and carries little risk.
    c. Most couples receive normal results from prenatal tests.
    d. Results of the tests will be provided before the delivery date.

25. Which one of the following considerations should the nurse deal with *first*?
    a. The couple believes that testing is used to identify anomalies in order to terminate pregnancies.
    b. The couple's clear-cut beliefs about pregnancy termination are very different from the reality of raising an abnormal child.
    c. The nurse believes that pregnancy termination for fetal abnormalities is often the best option.
    d. The nurse believes that raising a child with a terminal illness is extremely difficult.

26. Which one of the following goals is *most* appropriate for the nurse in this situation?
    a. To provide nonjudgmental supportive counseling
    b. To help Mr. and Mrs. Jones make their decision
    c. To provide follow-up care to the couple
    d. To educate the couple about neural tube defects

27. Which of the following statements by Mrs. Jones indicates that the nurse's goal was met?
    a. "I had no idea what was involved in raising a disabled child."
    b. "Your ideas have been very helpful. I think one of them will work."
    c. "We will discuss this and call you tomorrow with our decision."
    d. "I had no idea what neural tube defects were."

CHAPTER 6

Communication and Health Assessment of the Child and Family

1. Match each term with its description.

   a. Verbal communication
   b. Nonverbal communication
   c. Abstract communication
   d. Paralanguage
   e. Confirming behaviors
   f. Disconfirming behavior
   g. Triage
   h. Empathy
   i. Sympathy
   j. Family
   k. Family structure
   l. Genogram
   m. Family function
   n. Anthropometry

   _____ The pitch, pause, intonation, rate, volume, and stress apparent in speech

   _____ An essential parameter of nutritional status; the measurement of height, weight, head circumference, proportions, skinfold thickness, and arm circumference

   _____ The capacity to understand what another person is experiencing from within that person's frame of reference

   _____ Takes the form of play, artistic expression, symbols, photographs, and choice of clothing

   _____ Refers to the composition of the family

   _____ Involves having feelings or emotions in common with another person, rather than merely understanding those feelings

   _____ Often called *body language* and includes gestures, movements, facial expressions, postures, and reactions

   _____ Uses symbols to record data about family structure

   _____ Refers to all those individuals who are considered by the family member to be significant to the nuclear unit

   _____ Involves language and its expressions; vocalizations

   _____ Concerned with how family members behave toward one another and with the quality of the relationship

   _____ Response behavior that includes nodding the head and requesting clarification

   _____ Response behavior that includes tapping one's fingers and turning away from the speaker

   _____ Involves assessing symptoms and forming clinical judgment for further medical care

2. Which of the following would negatively affect the communication process between the nurse and the patient?
   a. The nurse delivers congruous messages to the patient.
   b. The nurse includes the child, as well as the parent, in the communication process.
   c. The nurse uses verbal and nonverbal communication to reflect approval of the patient's statement.
   d. The nurse uses a slow, even, steady voice to convey instruction.

3. Mrs. Green has brought her daughter Karen to the clinic where you work as a nurse. Karen, age 12 years, is a new patient and needs a physical exam so that she can play volleyball. Which of the following techniques would *not* be helpful to establish effective communication during the interview process?
   a. You introduce yourself and ask the name of all family members present.
   b. After the introduction, you are careful to direct questions about Karen to Mrs. Green since she is the best source of information.
   c. After the introduction and explanation of your role, you begin the interview by saying to Karen, "Tell me about your volleyball team."
   d. You choose to conduct the interview in a quiet area with few distractions.

4. List three reasons to include role clarification and explanation in the interview process.

5. The nurse says to 15 year-old Monique, "Tell me about your cough." This is an example of which type of communication technique?
   a. Direct
   b. Open-ended
   c. Reflective
   d. Closed

6. While conducting an assessment of the child, the nurse communicates with the child's family. Which one of the following does the nurse recognize as *not* productive in obtaining information?
   a. Obtaining verbal and nonverbal input from the child
   b. Observing the relationship between parents and child
   c. Using broad, open-ended questions
   d. Avoiding the use of guiding statements to direct the focus of the interview

7. The receptionist at the clinic where you are employed as a nurse has forwarded a call to you from Mrs. Garcia, mother of 4-year-old Maria. Mrs. Garcia tells you that Maria has had a fever all morning of around 100° F and that she now has diarrhea and vomiting. As you provide triage by phone, which one of the following actions is appropriate?
   a. Reassure Mrs. Garcia that Maria is not very sick and will be fine in a day or two.
   b. Confer with the practitioner at once.
   c. Wait to document in Maria's medical record until she comes in for a visit.
   d. Offer advice for home care and instruct Mrs. Garcia to call or come to the clinic if Maria's symptoms do not improve.

8. _____ is the capacity to understand what another person is feeling by experiencing from that person's frame of reference.
   a. Sympathy
   b. Empathy
   c. Reassurance
   d. Encouragement

9. The nurse is conducting an interview with 8-year-old Jesus and his mother, Mrs. Lopez. Mrs. Lopez is worried because Jesus has been acting up at home and at school and disrupting everyone. An interpreter has been requested since the mother speaks very little English. When using an interpreter for communication with Mrs. Lopez, the nurse realizes that:
   a. the interpreter will have very little to do because Jesus can interpret for his mother.
   b. when the interpreter and Mrs. Lopez speak for a long period, it will be necessary to interrupt to refocus the interview.
   c. the nurse will need to communicate directly with Mrs. Lopez and ignore the interpreter.
   d. the nurse will need to pose questions to elicit only one answer at a time from Mrs. Lopez.

10. Identify whether the following statements are true or false when planning how to communicate effectively with children.
   _____ Nonverbal components of the communication process do not convey significant message.
   _____ Children are alert to their surroundings and attach meaning to gestures.
   _____ Actively attempting to make friends with children before they have had an opportunity to evaluate an unfamiliar person will increase their anxiety.
   _____ The nurse should assume a position that is at eye level with the child.
   _____ Communication through transition objects, such as dolls or stuffed animals, delays the child's response to verbal communication offered by the nurse.

11. To effectively provide anticipatory guidance to the family, the nurse should:
   a. provide information to deal with each problem as it develops.
   b. provide teaching and interventions based on needs identified by the professional.
   c. be suspicious of the parent's ability to deal effectively with the child's needs.
   d. assist the parents in building competence in their parenting abilities.

12. Communication with children must reflect their developmental thought process. Match each developmental stage with the communication guidelines important at that stage. (Stages may be used more than once.)

   a. Infancy
   b. Early childhood
   c. School-age years
   d. Adolescence

   _____ Focus communication on the child; experiences of others are of no interest to children in this stage.
   _____ Children in this stage primarily use and respond to nonverbal communication.
   _____ Children in this stage interpret words literally and are unable to separate fact from fantasy.
   _____ Children in this stage assign human attributes to inanimate objects.
   _____ Children in this stage require explanations and reasons why procedures are being done to them.
   _____ Children in this stage have a heightened concern about body integrity, being overly sensitive to any activity that constitutes a threat to it.
   _____ Children in this stage are often willing to discuss their concern with an adult outside the family and often welcome the opportunity to interact with a nurse.

13. Which one of the following *best* describes the appropriate use of play as a communication technique with children?
    a. Small infants have little response to activities that focus on repetitive actions like patting and stroking.
    b. Few clues about intellectual or social developmental progress are obtained from the observation of child's play behaviors.
    c. Therapeutic play has little value in reduction of trauma from illness or hospitalization.
    d. Play sessions serve as assessment tools for determining children's awareness and perception of illness.

14. Several creative communication techniques may be used with children. Identify which technique is being used in each of the following examples.

    a. _____ The nurse shows Tina a picture of a child having an intravenous infusion started and asks Tina to describe the scene.

    b. _____ The nurse says to Tina, "I am concerned about how the medicine treatments are going because I want you to feel better."

    c. _____ The nurse reads Tina a story from a book and asks her to retell the story.

    d. _____ The nurse provides Tina with crayons and paper and asks her to draw a picture of her family.

    e. _____ The nurse gives Tina a doll and a stethoscope and allows her to listen to the doll's heart.

15. A complete pediatric health history includes ten expected components. List these components.

16. In eliciting the chief complaint, the nurse identifies which one of the following techniques as *not* appropriate?
    a. Limiting the chief complaint to a brief statement restricted to one or two symptoms
    b. Using labeling-type questions, such as "How are you sick?" to facilitate information exchange
    c. Recording the chief complaint in the child's or parent's own words
    d. Using open-ended neutral questions to elicit information

17. Read the following entry from a pediatric health history: "Nausea and vomiting for 3 days. Started with abdominal cramping past eating hamburger at home. No pain or cramping at present. Unable to keep any foods down but able to drink clear liquids without vomiting. No temperature elevation, no diarrhea." This entry represents which component of the health history?
    a. Chief complaint
    b. Past history
    c. Present illness
    d. Review of systems

18. Which one of the following is *not* part of the past history to be included in a pediatric health history?
    a. Symptom analysis
    b. Allergies
    c. Birth history
    d. Current medications

19. What are the *most* important previous growth patterns to record when completing a child's history of growth and development?

20. What are the *most* important developmental milestones to record when completing the child's health history?

21. The nurse knows that the *best* description of the sexual history for a pediatric health history:
    a. includes a discussion of the patient's plans for future children.
    b. allows the patient to introduce sexual activity history.
    c. includes a discussion of contraception methods only when the patient discloses current sexual activity.
    d. alerts the nurse to the need for sexually transmitted disease screening.

22. List five guidelines to include in an assessment of pain.

23. The _____ uses symbols to diagram data about the family structure. The _____ records the family medical history in chart form.

24. Indications for the nurse to conduct a comprehensive family assessment include which of the following?
    i.   Children with developmental delays
    ii. Children with history of repeated accidental injuries
    iii. Children with behavioral problems
    iv. Children receiving comprehensive well-child care

    a. i, ii, iii, and iv
    b. ii, iii, and iv
    c. i, ii, and iii
    d. ii and iii

25. Assessment of family structure is best conducted:
    a. after the first meeting with the patient.
    b. only when a problem is suspected within the family.
    c. towards the end of the interview when rapport has been established.
    d. by interviewing the patient about other family members' roles within the family.

26. Assessment of family interactions and roles, decision making and problem solving, and communication is known as assessment of:
    a. family structure.
    b. family function.
    c. family composition.
    d. home and community environment.

27. Describe the four principal areas of concern the nurse should focus on when assessing family structure.

28. The dietary history of a pediatric patient includes:
    a. a 12-hour dietary intake recall.
    b. a more specific, detailed history for the older child.
    c. financial and cultural factors that influence food selection.
    d. criticism of parents' allowance of nonessential foods.

Critical Thinking—Case Study

Mrs. Brown brings her 11-year-old son Kenny for a physical at the clinic where you work as a nurse. She is concerned because Kenny comes home from school "very tired and only wants to watch television." Kenny's bedtime has not changed, he performs well in school, and his mother denies stress or problems within the home. On physical exam, you discover Kenny is above the 90th percentile for weight by 25 pounds.

29. To effectively establish a setting for communication, you, upon entering the room, introduce yourself to Mrs. Brown and Kenny and explain your role and the purpose of the interview. You include Kenny in the interaction as you ask his name and age and what he is expecting at his visit today. You next inform Mrs. Brown and Kenny that he is 25 pounds overweight and that his diet and exercise plan must be "terrible" for Kenny to be in "such bad shape." Which aspect of effective communication have you, as a nurse, forgotten that will *most* significantly impact the exchange of information during this interview?
    a. Assurance of privacy and confidentiality
    b. Preliminary acquaintance
    c. Directing the focus away from the complaint of fatigue to one of obesity
    d. Injecting your own attitudes and feelings into the interview

30. Based on the information provided in the case study, you can correctly record which of the following?
    a. Chief complaint
    b. Present illness
    c. Past medical history
    d. Symptom analysis

31. Mrs. Brown, Kenny, and you agree to the need to conduct a more intensive nutritional assessment. Which one of the following ways to record Kenny's dietary intake would you suggest as *most* reliable in providing needed information to currently assess Kenny's dietary habits?
    a. 12-hour recall
    b. 24-hour recall
    c. Food diary for 3-day period
    d. Food frequency questionnaire

32. During the physical exam, which of the following physical findings could be consistent with excess carbohydrate nutrition?
    a. Caries
    b. Skin elastic and firm
    c. Hair stringy, friable, dull, and dry
    d. Enlarged thyroid

33. The physical exam has been completed to reflect that other than his obesity, Kenny is in excellent physical health with normal blood counts. The completed nutritional assessment reflects that Mrs. Brown has little knowledge about proper nutrition and that Kenny has a large intake of "junk" foods high in fat and calories but low in nutrients. Based on the data collected, which of the following nursing diagnoses is *most* appropriate?

    i.   Altered family process related to parent's knowledge deficit
    ii.   Altered family coping related to family's inability to purchase needed foods
    iii. Altered individual coping related to fatigue from poor dietary habits
    iv.   Altered nutrition: more than body requirements, related to eating practices
    v.   Altered nutrition: more than body requirements, related to knowledge deficit of parent

    a. i, ii, and iv
    b. iii and iv
    c. iii, iv, and v
    d. iv and v

34. Once the problem is defined, you include Mrs. Brown in the problem-solving process. Why is it important to include the parent in the problem-solving process?

CHAPTER 7

Physical and Developmental Assessment of the Child

1. In pediatric examinations, the normal sequence of head-to-toe direction is often altered to accommodate the patient's developmental needs. The nurse identifies which of the following goals as *least* likely to guide the examination process?
   a. Minimizing the stress and anxiety associated with the assessment of body parts
   b. Recording the findings according to the normal sequence
   c. Fostering a trusting nurse-child relationship
   d. Preserving the essential security of the parent-child relationship

2. Mr. Alls brings his 12-month-old son Keith in for his regular well-infant exam. The nurse knows that the *best* approach to the physical examination for this patient will be to:
   a. have the infant sit in the parent's lap to complete as much of the examination as possible.
   b. place the infant on the exam table with parent out of view.
   c. perform examination in head-to-toe direction.
   d. completely undress Keith and leave him undressed during the examination.

3. Behavior that signals the child's readiness to cooperate during the physical examination does *not* include:
   a. talking to the nurse.
   b. making eye contact with the nurse.
   c. allowing physical touching.
   d. sitting on parent's lap, playing with a doll.

4. The National Center for Health Statistics has growth charts available for pediatric patients. These

   growth charts have been revised to include _____,

   _____, and _____.

5. The assessment method that the nurse expects to provide the *best* information about the physical growth pattern of a preschool-age child is:
   a. recording height and weight measurements of the child.
   b. keeping a flow sheet for height, weight, and head circumference increases.
   c. obtaining a history of sibling growth patterns.
   d. measuring the height, weight, and head circumference of the child.

6. Describe how to measure recumbent length in a 24-month-old child.

7. Identify the following statements regarding the growth or development patterns of pediatric patients as true or false.

    _____ Normal growth patterns may vary among children of the same age group.

    _____ A sudden weight increase in a 10-year-old whose weight has been steady before is not an area for concern.

    _____ Growth is a continuous but uneven process, and the most reliable evaluation lies in comparison of growth measurements over a prolonged time.

    _____ Growth measurements during the physical examination should be age-specific and include length, height, weight, skinfold thickness, and arm and head circumference.

    _____ One convenient measurement of body fat is arm circumference.

8. Which one of the following findings for growth should be followed closely?
    a. Height and weight falls above the 5th percentile on the growth chart.
    b. Height and weight falls below the 5th percentile on the growth chart.
    c. Height and weight falls below the 95th percentile on the growth chart.
    d. Height and weight falls within the 50th percentile on the growth chart.

9. Head circumference is:
    a. measured in all children up to the age of 24 months.
    b. equal to chest circumferences at about 1 to 2 years of age.
    c. about 8 to 9 cm smaller than chest circumference during childhood.
    d. measured slightly below the eyebrows and pinna of the ears.

10. In infants and young children, the _____ pulse should be taken because it is the

    most reliable. This pulse should be counted for _____ because of the possibility of irregularities in rhythm. When counting respirations in infants, observe the

    _____ movements and count for _____ because their movements are irregular.

11. The nurse should obtain the vital signs of an infant in what order?
    a. Measure temperature, then count the pulse, and then count respirations.
    b. Count the pulse, then count respirations, and then measure the temperature.
    c. Count respirations, then count the pulse, and then measure the temperature.
    d. Measure the temperature, then count respirations, and then count the pulse.

12. Which one of the following findings should the nurse recognize as normal when measuring the vital signs of a 5-year-old child?
    a. Femoral pulses graded at +1
    b. Oral temperature of 100.9° F
    c. Blood pressure of 101/61
    d. Respiratory rate of 28

13. The nurse should eliminate which of the following observations when recording the general appearance of the child?
    a. Impression of child's nutritional status
    b. Behavior, interactions with parents
    c. Hygiene, cleanliness
    d. Vital signs

14. Match each term with its description or associated assessment findings. (Terms may be used more than once.)

a. Cyanosis
b. Pallor
c. Erythema
d. Ecchymosis
e. Petechiae

f. Jaundice
g. Plethora
h. Tissue turgor
i. Edema
j. Pitting edema

k. Koilonychia
l. Wryneck or torticollis
m. Opisthotonos
n. Genu valgum
o. Genu varum

_____ Appears in dark-skinned patients as ashen-gray lips and tongue

_____ Appears in light-skinned patients as purplish to yellow-green areas

_____ May be a sign of anemia, chronic disease, edema, or shock

_____ Redness of the skin that may be the result of infection, local inflammation, or increased temperature due to climatic conditions

_____ Large, diffuse areas, usually blue or black in color and the result of injury

_____ Small distinct pinpoint hemorrhages

_____ Yellow staining of the skin usually caused by bile pigments

_____ "spoon nails"; sometimes seen in iron deficiency anemia

_____ Injury to the sternocleidomastoid muscle with subsequent holding of the head to one side with the chin pointing toward the opposite side

_____ Hyperextension of the neck and spine

_____ Swelling or puffiness of skin

_____ Temporary indentation that occurs when the finger is pushed into the skin

_____ Intense redness of the lips or cheeks as a compensatory response to chronic hypoxia

_____ Amount of elasticity to the skin

_____ Lateral bowing of the tibia

_____ Knees are close together but feet are spread apart; "knock-knee"

15. You are assessing skin turgor in 10-month-old Ryan. You grasp the skin on the abdomen between the thumb and index finger, pull it taut, and quickly release it. The tissue remains suspended or tented for a few seconds, then slowly falls back on the abdomen. Which of the following evaluations can you correctly assume?
a. The tissue shows normal elasticity.
b. The child is properly hydrated.
c. The assessment was done incorrectly.
d. The child has poor skin turgor.

16. You are assessing 7-year-old Mary's lymph nodes. Using the distal portions of your fingers, you press gently but firmly in a circular motion along the occipital and postauricular node areas. You record the findings as "tender, enlarged, warm lymph nodes." Which of the following is true?
a. Your findings are within normal limits for Mary's age.
b. Your assessment technique was incorrect and should be repeated.
c. Your findings suggest infection or inflammation in the scalp area or external ear canal.
d. Your recording of the information is complete because it includes temperature and tenderness.

17. Which of the following assessment findings of the head and neck does *not* require a referral?
a. Head lag before 6 months of age
b. Hyperextension of the head with pain on flexion
c. Palpable thyroid gland, including isthmus and lobes
d. Closure of the anterior fontanel at the age of 9 months

18. Sinuses that are present soon after birth are the _____ and

    _____ sinuses.

19. Normal findings on examination of the pupils may be recorded as PERRLA, which means:

20. Match each term with its description.

    a. Hypertelorism   f. Hordeolum   k. Strabismus
    b. Ptosis   g. Blepharitis   l. Amblyopia
    c. Sunset eyes   h. Dacryocystitis   m. Chalazion
    d. Ectropion   i. Hyperopia   n. Binocularity
    e. Entropion   j. Myopia

    _____ Rolling out of the eyelid
    _____ Turning in of the eyelid
    _____ Inflammation and blockage of the lacrimal sac or duct
    _____ Farsightedness
    _____ Granuloma or cyst of the internal sebaceous glands
    _____ Large spacing between the eyes
    _____ Upper eyelid covering no part of the iris
    _____ Ability to focus on one visual field with both eyes at the same time
    _____ One eye deviating from point of fixation
    _____ Inflammation of the edge of the eyelid
    _____ Stye
    _____ Upper eyelid covering part of the pupil or the lower part of the iris
    _____ Nearsightedness
    _____ Type of blindness resulting from uncorrected "lazy" eye

21. Which one of the following assessments is an expected finding in the child's eye examination?
    a. Opaque red reflex of the eye
    b. Ophthalmoscopic exam reveals that veins are darker in color and about one fourth larger in size than the arteries.
    c. Strabismus in the 12-month-old infant
    d. A 5-year-old child who reads the Snellen eye chart at the 20/40 level

22. Match each type of eye chart with the procedure used for that chart.

    a. Snellen chart
    b. Tumbling chart
    c. HOTV chart

    _____ To pass line correctly, child must identify four out of six letters on the line; used for children who can read letters.
    _____ Child is asked to point in the direction the letter is facing.
    _____ Child is asked to point to the correct letter on a board held in the hands.

23. Which of the following children meet referral criteria?
    a. Jason, age 14 years, who identified fewer than four out of six correct letters with his right eye and five out of six correct with his left eye during visual acuity testing
    b. Sandra, age 3 years, who demonstrated eye movement with the unilateral cover test
    c. Tommy, age 4 years, who demonstrated a two-line difference between eyes on his visual acuity testing
    d. All of the above

24. When assessing the ear of a 2-year-old child, the nurse should:
    a. expect cerumen in the external ear canal.
    b. use the smallest speculum to prevent trauma to the ear.
    c. pull the pinna up and back to visualize the canal better.
    d. pull the pinna down and back to visualize the canal better.

25. The test that measures the compliance of the tympanic membrane and the middle ear pressure is:
    a. the Rinne test.
    b. the threshold acuity sweep test.
    c. vestibular testing.
    d. tympanometry.

26. Four-year-old Billy has been brought to the clinic by his parents because they have noticed a sudden foul odor in his mouth accompanied by a discharge from the right nares. The nurse knows that this is *most* likely to suggest:
    a. poor dental hygiene.
    b. foreign body in the nose.
    c. gingival disease.
    d. thumb-sucking.

27. The nurse is assessing the mouth and throat of 7-month-old Alex. Which of the following is recognized as a normal finding?
    a. Membranes are bright pink, smooth, and glistening.
    b. White curdy plaques are located on the tongue.
    c. Redness and puffiness are present along the gum line.
    d. Tip of the tongue extends to the gum line.

28. When assessing 4-year-old Gail's chest, the nurse should expect:
    a. movement of the chest wall to be symmetric bilaterally and coordinated with breathing.
    b. respiratory movements to be chiefly thoracic.
    c. anteroposterior diameter to be equal to the transverse diameter.
    d. retraction of the muscles between the ribs on respiratory movement.

29. The nurse asks 12-year-old Susan to repeat the word "ninety-nine" several times while the palmar surfaces of the nurse's hands are placed on the child's chest. The nurse is palpating for conduction of sound through the respiratory tract. What is this called?
    a. Pleural friction rub
    b. Crepitation
    c. Normal respiratory movements
    d. Vocal fremitus

30. On auscultation of 8-year-old Tammie's lung fields, the nurse hears inspiratory sounds that are louder, longer, and higher-pitched than on expiration. These sounds are heard over the chest, except over the scapula and sternum. These sounds are:
    a. bronchovesicular breath sounds.
    b. vesicular breath sounds.
    c. bronchial breath sounds.
    d. adventitious breath sounds.

31. The nurse is palpating for cardiac thrills, and knows that thrills are:
    a. vibrations caused by the flow of blood from one chamber to another through a narrowed opening.
    b. best felt with the dorsal surface of the hands.
    c. found at the point of maximum intensity.
    d. louder on inspiration than on expiration.

32. A heart sound that is the result of vibrations produced during ventricular filling and is normally heard in some children is:
    a. S_1.
    b. S_2.
    c. S_3.
    d. S_4.

33. When listening over the aortic area of the heart, the nurse should place the stethoscope where?
    a. Second right intercostal space close to sternum
    b. Second left intercostal space close to sternum
    c. Fifth left intercostal space close to sternum
    d. Fifth right intercostal space, left midclavicular line

34. Examination of the abdomen is performed correctly by the nurse in what order?
    a. Inspection, palpation, percussion, and auscultation
    b. Inspection, percussion, auscultation, and palpation
    c. Palpation, percussion, auscultation, and inspection
    d. Inspection, auscultation, percussion, and palpation

35. While assessing the male genitalia of 4-year-old Ben, the nurse notes that the urethral meatus is opening on the ventral side of the glans or shaft. Which of the following is true?
    a. This is a normal finding.
    b. This finding is consistent with hypospadias and needs referral.
    c. This finding is consistent with epispadias and needs referral.
    d. This finding is consistent with phimosis and needs referral

36. In performing an examination for scoliosis, the nurse understands that which one of the following is an *incorrect* method?
    a. The child should be examined only in his or her underpants (and a bra if an older girl).
    b. The child should stand erect with the nurse observing from behind.
    c. The child should squat down with hands extended forward so the nurse can observe for asymmetry of the shoulder blades.
    d. The child should bend forward with the back parallel to the floor so that the nurse can observe from the side.

37. How would the nurse test for the Brudzinski sign, and what would a positive sign in the presence of symptoms suggest?

38. Match each theory with its description.

    a. Freud's psychosexual theory
    b. Erikson's psychosocial theory
    c. Piaget's theory of cognitive development

    _____ Emphasizes the concept of critical periods in personality development, during which children strive to master conflicts

    _____ Based on the concept that during childhood certain regions of the body assume a prominent psychologic significance as the source of new pleasures

    _____ Describes children's progress through stages of mental activity in an orderly and sequential manner to allow adaptation to the environment

39. Complete the following statements about moral development.

    The _____ level of morality parallels the preconceptual level of cognitive development. At this level morality is external as children conform to rules imposed by authority

    figures. At the _____ level, children are concerned with conformity and loyalty.

    At the _____ level, children define moral values beyond the authority of the groups and persons holding these principles.

40. The Denver Developmental Screening test is limited by its inability to predict:
    a. developmental delays in children of cultural ethnic groups.
    b. gross motor delays.
    c. language delays.
    d. personal-social delays.

41. When discussing the results of an abnormal Denver Developmental Screening test with a parent, the nurse should:
    a. ask the parent whether the child's performance was typical behavior.
    b. emphasize the failed items first, delayed items second, and then the passed items.
    c. explain that referral for the child should be immediate.
    d. explain the necessity for testing all items to the right of the child's age line to determine developmental delays.

Critical Thinking—Case Study

Mary, a 13-year-old, has come to the clinic with her mother. Mary is complaining of right-side abdominal pain of 24 hours' duration. She tells you, the nurse, that she has had some nausea and vomiting but no diarrhea. Her appetite is depressed and she feels hot and feverish. Mary has taken Tylenol for pain but with little relief. A complete blood count has been ordered and results are pending.

42. You are preparing Mary for a physical exam. You know that during the examination, Mary, as an adolescent, will likely:
    a. prefer her parents to be present during the entire exam.
    b. desire to undress in private and will feel more comfortable when provided with a gown.
    c. prefer that traumatic procedures such as ear and mouth exams be performed last.
    d. need to have heart and lungs auscultated first.

43. You complete the physical exam and evaluate which one of the following as an abnormal finding?
    a. Bowel sounds are stimulated by stroking the abdominal surface with the fingernail.
    b. Mary has no abdominal discomfort when she is supine with the legs flexed at the hips and knees.
    c. Mary's eyes are open during palpation of the abdomen.
    d. When the nurse presses firmly over the area distal to the right side of the abdomen and quickly releases this pressure, pain is intensified in the lower right side.

44. Which one of the following organs is located in the lower right quadrant of the abdomen?
    a. Bladder
    b. Liver
    c. Ovaries
    d. Appendix

45. Mary's mother is apprehensive about her daughter's condition and asks you whether "it is serious." Which one of the following is your *best* response?
    a. "Mary has appendicitis and will need to have surgery immediately."
    b. "You will have to ask the doctor about her condition."
    c. "Mary has some abdominal pain that is not normal. We are watching her very carefully and will be able to tell you more when the laboratory tests are completed."
    d. "Mary should be able to go home as soon as the doctor finishes with the examination and the laboratory tests are completed."

46. While inspecting the abdomen, you should recognize which one of the following as a normal finding?
    a. Peristaltic waves
    b. Silvery, whitish lines when the skin is stretched out
    c. Bulging at the umbilicus
    d. Protruding abdomen with skin pulled tight

47. Two-year-old Drew is brought to the clinic by his mom. She tells the nurse that his eyes "look funny." What tests should the nurse use to determine ocular alignment? What findings in each test would indicate abnormal findings?

Gerald, age 16, has been complaining to the school nurse of chest pain during physical exercise class at school. The nurse is performing an assessment of the heart.

48. _____ is the sound caused by the closure of the tricuspid and mitral valves. It is

    heard loudest at the _____ of the heart. _____ is the sound heard as a result of the closure of the pulmonic and aortic valves. It is heard loudest at the

    _____ of the heart.

49. During S_2 a split is heard that does not change during inspiration. Based on this, the nurse should suspect:
    a. a normal finding referred to as *physiologic splitting*.
    b. mitral valve prolapse.
    c. that no anatomic cardiac defect exists, but that a physiologic abnormality such as anemia is likely to be present.
    d. fixed splitting, which can be a diagnostic sign of atrial septal defect.

CHAPTER 8

Health Promotion of the Newborn and Family

1. The chemical factors in the blood that stimulate the initiation of the first respiration in the neonate are

_____ _____, _____ _____ _____,

and _____ _____.

2. The primary thermal stimulus that helps initiate the first respiration is

_____.

3. The nurse recognizes that tactile stimulation probably has some effect on initiation of respiration in the neonate. Which one of the following is of *no* beneficial effect?
   a. Normal handling of the neonate
   b. Drying the skin of the neonate
   c. Slapping the neonate's heel or buttocks
   d. Placing the infant skin-to-skin with the mother

4. Which one of these neonates will *most* likely need additional respiratory support at birth?
   a. The infant born by normal vaginal delivery
   b. The infant born by cesarean birth
   c. The infant born vaginally after 12 hours of labor
   d. The infant born with high levels of surfactant

5. During the transition from fetal to neonatal circulation, the newborn's cardiovascular system accomplishes which of the following anatomic and physiologic alterations?
   i.   Closure of the ductus venosus
   ii. Closure of the foramen ovale
   iii. Closure of the ductus arteriosis
   iv. Increased systemic pressure and decreased pulmonary artery pressure

   a. i, ii, iii, and iv
   b. i, ii, and iii
   c. ii, iii, and iv
   d. i, iii, and iv

6. Identify the following statements about infant adjustments to extrauterine life as either true or false.

   _____ Factors that predispose the neonate to excessive heat loss are large surface area, thin layer of subcutaneous fat, and the lack of shivering to produce heat.

   _____ Nonshivering thermogenesis is an effective method of heat production in the neonate since it is able to produce heat with little use of oxygen.

   _____ Brown fat or brown adipose tissue has a greater capacity to produce heat than does ordinary adipose tissue.

   _____ The longer the infant is attached to the placenta, the less blood volume will be received by the neonate.

   _____ Deficient production of pancreatic amylase impairs utilization of complex carbohydrates.

_____ Deficiency of pancreatic lipase assists the neonate in the digestion of cow's milk.

_____ Most salivary glands are functioning at birth even though most infants do not start drooling until teeth erupt.

_____ The stomach capacity for most newborn infants is about 90 ml.

_____ The newborn should be expected to void within the first 48 hours.

_____ The liver is the most mature of the gastrointestinal organs at birth.

_____ At birth the skeletal system contains larger amounts of ossified bone than cartilage.

_____ After birth, development of the nervous system is from a cephalocaudal-proximodistal pattern.

7. What three factors make the infant more prone to problems of dehydration, acidosis, and overhydration?

8. Match each term with its description.

   a. Meconium
   b. Breast-fed infant stools
   c. Formula-fed infant stools

   _____ Pale yellow to golden; pasty consistency
   _____ First stool; dark green with pasty, sticky consistency
   _____ Pale yellow to light brown; firmer in consistency with more offensive odor

9. Newborns receive passive immunity in the form of IgG from the _____

   and _____.

10. The nurse recognizes that all of the following effects of maternal sex hormones in the newborn are normal _except_:
    a. hypertrophied labia.
    b. secretion of "witch's milk" from the newborn breasts.
    c. pseudomenstruation.
    d. bleeding from the breast nipples.

11. Fill in the blanks in the following statements as they pertain to sensory functions in the normal newborn.

    a. The newborn can fixate on a bright object that is within _____ and in the midline of the visual field.

    b. Infants have visual preferences for the colors of _____, _____, and

       _____ and for designs such as _____ _____ and _____.

    c. The newborn's response to _____-frequency sounds is one of decreased motor activity, and

       crying during exposure to _____-frequency sound elicits an alerting reaction.

12. The nurse is performing the 5-minute Apgar on a newborn. Which one of the following observations is included in the Apgar score?
    a. Blood pressure
    b. Temperature
    c. Muscle tone
    d. Weight

13. Match each period of reactivity with the observations the nurse is likely to make during that period.

    a. First period of reactivity
    b. Second stage of first period of reactivity
    c. Second period of reactivity

    _____ This is an excellent bonding period and the best time to start breast-feeding.
    _____ During this period, infant sleep lasts 2 to 4 hours; heart rate and respiratory rate decrease.
    _____ Gastric and respiratory secretions are increased; passage of meconium commonly occurs.

14. The nurse is using the Brazelton Neonatal Behavioral Assessment Scale to assess the newborn's behavioral responses. How should the nurse define *habituation*?
    a. Responsiveness of the newborn to auditory and visual stimuli
    b. Process whereby the newborn becomes accustomed to stimuli
    c. The ability of the infant to be easily aroused from sleep state
    d. A reactive Moro reflex by the infant, with good muscle tone and coordination

15. Which of the following is *not* correct about the relationship of newborn weight to gestational age?
    a. All infants below the weight of 2500 g (5 1/2 pounds) are premature by gestational age.
    b. Gestational age is more closely related to fetal maturity than is birth weight.
    c. Classification of infants by both weight and gestational age can be beneficial for predicting mortality risks.
    d. Hereditary influences are a normal part of assessment.

16. On assessment of a 24-hour newborn, the nurse makes the following observations. Which is normal?
    a. Cyanotic color centrally and peripherally
    b. Axillary temperature of 96° F
    c. Flexion of the infant's head and extremities, which rest on the chest and abdomen
    d. Respirations of 68

17. Match each term with its description.

    a. Milia   e. Acrocyanosis   i. Caput succedaneum
    b. Erythema toxicum   f. Cutis marmorata   j. Cephalhematoma
    c. Harlequin color change g. Mongolian spots   k. Vernix caseosa
    d. Nevus flammeus   h. Telangiectatic nevi   l. Lanugo

    _____ Irregular areas of deep blue pigmentation, usually in sacral and glutteal regions seen in the newborn
    _____ Distended sebaceous glands that appear as tiny white papules on the cheeks, chin and nose in the newborn
    _____ Condition in which the lower half of the body becomes pink and upper half is pale when the newborn lies on side
    _____ Edema of the soft scalp tissue

_____ Pink papular rash with vesicles superimposed on thorax, back, buttocks, and abdomen in the newborn

_____ Port-wine stain

_____ Hematoma between periosteum and skull bone

_____ Cyanosis of hands and feet

_____ "stork bites"; flat, deep pink, localized areas usually seen at back of neck

_____ Transient mottling when infant is exposed to decreased temperature, stress, or overstimulation

_____ Fine downy hair present on the newborn's skin

_____ Cheese-like substance; mixture of sebum and desquamating cell covering the skin at birth

18. Newborns lose up to 10% of their birth weight by 3 to 4 days of age. The factor that does *not* contribute to this process is:
    a. limited fluid intake in breast-fed infants.
    b. incomplete digestion of complex carbohydrates.
    c. loss of excessive extracellular fluid.
    d. passage of meconium.

19. When assessing blood pressure in the newborn, the nurse knows which of the following is true?
    a. A referral is needed with a difference in systolic BP in which the BP in the calf is 10 mm Hg less than in the upper arm.
    b. Routine BP measurements of full-term neonates are an excellent predictor of hypertension.
    c. A normal BP reading for a 3-day-old infant is approximately 90/60.
    d. BP should be measured routinely on all healthy newborns as recommended by the American Academy of Pediatrics.

20. A widened, tense, bulging fontanel can be a sign of _____ _____

    _____, whereas a markedly sunken, depressed fontanel is a sign of _____.

21. Assessment of the newborn includes which of the following?
    i.   Clinical gestational age assessment
    ii.   General measurements
    iii. General appearance
    iv.   Head-to-toe assessment
    v.   Parent-infant attachment

    a. i, ii, iii, iv, and v
    b. i, ii, iii, and iv
    c. ii, iii, iv, and v
    d. ii, iii, and iv

22. Which of the following observations from the eye assessment of a newborn is recognized as normal?
    a. Purulent discharge at age 48 hours
    b. Absence of the red reflex at age 24 hours
    c. No pupillary reflex at age 3 weeks
    d. Presence of strabismus at age 48 hours

23. How should the nurse assess auditory ability in the newborn?

24. It is important to assess for nasal patency in the newborn, because newborns are usually

_____.

25. The nurse correctly identifies the need to notify the physician for which of the following neonates?
    a. The 24-hour-old neonate found to have Epstein pearls on the side of the hard palate
    b. The 2-day-old neonate with periodic breathing
    c. The 24-hour-old neonate who has nasal flaring
    d. The 2-hour-old neonate who has a bluish, white, moist, umbilical cord with one vein and two arteries visible

26. Match each term with its description.

    a. Anal patency   e. Moro reflex
    b. Down syndrome   f. Tonic neck
    c. Rooting reflex   g. Grasp reflex
    d. Babinski reflex

    _____ Touching cheek along the side of the mouth causes infant to turn head toward that side and begin to suck.
    _____ Fanning of the toes and dorsiflexion of the great toe; disappears after 1 year of age
    _____ Symmetric abduction and extension of the arms; fingers fan out; thumb and index finger form a C
    _____ Passage of meconium from rectum during first 48 hours of life
    _____ Flexion caused by touching soles of feet near bases of digits or palms of hands
    _____ Transverse palmar crease
    _____ Response in which an infant in supine position extends the arm and leg on the side to which the head is turned and flexes the limbs of the opposite side

27. Fill in the blanks in the following statements.

    a. The loss of heat to cooler solid objects in the environment that are not in direct contact with an

       infant is called _____.

    b. Heat loss from the body through direct contact of the skin with a cooler solid object is termed

       _____.

    c. Placing an infant in the direct flow of air from a fan causes rapid heat loss through

       _____.

    d. Loss of heat through skin moisture is termed _____.

28. The nurse implements all of the following actions to maintain a patent airway in a newborn. Which one will be *least* effective?
    a. Maintaining the infant in a supine position during sleep
    b. Performing oropharyngeal suctioning for 5 seconds with sufficient time between attempts to allow infant to reoxygenate
    c. In the delivery room, suctioning the infant's pharynx first, then the nasal passages
    d. Continuing oral feedings for the infant with nasal flaring and intercostal retractions

29. Identify the following medications to be given as preventive care.

    a. _____ Prophylactic eye treatment against ophthalmia neonatorum

    b. _____ Administered by injection to prevent hemorrhagic disease
       of the newborn

    c. _____ First dose given between birth and 2 days of age to
       decrease incidence of hepatitis B (HBV)

30. In screening for phenylketonuria (PKU), the nurse knows:
    a. blood samples should be taken after 24 hours of age and again at 2 weeks of age.
    b. blood should be drawn using a venous blood sample.
    c. preparation includes instructing parents to keep the infant NPO for 2 hours before the test.
    d. to completely saturate the filter paper by applying blood to both sides of the paper.

31. The nurse should involve the parents in the care of their newborn. Teaching is *least* likely to include:
    a. the use of Ivory soap, oils, powder, and lotions with each bath.
    b. cleaning the vulva in a front-to-back direction or cleaning the foreskin by wiping around the glans.
       (If the foreskin is retracted, it must be by gentle retraction only as far as it will go with gentle
       return to normal position as necessary. The foreskin is not retracted in the newborn because it is
       normally tight.)
    c. care of the umbilical stump, including placing the diaper below the cord to avoid irritation and wet-
       ness of the site.
    d. care of the circumcision site, explaining that on the second day a yellowish white exudate forms
       normally as part of the granulating process.

32. Describe the current policy of the American Academy of Pediatrics on circumcision of newborn male
    infants.

33. Human milk is preferable to cow's milk because:
    a. human milk has a nonlaxative effect.
    b. human milk has more calories per ounce.
    c. human milk has greater mineral content.
    d. human milk offers greater immunologic benefits.

34. The nurse is instructing new parents about proper feeding techniques for their newborn. Indicate
    whether the following statements are true or false.

    _____ Infants need at least 2 hours of sucking daily.
    _____ After feeding, infants should be placed on the right side to prevent regurgitation and dis-
             tention.
    _____ Breast-fed infants tend to be hungry every 2 to 3 hours.
    _____ Supplemental feedings should not be offered to the breast-fed infant because this causes
             nipple confusion.
    _____ Supplemental water is not needed in breast-fed infants, even in hot climates.
    _____ Five behavioral stages occur during successful feeding. These are prefeeding, approach,
             attachment, consummatory, and satiety behaviors.

35. Mrs. Gonzalez is a first-time mother. She comes to the clinic because of painful nipples and is afraid she will have to terminate breast-feeding. The breast physical exam is normal. Which of the following actions does the nurse recognize as *most* likely causing the painful nipples?
    i.   Using an electric pump to express milk for the infant to drink when Mrs. Gonzalez is away from home
    ii.   Washing the nipples before and after each feeding with soap and applying aloe vera gel
    iii. Using plastic-backed nipple pads
    iv.   Letting warm water flow directly over the breast in the shower
    v.   Leaving breast milk on the areola after feedings and letting it dry
    vi.   Letting the infant breast-feed every 2 hours

    a. i and v
    b. iv and v
    c. iii and vi
    d. ii and iii

36. Which one of the following actions by the nurse will *least* likely promote the attachment process between the infant and parent?
    a. Recognizing individual differences present in the infant and explaining these normal characteristics to the parent
    b. Assisting the mother to assume the en face position when she is presented with her infant
    c. Explaining to the parents how to respond to their infant with the use of reciprocal interacting
    d. Explaining to the parents the need for infants to have an organized schedule of daily activities that allows them to remain in their crib during awake periods

Critical Thinking—Case Study

Michael was born by normal vaginal delivery to Marilyn and Doug Madison. Assessment at birth reflects the following: heart rate of 120; respiratory effort good with a strong cry, well-flexed muscle tone with active movement and reflex irritability; turns head away when nose is suctioned; and color assessment of body pink with feet and hands blue. Michael's weight is 6 pounds, and his length is 21 inches. Mrs. Madison is allowed to hold Michael and put him to breast in the delivery room. The Madisons do not plan to have Michael
circumcised.

37. What is the Apgar score for Michael?
    a. 8
    b. 10
    c. 9
    d. 7

38. The nurse is conducting a gestational age assessment of Michael based on the six neuromuscular signs. What are these signs, and what results would indicate a higher maturity rating?

39. Listed below are nursing actions that the nurse would perform during the transitional period. Arrange these actions in order of highest to lowest priority.

   i.   Taking head and chest circumference measurements
   ii. Assessing for neonatal distress
   iii. Administering prophylactic medications
   iv. Scoring for gestational age
   v.   Assessing vital signs

   a. ii, v, i, iii, iv
   b. i, ii, v, iii, iv
   c. ii, iii, i, v, iv
   d. ii, v, iv, i, iii

40. Identify, in order of highest to lowest priority, four nursing goals that are considered the basics for safe and effective care of the newborn.

41. You are assigned to care for 1-day-old Michael in the newborn nursery. List six daily assessments that should be conducted and documented.

42. Mrs. Madison and Michael are being discharged tomorrow. You are preparing to provide Mrs. Madison with the newborn discharge teaching plan. Michael is Mrs. Madison's first infant, and on assessment you find that she has several questions about her techniques of breast-feeding. You show her how to hold Michael for feeding, how to position him properly to facilitate sucking, and how to care for her breast. You also provide her with a video to reinforce your instruction. When you return later, Mrs. Madison asks you about the use of supplemental feedings. Which of the following is your best response?
   a. "It is okay to give Michael supplements but only after he is put to the breast."
   b. "Why would you think about that now? We'll discuss it tomorrow when you are ready to go home."
   c. "There is no need to give Michael supplemental feedings. Supplemental feeding may decrease your milk production."
   d. "You will need to give Michael supplemental feedings sometimes because you may not have enough milk."

43. You correctly evaluate the teaching plan you provided in question 42 as effective when:
    a. Mrs. Madison is discharged to take Michael home.
    b. Mrs. Madison explains to the nurse how to successfully breast-feed Michael.
    c. Mrs. Madison is seen by the nurse successfully breast-feeding Michael. Additionally, Mrs. Madison discusses with the nurse the information that the nurse had previously shared with her on breast-feeding.
    d. Mrs. Madison verbalizes that she has no further questions about breast-feeding and is able to describe to the nurse the teaching that had been provided.

44. Mrs. Madison and Michael are being discharged just 24 hours after birth. What should the nurse include in the early discharge newborn home care instructions for each of the following areas?

    Wet diapers

    Stools

    Activity

    Cord

    Position of sleep

45. Mrs. Madison is concerned because she feels Michael is getting a cold. She tells you that he is "sneezing a lot." Your *best* response would be:
    a. "It is because the nose has been flattened while going through the birth canal. It will go away in another day or two."
    b. "Michael cannot get a cold; he is breast-feeding and this gives him a natural immunity."
    c. "Sneezing is abnormal and you will need to watch Michael for fever development and decreased sucking."
    d. "Most newborns are obligatory nose breathers, and sneezing is very common."

46. You are a nurse assigned to the newborn nursery. While assessing a newborn, you see white patches on the inside of the mouth. How would you correctly determine whether this is a normal or abnormal finding?

47. A nursing assistant has been assigned to work with you. Summarize what you would tell him or her about each of the following issues.

The most important way to prevent cross-infection:

Preventing transmission of pseudomonas:

Handling newborn infants before the first bath:

CHAPTER 9

Health Problems of the Newborn

1. Match each term with its description or associated term.

   a. Cephalopelvic disproportion

   b. Crepitus

   c. Moniliasis

   d. *Staphylococcus aureus*

   e. Icterus

   f. Hemolytic

   g. Fiberoptic blanket

   h. Bronze-baby syndrome

   i. Heterozygous

   j. Homozygous

   _____ Causes impetigo

   _____ Suited for home phototherapy

   _____ Results in fetal head not being able to pass through the maternal pelvis

   _____ Rare reaction to phototherapy in which the serum, urine, and skin turn grayish brown

   _____ Candidiasis

   _____ Having dissimilar genes at a given position on a pair of chromosomes

   _____ Coarse, crackling sensation that can be produced by rubbing together fractured bone fragments

   _____ Having the same genes at a given point on a pair of chromosomes

   _____ Related to destruction of red blood cells

   _____ Jaundice

2. Birth injuries may occur during the delivery of the infant. Birth injuries are *not* usually the result of:
   a. forceful extraction deliveries.
   b. dystocia.
   c. excess amniotic fluid.
   d. breech presentations.

3. Which one of the following soft tissue birth injuries is *most* likely to need further evaluation?
   a. Subcutaneous fat necrosis
   b. Ecchymoses
   c. Petechiae appearing in areas other than the presenting part
   d. Petechiae appearing on the areas of the presenting part

4. Nursing care for soft tissue injury is *not* usually directed toward:
   a. assessing the injury.
   b. preventing breakdown and infection.
   c. providing explanations and reassurance to the parents.
   d. explaining the need for careful follow-up of injury after the infant's discharge.

5. Match each type of extracranial hemorrhagic injury with its description.

   a. Caput succedaneum

   b. Subgaleal hemorrhage

   c. Cephalhematoma

      _____ Bleeding into the area between the periosteum and bone; does not cross the suture line

      _____ Bleeding into the potential space that contains loosely arranged connective tissue

      _____ Edematous tissue above the bone; extends across sutures

6. An infant suffers a fracture of the clavicle during birth. Which one of the following would the nurse expect to observe on the physical examination of this infant?
   a. Crepitus felt over the affected area
   b. Symmetric moro reflex
   c. Complete fracture with overriding fragments
   d. Positive scarf sign

7. Match each type of paralysis with its correct description. (Types of paralysis may be used more than once.)

   a. Facial paralysis

   b. Brachial palsy

   c. Phrenic nerve paralysis

      _____ Arm hangs limp with the shoulder and arm adducted and internally rotated.

      _____ The eye cannot close completely on the affected side; the corner of the mouth droops, and an absence of forehead wrinkling occurs. This type of paralysis is caused by injury to cranial nerve VII.

      _____ This usually disappears spontaneously in a few days but may take several months.

      _____ This causes diaphragmatic paralysis, with respiratory distress as the most common sign of injury; injury is usually unilateral, with affected side of lung not expanding.

      _____ Nursing care includes maintaining proper positioning and preventing contractures.

      _____ Nursing care is aimed at aiding the infant in sucking and the mother with feeding techniques.

      _____ Undressing begins with the unaffected side, whereas dressing begins with the affected side.

      _____ Artificial tears are instilled to prevent drying.

8. Which of the following is *not* correct in describing erythema toxicum neonatorium?
   a. It is a benign, self-limiting rash that appears within the first 2 days of life.
   b. The rash is most obvious during crying episodes.
   c. The rash may be located on all areas of the body, including the soles of the feet and the palms of the hands.
   d. Lesions appear as 1- to 3-mm, white or pale yellow pustules with an erythematous base. Smears of the pustules show increased numbers of eosinophils and lowered numbers of neutrophils.

9. You are preparing to teach a class to new parents about candidiasis. Identify whether each of the following statements is true or false.

      _____ Candidiasis is a yeast-like fungus that can be transmitted by maternal vaginal infection during delivery, through person-to-person contact, and from contaminated articles.

      _____ In the neonate, candidiasis is usually found in the oral and diaper areas.

      _____ It is difficult to distinguish between oral candidiasis and coagulated milk in the infant's mouth because both are easily removed by simple wiping.

_____   Thrush appears when the oral flora are altered as a result of antibiotic therapy or poor handwashing by the infant's caregiver.

_____   Oral candidiasis is treated with the administration of oral nystatin four times a day, before feedings and at night.

_____   The infant can spread candidial dermatitis into the mouth with contaminated hands; therefore, the parents should be taught to place clothes over the diaper to break this cycle.

_____   It is not necessary to boil bottles or nipples for infants with oral candidiasis, because the fungus is heat-resistant.

_____   Oral nystatin should be placed in the far back of the throat to allow the infant to swallow it easily.

10. Which one of the following statements concerning impetigo is *not* correct and should be omitted by the nurse from the teaching plan?
    a. Impetigo is caused by *Staphylococcus aureus*.
    b. Impetigo is an eruption of vesicular lesions that occur on skin that has not been traumatized.
    c. Distribution of impetigo lesions usually occurs on the perineum, trunk, face, and buttocks.
    d. The infected child or infant must be isolated from others until all lesions have healed.

11. Identify the type of birthmark described by each of the following statements.

    a. _____ These lesions are pink, red, or purple and often thicken, darken, and proportionately enlarge as the child grows.

    b. _____ These are red, rubbery nodules with a rough surface that are recognized as tumors that involve only capillaries.

    c. _____ These are multiple flat, light brown marks that are often associated with the autosomal-dominant hereditary disorder neurofibromatosis.

12. Treatment for port-wine stain includes laser therapy. The teaching plan for treatment expectations includes which of the following?
    a. The lesion will have a bright pink appearance for 10 days after treatment.
    b. Expose the infant to sunlight for 15 minutes daily after treatments.
    c. Administer salicylates before each treatment for pain.
    d. After treatment, gently wash the area daily with soap and dab it dry.

13. _____ is an excessive accumulation of bilirubin in the blood and is

    characterized by _____, a yellow discoloration of the skin.

14. In discussing the pathophysiology of bilirubin, the nurse knows that red blood cell destruction results

    in _____ and _____. _____

    _____ is an insoluble substance bound to albumin. In the liver this is changed to a

    soluble substance, _____ _____.

15. _____ is the term used to describe the yellow staining of the brain cells that can result in bilirubin encephalopathy.
    a. Jaundice
    b. Physiologic jaundice
    c. Kernicterus
    d. Icterus neonatorum

16. Which one of the following statements about bilirubin encephalopathy is true?
    a. Development may be enhanced by metabolic acidosis, lowered albumin levels, intracranial infections, and increases in the metabolic demands for oxygen or glucose.
    b. It produces no permanent neurologic damage.
    c. Serum bilirubin levels alone can predict the risk for brain injury.
    d. It produces permanent liver damage by deposits of conjugated bilirubin within the cell.

17. A newborn develops hyperbilirubinemia at 48 hours of age. The condition peaks at 72 hours and declines at about age 7 days. The *most* likely cause of this hyperbilirubinemia is:
    a. physiologic jaundice.
    b. pathologic jaundice.
    c. hemolytic disease of the newborn.
    d. breast milk jaundice.

18. Of the four infants described below, which one should the nurse recognize as being *least* likely to develop jaundice?
    a. An infant with subgaleal hemorrhage that is now resolving
    b. An infant with cephalhematoma that is now resolving
    c. The infant who has feedings started early, which will stimulate peristalsis and rapid passage of meconium
    d. The infant who is of Native American descent

19. Which one of the following therapies should the nurse expect to implement for jaundice associated with breast-feeding?
    a. Increased frequency of breast-feedings
    b. Permanent discontinuation of breast-feedings
    c. Discontinuation of breast-feedings for 24 hours with the use of home phototherapy
    d. Increased frequency of breast-feedings and addition of caloric supplements

20. Newborns are more prone to produce higher levels of bilirubin because they:
    i.   have higher concentrations of circulating erythrocytes.
    ii. have red blood cells with a shorter life span.
    iii. have reduced albumin concentrations.
    iv. have anatomically underdeveloped livers.

    a. i, ii, iii, and iv
    b. i, ii, and iii
    c. ii, iii, and iv
    d. iii and iv

21. Which one of the following is true regarding diagnostic evaluations for bilirubin?
    a. Newborn levels of unconjugated bilirubin must exceed 5 mg/dl before jaundice is observable.
    b. Hyperbilirubinemia is defined as a serum bilirubin value of above 8 mg/dl in full-term infants.
    c. When jaundice occurs before 24 hours of age, bilirubin level assessment is unnecessary.
    d. Transcutaneous bilirubinometry is an effective cutaneous measurement of bilirubin in full-term infants being treated with phototherapy.

22. The fiberoptic blanket is an alternative to the traditional "bililight" phototherapy. What are four advantages of its use?

23. Implementation of phototherapy for an infant with jaundice does *not* include:
    a. shielding the infant's eyes by an opaque mask.
    b. recognizing that once phototherapy has been started, visual assessment of jaundice increases in validity; therefore, fewer serum bilirubin levels will be necessary.
    c. repositioning infant frequently to expose all body surfaces to the light.
    d. assessing the infant for side effects, including loose, greenish stools, skin rashes, hyperthermia, dehydration, and increased metabolic rates.

24. Complete the following:

    a. Erythroblastosis fetalis is caused by _____ _____.

    b. Problems of Rh incompatibility may arise when the mother is _____ and the

       infant is _____. The most common blood group incompatibility in the neonate

       occurs when the mother has type _____ blood and the infant has either type _____ or

       type _____ blood.

    c. The nurse is reviewing maternal laboratory results. The nurse knows that the _____

       _____ test monitors anti-Rh antibody titers. The test performed postnatally to detect antibodies attached to the circulating erythrocytes of affected infants is called the

       _____ _____ test.

    d. To be effective in preventing maternal sensitization to the Rh factor, the nurse must administer Rho

       immune globulin (RhoGam) to the Rh-negative mother within _____ _____ after the first delivery or abortion and with each subsequent pregnancy. To further decrease the risk for

       Rh alloimmunization, RhoGam is administered at _____ weeks of gestation. RhoGam is

       administered by the _____ route.

25. Explain how the nurse is expected to assist the practitioner with a blood exchange transfusion in the newborn.

26. Which of the following statements about hypoglycemia in the newborn is true?
    a. Hypoglycemia is present when the newborn's blood glucose is lower than the baby's requirement for cellular energy and metabolism.
    b. In the healthy term infant who is born without complications, blood glucose is routinely monitored within 24 hours of birth to detect hypoglycemia.
    c. A plasma glucose less than 60 mg/dl requires intervention in the term newborn.
    d. Pregnancy-induced hypertension and terbulaline administration have not been found to alter infant metabolism or increase the hypoglycemia risk in the newborn.

27. What assessment finding is the nurse *most* likely to see in the infant as a result of hypoglycemia?
    a. Forceful, low-pitched cry
    b. Tachypnea
    c. Jitteriness, tremors, twitching
    d. Vomiting, refusal to eat

28. Which of the following nursing interventions are recognized as appropriate for the infant with hypoglycemia?
    i.   Institute early bottle-feeding or breast-feeding.
    ii. Increase environmental stimulants.
    iii. Protect from cold stress and respiratory difficulty that predispose the infant to decreased blood glucose levels.
    iv. Force early oral glucose feedings, avoiding formula and breast milk until newborn is stable.

    a. i, ii, iii, and iv
    b. i and iii
    c. iii and iv
    d. i, ii, and iii

29. Full-term infants at risk for hypoglycemia shortly after birth include which of the following?
    i.   Those born to diabetic mothers
    ii. Those that are small for gestational age
    iii. Those that are large for gestational age

    a. i, ii, and iii
    b. i and ii
    c. ii and iii
    d. i and iii

30. Hyperglycemia in the newborn is defined as a blood glucose concentration greater than

    _____ in the full-term infant and greater than _____ in the preterm infant.

31. Infants at risk for early-onset hypocalcemia include:
    a. postterm infants.
    b. infants that develop jaundice.
    c. infants born to hypertensive mothers.
    d. small-for-gestational-age infants who experience perinatal hypoxia.

32. The nurse caring for the infant who has hypocalcemia and is receiving intravenous calcium gluconate recognizes that which one of the following is included in the care plan?
    a. Scalp veins are the preferred site for intravenous administration of calcium gluconate.
    b. Observe for signs of hypercalcemia, including vomiting and bradycardia.
    c. Stimuli should be increased until calcium levels rise.
    d. Calcium gluconate is compatible with sodium bicarbonate.

33. The nurse is assessing Sarah, a neonate born at home, and observes slight blood oozing from the umbilicus. What is the *most* likely cause of Sarah's hemorrhagic disease?
    a. The neonate was born with an anatomically immature liver.
    b. Coagulation factors (II, VII, IX, X) are deactivated in the neonate.
    c. Vitamin K was administered to the neonate shortly after birth.
    d. The newborn was born with a sterile intestine and was unable to synthesize vitamin K until feedings began.

34. The goal is to prevent hemorrhagic disease in the newborn by prophylactic administration of vitamin K (AquaMEPHYTON). How does the nurse correctly administer this drug?

35. Lucy has been diagnosed with congenital hypothyrodism. The nurse is instructing the parents on how to care for Lucy. Which one of the following is the nurse *least* likely to include in the plan?
    a. The drug of choice is synthetic levothyroxine sodium.
    b. The drug is tasteless and can be crushed and added to formula, water, or food.
    c. If the dose is missed, twice the dose should be given the next day.
    d. Signs of overdose of the drug include slow pulse rate, lethargy, cool skin, and excessive weight gain.

36. When teaching the parents of the newborn about testing for PKU, the nurse should include which one of the following key points?
    a. The test is performed only on infants expected to have the disorder.
    b. The test is performed on cord blood.
    c. The test is not reliable if the blood sample is taken after the infant has ingested a source of protein.
    d. The test should be performed on all newborns before they leave the hospital, and a repeat blood specimen should be obtained by 2 weeks of age if the first test was taken within the first 24 hours of life.

37. Dietary instructions for the parents of a child with phenylketonuria include which of the following?
    i.   Maintain a low-phenylalanine diet through adolescence.
    ii.   Increase intake of high-protein foods such as meat and dairy products.
    iii. Measure vegetables, fruits, juices, breads, and starches.
    iv.   Tang or strawberry or chocolate Quik may be added to alter the flavor of formula without greatly altering phenylalanine content.
    v.   Introduce solid foods such as cereal, fruits, and vegetables during infancy as usual.
    vi.   Use soy formula during infancy.

    a. i, ii, iii, and iv
    b. i, iii, iv, v, and vi
    c. iii, iv, and v
    d. i, iii, iv, and v

38. In educating the parents of a newborn with galactosemia, the nurse includes which one of the following in the plan?
    a. All food labels should be read carefully for the presence of lactose.
    b. Once the diagnosis is made and the diet is altered, little follow-up of these infants is necessary.
    c. Breast milk is acceptable for infants with galactosemia.
    d. Signs of visual impairment are unlikely in children with this disorder.

39. Diagnostic evaluation testing for congenital hypothyroidism in the newborn includes which of the following?
    i.   A low level of T4
    ii.   A high level of TSH
    iii. Mandatory testing of all newborns within the first 24 to 48 hours or before discharge
    iv.   Venous blood samples taken on two separate occasions

    a. i and iii
    b. i, ii, and iii
    c. i, ii, and iv
    d. ii and iv

40. TORCH complex is a group of microbial agents that cause similar manifestations in the neonate. Identify what each letter stands for.

    T

    O

    R

    C

    H

41. The nurse can expect the infant with fetal alcohol syndrome to exhibit which of the following on assessment?
    a. Normal prenatal growth patterns
    b. Normal feeding patterns
    c. Thicker upper lip and longer palpebral fissures
    d. Irritability

42. How can HIV be transmitted from the mother to the infant?

Critical Thinking—Case Study

Mrs. Becker had a normal pregnancy and delivery without complications at 39 weeks gestation. She is breast-feeding her 2-day-old neonate, Ben, when she notices that Ben's skin looks yellow. Tests reveal that Ben's total serum bilirubin level is 13 mg/dl.

43. Mrs. Becker asks the nurse about Ben's condition and the seriousness of his illness. Which one of the following is the *best* response?
    a. "Ben has pathologic jaundice, a serious condition."
    b. "Ben has breast milk jaundice, and you will need to stop breast-feeding."
    c. "Ben probably has physiologic jaundice, a normal finding at his age."
    d. "Infants with serum bilirubin levels of 13 mg/dl will develop bilirubin encephalopathy and severe brain damage."

44. The physician tells Mrs. Becker to increase her frequency of breast-feeding to every 2 hours and to avoid supplementation. The nurse is discussing the rationale for this management with Mrs. Becker. Which one of the following is the basis for the ordered treatment?
    a. The jaundice is related to the process of breast-feeding, probably from decreased caloric and fluid intake by breast-fed infants.
    b. The jaundice is caused by a factor in the breast milk that breaks down bilirubin to a lipid-soluble form, which is reabsorbed in the gut.
    c. The jaundice is caused by the mother's hemolytic disease.
    d. The jaundice is increased because the infant was put to breast early, which increases the amount of time meconium is kept in the gut before excretion.

45. Ben's serum bilirubin level has not decreased as the physician hoped, and phototherapy has been ordered. Which of the following is the priority goal at this time?
    a. The family will be prepared for home phototherapy.
    b. The infant will receive adequate intravenous hydration.
    c. The infant will experience no complications from phototherapy.
    d. The infant will have hourly bilirubin level testing completed.

46. When caring for Ben, the nurse should take all the following actions to prevent complications *except*:
    a. making certain that eyelids are closed before applying eye shields; checking eyes at least every shift for discharge or irritation.
    b. monitoring axillary temperature closely to detect hyperthermia and/or hypothermia.
    c. maintaining an 18-inch distance between infant and light.
    d. applying oil daily to skin to avoid breakdown.

47. Which of the following is the *best* expected patient outcome for Ben while he is on phototherapy?
    a. Newborn begins feeding soon after birth.
    b. Family demonstrates an understanding of therapy and prognosis.
    c. Newborn displays no evidence of infection.
    d. Newborn displays no evidence of eye irritation, dehydration, temperature instability, or skin break-down.

48. Accurate charting is an important nursing responsibility when caring for the newborn receiving phototherapy. What is included in the charting?

49. Once phototherapy is considered permanently completed, the nurse should expect what occurrence related to the bilirubin level?

CHAPTER 10

The High-Risk Newborn and Family

1. Provide the correct term for each of the following descriptions.

   a. _____
   An infant whose birth weight is less than 2500 g, regardless of gestational age

   b. _____
   An infant whose birth weight is less than 1000 g

   c. _____
   An infant whose birth weight falls below the 10th percentile on intrauterine growth curves

   d. _____
   An infant whose birth weight falls above the 90th percentile on intrauterine growth curves

   e. _____
   An infant born before completion of 37 weeks of gestation

   f. _____
   An infant born between the 38th week and completion of the 42nd week of gestation

   g. _____
   An infant born after 42 weeks gestation

   h. _____
   Death of a fetus after 20 weeks of gestation

   i. _____
   Death that occurs in the first 27 days of life

   j. _____
   Describes the total number of fetal and early neonatal deaths per 1000 live births

   k. _____
   The capacity to balance heat production and conservation and heat dissipation

   l. _____
   An environment that permits the infant to maintain a normal core temperature with minimum oxygen consumption and caloric expenditure

   m. _____
   Heat loss that occurs when infants are exposed to drafts or increased air flow

   n. _____
   Type of heat loss that can be effectively reduced by use of double-walled incubator in high-risk newborn

   o. _____
   Type of heat loss that can be reduced by warming all items that come into direct contact with newborn

2. Which one of the following is *not* used as a category in the classification of high-risk newborns?
   a. Birth size
   b. Gestational age
   c. Mortality
   d. Birth age

3. Which of the following is a neonatal intensive care facility that provides a full range of maternal new-born services, has the capacity to provide care for the most complex neonatal complications, and has at least one full-time neonatologist on staff?
   a. Level I facility
   b. Level II facility
   c. Level III facility
   d. Level IV facility

4. When the high-risk neonate needs transportation to a facility that can provide intensive care, the nurse recognizes that priority care for this neonate must include:
   a. transfer of both the mother and infant.
   b. immediate transport often before stabilization of the neonate.
   c. complete life support system available during transport.
   d. prevention of transport delay by carrying the infant in the nurse's arms to the waiting transport vehicle.

5. A thorough systematic physical assessment is a must in the care of the high-risk neonate. Subtle

   changes in _____ _____, _____, _____ or

   _____ _____ often indicate an underlying problem.

6. At birth the newborn is immediately assessed to determine any apparent problems and to identify those that demand immediate attention. The assessment *not* usually conducted at birth or immediately after birth is:
   a. assignment of a gestational age score.
   b. assignment of an Apgar score.
   c. evaluation for obvious congenital anomalies.
   d. evaluation for neonatal distress.

7. Identify whether the following statements about high-risk care of the neonate are true or false.

   _____ Neonates under intensive observation are placed in a controlled environment and monitored for heart rate, respiratory activity, and temperature.

   _____ Sophisticated monitoring and life-support systems can replace the observations of the infant by nursing personnel.

   _____ Electrodes for cardiac monitors should not be applied to the back or upper arms of the neonate.

   _____ Infants who are mechanically ventilated and have low Apgar scores can have lower blood pressures.

   _____ An accurate output measurement can be obtained in the neonate by using a urine collecting bag or by weighing the infant's diaper. Regardless of the method used, a 40-g weight of urine would be recorded as 40 ml of urine.

   _____ The nurse is preparing the infant for a heel stick. This preparation is done to create adequate vasodilation and is accomplished by placing a heating pad on the infant's heel.

   _____ Nurses are allowed to turn off alarm systems for electronic monitoring devices when their sounds disturb the infant's parents.

8. Identify the two *most* critical goals in caring for the high-risk infant.

9. The major source of increased production of heat during cold stress in the high-risk neonate is

_____ _____.

10. Low-birth-weight infants are at a disadvantage for heat production when compared with full-term infants because they have:
   i.   small muscle mass.
   ii. fewer deposits of brown fat.
   iii. less insulating subcutaneous fat.
   iv. poor reflex control of skin capillaries.

   a. i, ii, iii, and iv
   b. ii, iii, and iv
   c. i, ii, and iii
   d. i, iii, and iv

11. Identify three major consequences produced by cold stress that create additional hazards for the neonate.

12. Match each term with its description.

   a.   Thermal stability
   b.   Neutral thermal environment
   c.   Convective heat loss

   d.   Radiant heat loss
   e.   Conductive heat loss
   f.   Evaporative heat loss

   _____ Capacity to balance heat production, heat conservation, and heat dissipation
   _____ Allows one to maintain normal core temperature with minimal oxygen consumption and caloric use
   _____ Occurs by transfer of body heat to a cooler solid object not in direct contact
   _____ Occurs when infants are exposed to drafts or when surrounding air is cool
   _____ Can be decreased by drying the neonate thoroughly with warm towels
   _____ Loss of heat through direct contact with a cooler surface

13. Which of the following interventions is *least* likely to be effective for high-risk neonates?
   a. Maintaining a neutral thermal environment
   b. Placing the heat-sensing probe on the infant's abdomen when the infant is in the prone position
   c. Ensuring that the oxygen supplied to the infant via a hood around the head is warmed and humidified
   d. Warming all items that come in direct contact with the infant, including the hands of caregivers

14. A primary objective in the care of high-risk infants is to maintain respiration. Describe how the nurse should complete the respiratory assessment.

15. The best way to prevent infection in the high-risk neonate begins with:
    a. meticulous and frequent handwashing of all persons coming in contact with the infant.
    b. observing continually for signs of infection.
    c. requiring everyone working in the NICU to put on fresh scrub clothes before entering the unit.
    d. performing epidemiologic studies at least monthly.

16. Baby girl Miller has been admitted to the NICU with low birth weight and possible infection. Parenteral fluids have been ordered for hydration and antibiotic administration.

    What are the preferred sites for peripheral IV infusions for this infant?

    In many neonatal centers a specially inserted catheter is used for IV hydration and medication administration because it is less expensive and decreases trauma to the neonate. What is this catheter called?

    The nurse starts a peripheral line and places the neonate on an infusion pump to regulate the rate of IV administration. Ten minutes later the nurse observes for signs of infiltration. What signs should the nurse be looking for?

17. A complication that develops with the use of the umbilical catheter is thrombi. This complication is *best* recognized by the appearance of:
    a. blanching of the buttocks and genitalia.
    b. bluish discoloration seen in the toes, called "cath toes."
    c. bounding pedal pulses.
    d. hemorrhage from the umbilical catheter area.

18. Introduction of minimal enteral feedings in the metabolically stable preterm infant:
    a. increases incidence of necrotizing enterocolitis.
    b. increases mucosal atrophy incidence.
    c. stimulates the infant's GI tract.
    d. maintains serum glucose homeostasis.

19. Identify whether the following statements are true or false.

    _____ Premature infants receiving continuous feedings show better weight gain than those receiving intermittent bolus feedings.

    _____ Milk produced by mothers of preterm infants changes in content over the first 30 days postnatally, until its content is similar to that of full-term human milk.

    _____ Milk produced by mothers whose infants are born at term contains higher concentrations of protein, sodium chloride, and IgA.

    _____ LBW infants (<1500 g) who are fed only human milk demonstrate decreased growth rates and nutritional deficiencies.

    _____ Preterm infants who are fed fortified human milk have shorter hospital stays and less infection than infants given preterm formulas.

    _____ Fortified human milk is mixed daily, stored in the refrigerator, and used within 24 hours.

    _____ IgA concentration is higher in the milk of mothers of term infants as compared with mothers of preterm infants.

    _____ Pasteurization of donor human milk kills HIV without harming leukocytes and milk lipids.

20. The amount to be fed to the infant by nipple is:
    a. determined by the infant's tolerance to previous feedings.
    b. increased when the infant requires 25 minutes or more for feeding completion.
    c. increased when the infant reaches the postnatal age of 34 weeks.
    d. increased when prodding techniques are used to increase sucking and decrease aspiration.

21. Feeding facilitation techniques for preterm infants include:
    a. using a pliable nipple with faster flow.
    b. using a slightly firm nipple with slow flow.
    c. manipulating the nipple frequently by twisting and turning when the infants stops sucking.
    d. positioning the infant on the back with the head supported.

22. What is the *best* measurement of feeding success in the infant?
    a. Soft abdomen
    b. No aspirated gastric residual
    c. Ability to suck on pacifier
    d. Coordinated sucking and swallowing ability

23. An infant who weighs 1400 g appears to be ready for enteral feedings. Which one of the following should the nurse include in the implementation of gavage feedings?
    a. Insert the tube into the unobstructed nares.
    b. Perform the procedure with the infant in a supine position with the head elevated 45 degrees.
    c. Aspirate the contents of the stomach, measure these contents, and replace the residual before beginning the feeding. The amount of residual is subtracted from the total feeding to prevent overdistending the stomach.
    d. Allow the feeding to flow by gravity; then push a small amount of the feeding into the stomach; then allow the remainder of the feeding to flow by gravity.

24. _____ _____ increases oxygenation during tube feeding and has been shown to increase readiness in low-birth-weight infants for bottle-feeding.

25. In caring for a preterm infant's skin, the nurse knows to:
    a. use scissors to remove dressings or tape from the infant's extremities.
    b. use solvents to remove tape from the neonate's skin.
    c. use alkaline-based soaps in removal of stool.
    d. use transparent adhesive dressings to secure and protect central lines.

26. Which of the following is a correct nursing intervention to prevent skin damage in the neonate?
    a. Instruct parents before discharge on regular use of sunscreen for all infants under 6 months of age.
    b. Apply adhesive tape to protect arms, elbow, and knees from friction rubs.
    c. Use powders on diaper dermatitis areas to promote moisture barrier.
    d. Use water, air, or gel mattresses to decrease skin breakdown.

27. Manifestations of acute pain in the neonate include:
    a. increased transcutaneous oxygen saturation.
    b. increased heart rate and rapid, shallow respirations.
    c. hypoglycemia.
    d. all of the above.

28. Identify the following as true or false.
    _____ Each infant is different; therefore, supportive developmental care requires ongoing data collection by the nurse.
    _____ Developmentally supportive care uses both physiologic and behavioral information to evaluate the needs of the infant in an NICU setting.

_____   Developmental maturation for the young preterm infant is seen by a decrease in quiet sleep.

_____   Nursing care for the neonate should include modification of care to provide longer episodes of undisturbed sleep.

_____   Prolonged "clustering" of care for the ill infant promotes physiologic stability.

_____   The best time for care of an infant is when the infant is awake.

_____   Containment or facilitated tucking positioning of the infant during procedures has been shown to increase physiologic and behavioral stressors.

_____   Stroking a preterm infant who is not physiologically stable can result in distress, including oxygen desaturation.

_____   Bed sharing after discharge, whether with parent or siblings and regardless of infant sleep position, has been associated with increased incidence of sudden infant death syndrome.

_____   Therapeutic positioning for preterm and high-risk infants should provide support to maintain flexed and midline postures.

_____   Using earmuffs in the NICU is an important intervention to prevent later speech and language difficulties.

_____   UV radiation from fluorescent fixtures in the NICU should be reduced by using plastic or glass shields because it is potentially damaging to the retina.

29. The _____ sleeping position is recommended by the American Academy of Pediatrics for healthy infants in the first year of life as a preventive measure for SIDS.

30. What is the most widely used narcotic analgesic for pharmacologic management of neonatal pain?

31. Which of the following is the *best* way for the nurse to promote a healthy parent-child relationship for the family with a high-risk neonate?
    a. Reinforce parents during their caregiving activities and interactions with their infant.
    b. Discourage parents from talking about the baby.
    c. Reassure parents that the infant is doing well.
    d. Encourage the mother to stay by the infant's bedside to promote bonding.

32. The term _____ _____ _____ is applied to physically healthy children who are perceived by parents to be at high risk for medical or developmental problems.

33. Discharge instructions for the parents of the preterm infant should *not* include:
    a. warning parents that their infant may still be in danger and will need constant attention.
    b. providing information to the parents on how to contact personnel for later questions.
    c. instructions about car safety seats, including how these seats can be adapted for smaller children with the placement of blanket rolls on each side of the infant to support the head and trunk.
    d. providing adequate information about immunization needs.

34. To help parents deal with neonatal death, the nurse should:
    a. discourage the parent from staying with the infant before death to prevent overattachment.
    b. explain to the parents that the infant would have had many developmental problems and it is better that the infant did not suffer.
    c. give the parents the opportunity to hold and talk with the infant before and after death.
    d. force the parents to see the infant after death because closure is necessary.

35. A physical characteristic usually observed in the preterm infant and *not* observed in the full-term infant is:
    a. proportionately equal head in relation to the body.
    b. skin that is translucent, smooth, shiny with small blood vessels clearly visible underneath the epidermis.
    c. distinct creases extending across the entire palms of the hands and down the complete soles of the feet.
    d. absence of lanugo and little vernix caseosa.

36. Apnea in the preterm infant is defined as a lapse of spontaneous breathing lasting for how many seconds?
    a. 5
    b. 10
    c. 15
    d. 20

37. Bryan, a 2-day-old preterm infant being cared for in the NICU, had some periods of apnea yesterday. Today when you arrive to work, you learn in report that the infant has had no further apneic episodes since yesterday. However, shortly after you begin your shift, Bryan's apnea monitor alarm sounds. What should you do *first*?
    a. Use tactile stimulation, rubbing on the infant's back to stop the apneic spell.
    b. Suction his nose and oropharynx.
    c. Assess the infant for color and for presence of respiration.
    d. Place the infant on his abdomen.

38. The preterm infant is having respirations with absence of diaphragmatic muscle function. This is causing a lack of respiratory effort because the CNS is not transmitting signals to the respiratory muscles. What is this type of apnea called?
    a. Obstructive apnea
    b. Central apnea
    c. Periodic apnea
    d. Mixed apnea

39. A late and serious sign of respiratory distress in the neonate is:
    a. central cyanosis.
    b. respiratory rate of 90 breaths/minute.
    c. substernal retractions.
    d. nasal flaring.

40. Which one of the following is a correct procedure to use when suctioning the nasopharyngeal passages, trachea, or ET tube in a newborn?
    a. Pulse oximeter is observed before, during, and after suctioning to provide an ongoing assessment of oxygenation status.
    b. Continuous suction is applied as the catheter is withdrawn.
    c. The catheter is inserted gently and slowly, and suction is conducted to a point where the catheter meets resistance before the catheter is withdrawn.
    d. The time the airway is obstructed by the catheter is limited to no more than 10 seconds.

41. Discuss the importance of surfactant to the preterm infant's lungs.

42. Match each term with its description.

    a. Pulmonary interstitial emphysema

    b. Lung compliance

    c. Continuous positive airway pressure (CPAP)

    d. Intermittent mandatory ventilation (IMV)

    e. Positive end-expiratory pressure (PEEP)

    f. Nasal flaring

    g. Grunting

    h. Synchronized intermittent mandatory ventilation (SIMV)

    i. High-frequency ventilation (HFV)

    _____ Method that infuses air or oxygen under a preset pressure by means of nasal prongs, a face mask, or an endotracheal tube

    _____ Method that allows infant to breathe spontaneously at his or her own rate but provides mechanical cycled respirations and pressure at regular preset intervals by means of a endotracheal tube and ventilator

    _____ Condition that develops in the preterm infant with RDS and immature lungs as a result of overdistention of distal airways

    _____ Method that provides increased end-expiratory pressure during expiration and between mandatory breaths, preventing alveolar collapse

    _____ Lung distensibility

    _____ Abnormal sounds made on respiration as a result of increased effort required to fill the lungs; associated with atelectasis

    _____ Widening of the nostril during inspiration; signals respiratory distress

    _____ Infant-triggered ventilator with signal detector and assist/control mode

    _____ Method that delivers gas at very rapid rates to maintain adequate minute volumes using lower proximal airway pressures

43. Susie, a neonate born 20 minutes ago, was observed at birth to have meconium staining. If Susie has meconium in the lungs, this *most* likely will:
    a. prevent air from entering the lungs.
    b. trap inspired air in the lungs.
    c. cause no problems with breathing.
    d. lead to respiratory alkalosis.

44. An important nursing function is close observation of neonates at risk for developing air leaks. These infants include:
    a. those with respiratory distress syndrome (RDS).
    b. those with meconium-stained amniotic fluid.
    c. those receiving CPAP or positive-pressure ventilation.
    d. all of the above.

45. Infants diagnosed with bronchopulmonary dysplasia have special care needs. These needs include:
    a. opportunities for adequate rest.
    b. increases in environmental stimuli.
    c. decreases in caloric intake.
    d. rapid weaning from ventilators.

46. Why is diagnosis and treatment of sepsis sometimes delayed in the neonate?

47. The laboratory evaluation for the diagnosis of sepsis is *least* likely to include:
    a. blood cultures.
    b. spinal fluid culture.
    c. urine culture.
    d. gastric secretions culture.

48. Clinical signs seen in necrotizing enterocolitis are:
    a. increased abdominal girth.
    b. increased gastric residual.
    c. positive stool hematest.
    d. all of the above.

49. Clinical manifestations of patent ductus arteriosus (PDA) include which of the following?
    a. Increased $PaCO_2$, decreased PaO_2, and decreased FiO_2
    b. Narrow pulse pressure with increased diastolic blood pressure
    c. Systolic or continuous murmur heard as a "machinery-type" sound
    d. All of the above

50. Therapy for preterm infants who develop PDA often includes the administration of:
    a. theophyllin.
    b. indomethacin.
    c. digoxin.
    d. heparin.

51. Which of the following is a correct statement about persistent pulmonary hypertension of the newborn (PPHN)?
    a. PPHN is primarily a condition of premature infants.
    b. PPHN is rarely associated with meconium aspiration.
    c. A loud pulmonary component of the second heart sound and often a systolic ejection murmur are present with PPHN.
    d. Vasodilators, such as tolazoline, are used to decrease cardiac output.

52. Why does the nurse carefully monitor and record amounts of all blood drawn for tests in the preterm infant?
    a. Early prevention of anemia
    b. Prevention of infection
    c. Prevention of polycythemia
    d. Detection of factors that contribute to hypothermia

53. Define polycythemia and identify the infants who are most at risk for this condition.

54. The treatment of retinopathy of prematurity (ROP) includes _____ and _____ _____ by a pediatric ophthalmologist.

55. Brenda is a 1-hour-old newborn who suffered asphyxia before birth, resulting in hypoxic-ischemic brain injury. What signs can the nurse expect to see indicating encephalopathy?

56. Which of the following interventions is *contraindicated* in the preterm infant with increased intracranial pressure?
    a. Avoiding interventions that produce crying
    b. Administration of hyperosmolar solutions
    c. Administering analgesics to reduce discomfort
    d. Turning the head to the right without body alignment

57. The nurse must be able to distinguish between seizures and jitteriness in the neonate. Which of the following is true about seizures?
    a. Seizures are not accompanied by ocular movement.
    b. Seizures have their dominant movement as tremor.
    c. In seizures the dominant movement cannot be stopped by flexion of the affected limb.
    d. Seizures are highly sensitive to light manual stimulation.

58. John is a newborn just delivered of a diabetic mother. The nurse will watch John for signs that he is rapidly developing:
    a. hyperglycemia.
    b. hypoglycemia.
    c. failure of the pancreas.
    d. dehydration.

59. Infants born to narcotic-addicted mothers may exhibit all of the following clinical manifestations *except*:
    a. tremors and restlessness.
    b. frequent sneezing.
    c. coordinated suck and swallow reflex.
    d. high-pitched, shrill cry.

Critical Thinking—Case Study

Baby Mark was born at 36 weeks gestation and weighed 2300 g at birth. At 1 minute of age, his Apgar score was 5. Mark was suctioned, and oxygen administration was started. He responded with spontaneous respirations. You are the nurse who has been assigned to care for Mark in the special care nursery. His admission vital signs are heart rate 150, respirations 56, and axillary temperature of 96.4° F. Mark is placed in a radiant warmer and oxygen administration is continued by oxygen hood.

60. You would classify Baby Mark as a:
    i.   full-term infant.
    ii. preterm infant.
    iii. low-birth-weight infant.
    iv. small-for-gestational-age infant.

    a. i and iv
    b. ii and iv
    c. ii and iii
    d. i and iii

61. You identify Mark as being at risk for developing respiratory distress syndrome based on his:
    i. gestational age.
    ii. low Apgar score.
    iii. hypothermia.
    iv. respiratory rate of 56.

    a. i, ii, iii, and iv
    b. i, ii, and iii
    c. ii, iii, and iv
    d. ii and iii

62. The nurse's plan for oxygen administration includes:
    a. frequent suctioning.
    b. frequent assessment to include unobstructed nares.
    c. nipple feeding with respiratory rates of 70 and below.
    d. turning off monitor alarms to allow the neonate to rest.

63. Baby Mark's parents are visiting him for the first time. How can the nurse assist the parents in feeling more comfortable in the NICU atmosphere?
    a. Discourage questions of a technical nature.
    b. Tell the parents that Mark is going to be fine.
    c. Explain what is happening with Mark and why he is receiving this type of care.
    d. Leave the parents alone with the infant.

64. The nurse will develop a plan of care for Mark that recognizes which of the following as the *best* expected outcome?
    a. Oxygen is administered correctly, and arterial blood gases are within normal limits.
    b. Monitor for changes in thermal environment.
    c. Record oxygen delivery rates every 2 hours.
    d. Assess respiratory status every hour.

65. Mark has had an apneic episode. What should the nurse include in the documentation of this episode?

66. As a nurse in the NICU, you are assigned to care for a 4-pound preterm infant named Maria. In report you learn that Maria is still on gavage feedings and that tomorrow she is scheduled to begin bottle-feeding. If Maria tolerates her bottle-feedings well, she is scheduled to go home in a few days. You observe the infant closely for behaviors that indicate readiness for bottle-feedings. Name these behaviors.

67. The nurse in the special care nursery should position the preterm infant in the _____ position to improve oxygenation. On discharge from the nursery to home, the nurse instructs the parents to

    place the infant in the _____ position while sleeping.

CHAPTER 11

Conditions Caused by Defects in Physical Development

1. Match each term with its description.

   a. Growth
   b. Hyperplasia
   c. Hypertrophy
   d. Differentiation

   e. Organogenesis
   f. Teratogenesis
   g. Sensitive or critical period

   _____ Prenatal growth process disturbed to produce a structural or functional defect
   _____ Period with which the major impact of environmental factors coincides
   _____ Beginning of all major organ systems
   _____ Process during which cells divide and synthesize new proteins
   _____ Increase in cell number
   _____ Increase in cell size
   _____ Modification and specialization of early cells to form the individual

2. The most typical parental response to the birth of an infant with a physical disability includes:
   a. hostility and bitterness.
   b. disbelief and denial.
   c. strengthening of the psychologic attachment the mother has formed during pregnancy with the unborn child.
   d. establishment of realistic goals.

3. The nurse can independently implement which one of the following actions in the preoperative neonate?
   a. Start a peripheral intravenous line.
   b. Begin administration of prophylactic antibiotics.
   c. Provide accurate information to the newborn's parents regarding what to expect postoperatively.
   d. Begin pain management control.

4. Primary roles of the nurse in the care of an infant born with a physical defect include:
   a. discouraging the parents from talking about the infant.
   b. showing the parents photographs of other infants with similar defects and assure them the defect can be corrected.
   c. supplying information only as requested by the parents.
   d. supporting and encouraging the parents in their caregiving tasks.

5. Identify the following statements about postoperative care of the neonate as true or false.
   _____ The newborn's poor chest wall stability, along with smaller and more reactive airways, contributes to postoperative respiratory compromise.
   _____ Most postoperative neonates require mechanical ventilation.
   _____ Neonates are highly subject to acidosis and hypoxia and require continuous monitoring of acid-base balance and oxygen status.
   _____ The preterm infant is at high risk for developing respiratory complications from general anesthesia.

85

_____ The neonate is particularly sensitive to vagal stimulation, which can be induced by post-operative nasogastric tubes, endotracheal tubes, and suctioning.

_____ The neonate's risk for rapid fluid shifts can be intensified by stress and loss of fluid during surgical procedures.

_____ The more preterm or physiologically immature the infant, the more difficult to measure pain response.

6. Critical guidelines for neonatal postoperative care include continuous monitoring of oxygen and acid-base status. What actions would the nurse expect to take to achieve this goal?
   a. Monitor neonatal weight postoperatively and keep accurate intake and output record.
   b. Monitor axillary temperature, blood pressure, and heart rate every 15 minutes x 4, every 30 minutes x 2, every 1 hour x 6, and then every 2 hours for 24 hours.
   c. Monitor surgical site/skin status for drainage, bleeding, and amount of output from tubes.
   d. Monitor pulse oximetry and arterial blood gases.

7. The nurse has completed the physical assessment of an infant and has noticed a cutaneous dimple with dark tufts of hair between L5 and S1. Which of the following medical conditions should the nurse suspect?
   a. Spina bifida occulta
   b. Spina bifida cystica
   c. Meningocele
   d. Cranioschisis

8. Research has shown that supplemental folic acid can reduce the recurrence rates of spina bifida, anencephaly, or encephalocele. How should this supplement be administered?
   a. Daily folic acid dose to 4 mg beginning 1 month before conception and during the first trimester
   b. Daily folic acid dose of 0.4 mg as soon as pregnancy is confirmed
   c. Daily folic acid dose of 4 mg given through the use of multivitamin preparations beginning 1 month before conception and throughout the first trimester
   d. Daily folic acid dose of 4 mg beginning with the confirmation of pregnancy and continuing throughout pregnancy

9. Match each medical condition with its description.

   a. Anencephaly   e. Cranioschisis   h. Meningocele
   b. Myelodysplasia   f. Exancephaly   i. Setting-sun sign
   c. Myelomeningocele   g. Encephalocele   j. Congenital torticollis
   d. Hydrocephalus

   _____ Hernial protrusion of a saclike cyst, containing meninges, spinal fluid, and nerves
   _____ Condition that results from disturbances in the dynamics of CSF absorption and flow
   _____ Congenital malformation in which both cerebral hemispheres are absent
   _____ Any malformation of the spinal canal and cord
   _____ Marked by eyes rotated downward with sclera visible above the iris
   _____ Herniation of brain and meninges through a defect in the skull, resulting in fluid-filled sac
   _____ Total exposure of the brain through a skull defect
   _____ Condition resulting from sustained contraction of the sternocleidomastoid muscle
   _____ Hernial protrusion of saclike cyst of meninges filled with spinal fluid
   _____ Skull defect with tissues protruding

10. The major complications of myelomeningocele are _____ _____

   _____ and _____.

11. a. Name two methods by which prenatal neural tube defects can be diagnosed.

    b. When is the best time to perform these diagnostic tests?

12. Therapeutic management that provides the most favorable morbidity and mortality outcomes for the child born with myelomeningocele is:
    a. early physical therapy.
    b. closure of the defect within first 24 hours.
    c. vigorous antibiotic therapy.
    d. splint application to lower extremities.

13. a. What is the management goal for genitourinary function in the infant with myelomeningocele?

    b. What is the goal for the older child with the same condition?

14. Management of the genitourinary function in the patient with myelomeningocele includes clean intermittent catheterization (CIC) and anticholinergic medication. Which of the following statements about their use is correct?
    i.   CIC is used to prevent spontaneous voiding.
    ii. Parents are taught to catheterize the infant every 3 hours during the day and once each night.
    iii. Anticholinergic medications enhance sphincter competence.
    iv. Anticholinergic medications reduce detrusor muscle tone and reduce bladder pressure.

    a. i and iii
    b. i and iv
    c. ii and iii
    d. ii and iv

15. Myelomeningocele may be associated with hydrocephalus. What should the nurse assess to identify an infant with hydrocephalus?
    a. Upward eye slanting
    b. Strabismus
    c. Wide or bulging fontanels
    d. Decreased head circumference

16. Upon delivery of an infant with myelomeningocele, which one of the following nursing actions may be *contraindicated*?
    a. Examination of the membranous cyst for intactness
    b. Diapering the infant
    c. Keeping moist, sterile normal saline dressings on the defect
    d. Keeping infant in the prone position

17. An infant born with spina bifida who needs intermittent urinary catheterization has developed sneezing, wheezing, and a rash over his lower pelvic and genital area. The nurse should suspect this infant has developed:
    a. asthma.
    b. emphysema.
    c. latex allergy.
    d. anaphylaxis.

18. _____ hydrocephalus is caused by either maldevelopment or an intrauterine

    infection. _____ hydrocephalus is caused by infection, neoplasm, or
    hemorrhage. In infants with hydrocephalus, the first signs observed by the nurse may be

    _____.
    Signs and symptoms in late childhood are caused by increased ICP and are related to the focal lesion.

    They may include _____.

    Impaired absorption of CSF fluid within the subarachnoid space is termed _____
    hydrocephalus. Obstruction of the flow of CSF fluid through the ventricular system is termed

    _____ hydrocephalus.

19. Surgical shunts are often required to provide drainage in the treatment of hydrocephalus. What is the
    preferred shunt for infants?
    a. Ventriculoperitoneal shunt
    b. Ventriculoatrial shunt
    c. Ventricular bypass
    d. Ventriculopleural shunt

20. The nurse recognizes that which one of the following should be included in the postoperative care of a
    patient with a shunt?
    a. Positioning the patient in a head-down position
    b. Continuous pumping of the shunt to assess function
    c. Monitoring for abdominal or peritoneal distention
    d. Positioning the child on the side of the operative site to facilitate drainage

21. The major complications of VP shunts are _____ and _____.

22. Posterior fontanel is closed by age _____. Anterior fontanel is closed by age

    _____. Sutures are unable to be separated by ICP by age _____.

23. Identify the following statements about microcephaly as true or false.
    _____ Microcephaly is defined as a head circumference greater than 5 standard deviations below
             the mean.
    _____ Primary microcephaly can be caused by irradiation between 4 to 20 weeks of gestation.
    _____ Secondary microcephaly can be caused by infection during the third trimester, the perina-
             tal period, or early infancy.
    _____ All children with microcephaly are mentally retarded.
    _____ There is no treatment for microcephaly.
    _____ Nursing care is supportive and directed toward helping parents adjust to a child with cog-
             nitive impairment.

24. Therapeutic management for craniosynostosis is:
    a. placement of ventriculoperitoneal shunt.
    b. removal of neoplasm.
    c. release of fused sutures.
    d. supportive assistance for parents.

25. Nursing care after surgery for the infant with craniosynostosis includes:
    a. careful monitoring of hematocrit and hemoglobin because of expected large blood loss during surgery.
    b. applying ice compresses for 5 minutes every hour since eyelids are often swollen shut.
    c. avoiding sedation and pain medications because neurologic status may be falsely altered.
    d. avoiding supine positioning.

26. In preparing the nursing care plan for the infant born with craniofacial abnormalities, the nurse recognizes which of the following as true?
    a. Children with this deformity face erroneous assumptions of mental retardation.
    b. Abnormalities include deformities involving the skull and facial bones.
    c. A helmet is often required after surgery to protect the operative site and bone grafts for 6 months to 2 years.
    d. All of the above are true.

27. What positioning instructions should be given to parents of an infant with positional plagiocephaly?

28. In severe cases of positional plagiocephaly, helmet therapy is advised. Describe this.

29. Match each degree of developmental hip dysplasia with its description.

    a. Acetabular dysplasia

    b. Subluxation

    c. Dislocation

    _____   Femoral head remains in contact with the acetabulum, but the head of the femur is partially displaced.
    _____   Femoral head remains in the acetabulum (mildest form).
    _____   Femoral head loses contact with the acetabulum.

30. The nurse observes which of the following signs in the infant with developmental dysplasia?
    a. Negative Ortolani test
    b. Asymmetric folds in skin of legs
    c. Lengthening of the limb on the affected side
    d. Limitation in adduction of the leg

31. Match each age group with the expected therapeutic management for developmental hip dysplasia at that age.

    a. Newborn to 6 months

    b. 6 to 18 months

    c. Older child

    _____   More complex management including operative reduction and innominate osteotomy procedures designed to construct an acetabular roof
    _____   Use of abduction devices such as Pavlik harness; can also include skin traction, hip spica cast
    _____   Gradual reduction by traction and individualized home traction program followed by attempted closed reduction of the hip

32. Why is the practice of double or triple diapering an infant with developmental dysplasia of the hip no longer recommended?

33. Match each skeletal congenital defect with its description or common name.

a. Achondroplasia
b. Osteogenesis imperfecta
c. Pes planus
d. Pes valgus

e. Pes varus
f. Metatarsus valgus
g. Polydactyly
h. Genu varnum

i. Genu recurvatum
j. Klippel-Feil syndrome
k. Arachnodactyly (Marfan syndrome)

_____ Commonly called "flatfoot"

_____ Inversion of entire foot, with sole resting on the ground

_____ Inherited defect of ossification at the epiphyseal plate, resulting in short limbs, large head, and lordosis

_____ Eversion of entire foot with sole resting on the ground

_____ Eversion of forefoot with heel remaining straight

_____ Inherited condition characterized by fragile, brittle bones

_____ Inherited abnormal length of extremities, fingers, toes, hypermobility of joints; defects of chest (pigeon breast) and spine

_____ Commonly called "back knee"

_____ Commonly called "bowleg"

_____ Excessive number of fingers, toes or both

_____ Characterized by the absence of one or more cervical vertebrae and the fusion of two or more cervical vertebrae

34. Match each congenital clubfoot condition with its description.

a. Talipes varus
b. Talipes valgus

c. talipes equinus
d. talipes calcaneus

_____ Eversion, or bending outward

_____ Inversion, or bending inward

_____ Plantar flexion, in which the toes are lower than the heel

_____ Dorsiflexion, in which the toes are higher than the heel

35. Treatment of clubfoot includes:
a. correction of the deformity.
b. maintenance of the correction until normal muscle is gained, often accomplished by casts or orthoses.
c. follow-up observation to detect possible recurrence of the deformity.
d. all of the above

36. Match each term with its description.

    a. Metatarsus varus   d. Phocomelia
    b. Amelia   e. Atresia
    c. Meromelia

    _____ Deficiency of long bones, with development of hands and feet attached at or near the shoulders; sometimes called "seal limbs"
    _____ Absence of complete extremity
    _____ Medial adduction of the toes and forefoot
    _____ Partial absence of extremity
    _____ Absence of a normal opening

37. An important assessment for the nurse to perform in identifying cleft palate is to:
    a. assess sucking ability of infant.
    b. assess color of lips.
    c. palpate the palate with the gloved finger.
    d. do all of the above.

38. Describe long-term problems often experienced by children with cleft lip or cleft palate.

39. Which feeding practices should be used for the infant with a cleft lip or palate?
    a. Use a large, hard nipple with a large hole.
    b. Use a normal nipple and position it sideways in the mouth.
    c. Use a special nipple, positioned so it is compressed by the infant's tongue and existing palate.
    d. Hold breast feeding until after surgical correction of the defect

40. Which of the following is acceptable in providing postoperative care for the infant with a cleft lip or palate?
    a. Use of tongue depressor in the mouth to assess surgical site
    b. Continuous elbow restraints to prevent injury
    c. Placement of infant in the prone position after cleft lip repair
    d. Placement of the infant in the prone position after cleft palate repair

41. In preparing the parents of a child with cleft palate, the nurse includes which of the following in the long-term family teaching plan?
    a. Explanation that tooth development will be delayed
    b. Guidelines to use for speech development
    c. Use of decongestants and Tylenol to care for frequent upper respiratory symptoms
    d. All of the above

42. The priority nursing goal in the immediate care of a postoperative infant after repair of a cleft lip or cleft palate is to:
    a. keep the infant well hydrated.
    b. prevent vomiting.
    c. prevent trauma to operative site.
    d. administer medications to prevent drooling.

43. The nurse observes frothy saliva in the mouth and nose of the neonate, as well as frequent drooling. When fed, the infant swallows normally, but suddenly the fluid returns through the infant's nose and mouth. The nurse should suspect what medical condition?
    a. Esophageal atresia
    b. Cleft palate
    c. Anorectal malformation
    d. Biliary atresia

44. Discuss the nurse's role in the assessment of anorectal malformation.

45. The best definition of biliary atresia is:
    a. jaundice persisting beyond 2 weeks of age with elevated direct bilirubin levels.
    b. progressive inflammatory process causing intrahepatic and extrahepatic bile duct fibrosis.
    c. absence of bile pigment.
    d. hepatomegaly and palpable liver.

46. A hernia that is constricted and cannot be reduced manually is referred to as

    _____.

47. Identify the following statements about umbilical hernia as either true or false.
    _____ The disorder affects African Americans more often than it does Caucasians.
    _____ It affects preterm infants more than full-term infants.
    _____ It may be present in association with Down syndrome.
    _____ It is most prominent when the infant is crying.
    _____ It usually resolves spontaneously by 3 to 4 years of age.

48. Which one of the following is *contraindicated* as part of the therapeutic management for the neonate with congenital diaphragmatic hernia?
    a. Endotracheal intubation
    b. Gastrointestinal decompression
    c. Positioning the infant with the head and chest elevated above the abdomen
    d. Bag and mask ventilation

49. Match each condition with its description.

a. Gastroschisis	e. Femoral hernia	i. Hydrocele
b. Omphalocele	f. Cryptorchidism	j. Bladder exstrophy
c. Phimosis	g. Hypospadias	k. Hydronephrosis
d. Inguinal hernia	h. Epispadias	l. Paraphimosis

    _____ Prevents retraction of the foreskin
    _____ Herniation of the abdominal contents through the umbilical ring
    _____ Characterized by herniation lateral to the umbilical ring
    _____ Externalization of the bladder
    _____ Painless inguinal swelling
    _____ Swelling in the groin area associated with severe pain (most common in females)
    _____ Characterized by an inability to replace retracted foreskin in its normal position

_____ Fluid in the processus vaginalis

_____ Failure of one or both testes to descend

_____ Condition in which urethral opening is located below the glans penis or along the ventral surface of penile shaft

_____ Opening of the urethra on dorsum of penis

_____ Distension of the renal pelvis and calyces

50. Identify the primary criteria used to assign gender to an infant born with ambiguous genitalia.

Critical Thinking—Case Study

Jane Williams is a newborn diagnosed with myelomeningocele. She has been admitted to the NICU.

51. Which one of the following is the primary nursing goal for the care of Jane before surgical correction of the myelomeningocele?
    a. Observing for increasing paralysis
    b. Preventing infection
    c. Preventing skin breakdown
    d. Limiting environmental stimulus

52. Thirty-six hours after birth, the nurse notes that Jane is irritable and lethargic and has developed an elevated temperature. What should the nurse suspect?
    a. Hydrocephalus
    b. Infection
    c. Latex allergy
    d. Urinary retention

53. Which one the following nursing diagnoses is *most* relevant to Jane's care?
    a. Altered bowel elimination related to neurologic deficits
    b. High risk for infection related to the presence of infectious organisms
    c. Altered nutrition related to immobility
    d. Altered self-concept related to physical disability

54. Develop goals related to Jane's care in the NICU.

55. Which one of the following is the *best* way to meet Jane's tactile stimulation needs before repair of the myelomeningocele?
    a. Cuddling Jane frequently and encouraging parents to hold her in their arms
    b. Placing black and white drawings within Jane's view
    c. Caressing and stroking Jane frequently while she is placed on a pillow across her parent's lap
    d. Changing her diaper and dressing frequently

56. Jane has had corrective surgery and is now 6 hours postoperative. The nurse must observe her

abdomen closely for the development of _____ _____.

57. After closure of the meningomyelocele, Jane's nursing care should include which one of the following?
    a. Measuring the head circumference daily
    b. Keeping external stimulus at a minimum
    c. Keeping strict limitation of leg movement
    d. Withholding breast- or bottle-feedings

CHAPTER 12

Health Promotion of the Infant and Family

1. Match each biologic development term with its description or example.

   a. Binocularity
   b. Depth perception
   c. Visual preference
   d. Respiratory rate
   e. Heart rate
   f. Sinus arrhythmia
   g. Hemopoietic changes
   h. Physiologic anemia
   i. Digestive process
   j. Ptyalin

   k. Amylase
   l. Lipase
   m. Trypsin
   n. Suckling
   o. Sucking
   p. Swallowing
   q. Infantile swallow reflex
   r. Mature swallow reflex
   s. Santmyer swallow

   t. Immunologic system
   u. Thermoregulation
   v. Thermogenesis
   w. Total body fluid
   x. Renal structures
   y. Endocrine system
   z. Righting reflexes
   aa. Crawling
   bb. Creeping

   _____ Immature at birth; does not begin functioning until age 3 months

   _____ Stereopsis; begins to develop by age 7 to 9 months

   _____ Receives a significant amount of maternal protection until infant is about 3 months of age

   _____ Begins to slow in infants and is relatively stable

   _____ Heart rate that increases with inspiration and decreases with expiration

   _____ The fixation of two ocular images into one cerebral picture (fusion); begins to develop by 6 weeks of age and should be well established by age 4 months

   _____ The presence of fetal hemoglobin for the first 5 months

   _____ For infants, looking at the human face

   _____ Caused by high levels of fetal hemoglobin, which is thought to depress the production of erythropoietin

   _____ During infancy, this rate slows down with sinus arrhythmia commonly seen

   _____ Amylase; present in small amounts in the newborn but usually has little effect

   _____ Deglutition; the ability to collect the food and propel it into the esophagus

   _____ The term often used to denote breast-feeding; nutritive sucking; its primary purpose is the intake of food

   _____ Propelling forward on hands and knees with belly off floor

   _____ Enzyme needed to achieve adult levels of fat absorption

   _____ Pancreatic enzyme needed for digestion of complex carbohydrates

   _____ Secreted in sufficient quantities to catabolize protein into polypeptides and some amino acids in infants

   _____ Reflex that matures at about 35 weeks gestation; divided into nutritive and nonnutritive, the latter probably serving to satisfy a basic urge rather than a physical need

   _____ Somatic reflex in which the tongue remains behind the central incisors and the mandible no longer thrusts forward; tongue pressure and movement against the hard palate pushes the food back into the pharynx

_____ Elicit postural responses of flexion or extension that are responsible for motor activities such as rolling over, assuming the crawl position, and maintaining normal head-trunk-limb alignment during activities

_____ Visceral reflex in which food lies in a shallow groove on the top of the tongue and the fluid flows by gravity down the tongue and along the sides of the mouth; efficient for fluids but not for solids

_____ Complete maturity of this system occurs during the latter half of the second year

_____ Shivering

_____ A special reflex exhibited by infants when a puff of air is directed at the face

_____ Comprises 75% of the body weight at birth

_____ Propelling forward with belly on floor

_____ More efficient during infancy than in the newborn stage

_____ Adequately developed at birth but functions are immature

2. Match each psychosocial development term with its description.

a. Acquiring a sense of trust/overcoming a sense of mistrust
b. Narcissism
c. Grasping
d. Biting
e. Cognition
f. Sensorimotor phase
g. Separation
h. Object permanence
i. Symbols
j. Use of reflexes
k. Primary circular reactions
l. Secondary circular reactions
m. Imitation
n. Play
o. Affect
p. Secondary schemas
q. Reactive attachment disorder (RAD)
r. Solitary play
s. Revised Infant Temperament Questionnaire (ITQ)
t. Spoiled child syndrome
u. Weaning
v. Graduated extinction
w. Fluoride

_____ The third stage of the sensorimotor period; lasts until 8 months of age; characterized by repeated and prolonged reactions; phase in which grasping becomes pulling

_____ The phase with which the infant is concerned, according to Erikson

_____ Usually refers to relinquishing the breast or bottle for a cup

_____ Reaching out to others; initially reflexive; has powerful social meaning for the parents

_____ Total concern for oneself; at its height in the newborn

_____ The ability to know; most commonly explained by Piaget's theory of development

_____ Mental representations; a major intellectual achievement of the sensorimotor period

_____ Occurs in the second stage of infancy; a more aggressive and active way in which infants hold onto what is their own and attempt to more fully control their environment

_____ A crucial event in the sensorimotor phase, in which infants learn to detach themselves from other objects in the environment

_____ The term used by Piaget to describe the period from birth to 24 months

_____ Marks the beginning of the replacement of reflexive behavior with voluntary acts in the sensorimotor period; occurs from 1 to 4 months; sucking and grasping become deliberate acts to elicit certain responses

_____ The realization that objects which exit the visual field still exist; a major accomplishment for the infant in the sensorimotor phase

_____ Identifies the first stage of the sensorimotor period; the experience of perceiving patterns or ordering; provides a foundation of the subsequent stages

_____ Occurs during the fourth sensorimotor stage of Piaget; characterized by infants using previous behavior achievements as the foundation of adding new skills

_____ Ability that requires the differentiation of selected acts from several events; developed by infants in the second half of the first year

_____ The type of play that infants engage in; denotes one-sided play

_____ Activity in which infants take pleasure in performing acts after they have mastered them; consumes most of the infant's waking hours

_____ Excessive self-centered and immature behavior resulting from the failure of parents to enforce consistent age-appropriate limits

_____ Outward manifestation of emotion and feeling; seen as infants begin to develop a sense of permanency

_____ A psychologic and developmental problem that stems from maladaptive or absent attachment between the infant and parent

_____ Approach to dealing with night crying; to let the child cry for progressively longer times between brief parental interventions that consist only of reassurance

_____ A screening tool that focuses on nine temperament variables

_____ An essential mineral for building caries-resistant teeth; needed beginning at 6 months of age if the infant does not receive water with an adequate fluoride content

3. Match each child care term with its description.

a. In-home child care
b. Family daycare home
c. Center-based child care
d. Work-based group child care
e. Sick-child care

_____ Available for times when the child is ill and often located in community hospitals

_____ Usually refers to a licensed daycare facility that provides care for six or more children, for 6 or more hours in a 24-hour day

_____ May consist of a full-time babysitter who lives in the home or comes to the home

_____ An option that is becoming increasingly popular to provide quality and convenient child care to employees

_____ Typically provides child care and protection for up to five children for part of a 24-hour day

4. Match each immunization term with its description.

a. Attenuate
b. Whole-cell pertussis vaccine
c. Acellular pertussis vaccine
d. Vaccine associated polio paralysis (VAPP)
e. Vaccination
f. ComVax
g. Vaccine
h. Toxoid
i. Vaccine Adverse Event Reporting System (VAERS)
j. National Childhood Vaccine Injury Act (NCVIA) of 1986/ Vaccine Compensation Amendments of 1987

_____ Contains one or more immunogens derived from the _Bordetella pertussis_ organism; highly purified; associated with fewer local and system reactions

_____ Originally meant inoculation with vaccinia small pox virus to render a person immune to smallpox; now denotes the physical act of administering any vaccine or toxoid

_____ To reduce the virulence of a pathogenic microorganism by treating it or cultivating it on a certain medium

_____ A rare complication of the oral polio vaccine (OPV); prompted the change from the exclusive use of OPV to the exclusive use of IPV

_____ Combines Hib and hepatitis B in one vaccine

_____ A modified bacterial toxin that has been made nontoxic but retains the ability to stimulate the formation of antitoxin

_____ A suspension of live (usually attenuated) or inactivated microorganisms (e.g., bacteria, viruses, or rickettsiae) or fractions of the microorganisms administered to induce immunity

_____ Laws passed to provide compensation for children who are inadvertently injured by vaccines and to provide greater protection from liability for vaccine manufacturers

_____ Agency to which any adverse reactions after administration of any vaccine are reported

_____ Prepared from inactivated cells of *Bordetella pertussis*; contains multiple antigens

5. Match each injury prevention term with its description.

   a. Clothing closures, food items, pacifiers
   b. Syringe cap
   c. Easy-open tear-down strip
   d. Baby powder
   e. Latex balloons
   f. Bed/crib safety hazards
   g. Plastic bag
   h. Cords
   i. Changing tables, infant seats, high chairs, walkers

   _____ Poses a suffocation danger because it is light-weight and can be easily become wrapped around the head of an active infant

   _____ The leading cause of pediatric choking deaths from children's products

   _____ Common causes of aspiration in infants, because they are often small, cylindrical, and/or pliable

   _____ A tamper-resistant safety device that can be aspirated and is very difficult to locate because it is clear

   _____ A potential aspiration hazard when using a syringe to accurately measure and dispense oral liquid medication to young children

   _____ Items that present opportunities for the danger of falling

   _____ A mixture of talc and other silicates that is hazardous if aspirated

   _____ Should be less than 30 cm (12 in) to decrease the risk for strangulation

   _____ Items that pose a number of hazards from suffocation to strangulation

6. If the infant weighs 7.5 kg at age 5 months, about how many kilograms was his or her probable birth weight?
   a. 7.0
   b. 4.0
   c. 3.3
   d. 15.4

7. If the infant's head circumference is 46 cm at 6 months, how many centimeters would you expect his or her head circumference to be at 8 months?
   a. 46.5
   b. 47
   c. 47.5
   d. 49

8. The infant's posterior fontanel usually closes by:
   a. 6 to 8 weeks.
   b. 3 to 6 months.
   c. 12 to 18 months.
   d. 9 to 12 months.

9. Match each neurologic reflex with its expected behavioral response *and* with the age of its appearance in infancy. (Each reflex will be used twice.)

a. Labyrinth righting
b. Neck righting
c. Body righting

d. Otolith righting
e. Landau
f. Parachute

Expected Behavioral Response

_____ When infant is suspended in a horizontal prone position and suddenly thrust downward, hand and fingers extent forward as if to protect against falling.

_____ When body of an erect infant is tilted, head is returned to upright erect position.

_____ This is a modification of the neck righting reflex in which turning hips and shoulders to one side causes all other body parts to follow.

_____ When infant is suspended in a horizontal prone position, the head is raised and legs and spine are extended.

_____ While infant is supine, head is turned to one side. Shoulder, trunk, and finally pelvis will turn toward that side.

_____ Infant in prone or supine position is able to raise head.

Age of Appearance

_____ 7 to 12 months; persists indefinitely
_____ 6 months; persists until 24 to 26 months
_____ 2 months; strongest at 10 months
_____ 6 to 8 months; persists until 12 to 24 months
_____ 7 to 9 months; persists indefinitely
_____ 3 months; persists until 24 to 36 months

10. Which one of the following statements is true about the proportion of the chest at the end of the infant's first year?
    a. The contour of the chest is more like a neonate's than an adult's.
    b. The anteroposterior diameter is larger than the lateral diameter.
    c. The chest is small in relation to the size of the heart.
    d. The chest circumference is about equal to the head circumference.

11. Of the following characteristics of vision, the one that is developed at the earliest age is:
    a. binocularity.
    b. stereopsis.
    c. corneal reflex.
    d. convergence.

12. The characteristic of respiratory system that predisposes the infant to middle ear infection is the:
    a. short, angled eustachian tube.
    b. short, straight eustachian tube.
    c. close proximity of the trachea to the bronchi.
    d. size of the lumen of the eustachian tube.

13. The nurse can expect that an infant will respond to the sound of a human voice by about:
    a. 3 months of age.
    b. 4 months of age.
    c. 6 months of age.
    d. 10 months of age.

14. Of the following hemopoietic changes, the one that is considered abnormal in the first 5 months of life is:
    a. low iron levels.
    b. physiologic anemia.
    c. presence of fetal hemoglobin.
    d. low hemoglobin level.

15. All of the following digestive processes are deficient in an infant until about 3 months *except*:
    a. amylase.
    b. lipase.
    c. saliva.
    d. trypsin.

16. The _____ is the most immature of all the gastrointestinal organs throughout infancy.

17. The purpose of nonnutritive sucking is to:
    a. satisfy the basic sucking urge.
    b. take in food.
    c. collect food and propel it into the esophagus.
    d. provide an efficient way to process fluids.

18. Which of the following is a characteristic of the somatic swallow reflex?
    a. The mandible does not thrust forward.
    b. The tongue remains in front of the central incisors.
    c. The tongue is concave and inclined against the palate.
    d. It is efficient for fluids but not for solids.

19. After birth, normal levels of immunoglobulin in humans are:
    a. reached by 1 year of age.
    b. reached in early childhood.
    c. transferred from the mother.
    d. reached by 9 months of age.

20. Of the following mechanisms, the one that decreases the newborn's thermoregulation efficiency is:
    a. shivering.
    b. limited adipose tissue.
    c. dilation of the capillaries.
    d. constriction of the capillaries.

21. The infant is predisposed to a more rapid loss of total body fluid and dehydration because:
    a. of a high proportion of extracellular fluid.
    b. of a high proportion of intracellular fluid.
    c. total body water is at about 40%.
    d. extracellular fluid is 20% of the total.

22. Complete maturity of the kidney occurs:
    a. at birth.
    b. by 6 months.
    c. by 1 year.
    d. by 24 months.

23. Until the renal structures mature, the range of specific gravity for the infant ranges from 1.__ __ __ to 1.__ __ __ .

24. The expected immaturity of the infant's functioning endocrine system will be demonstrated in the infant's:
    a. growth patterns.
    b. thyroid levels.
    c. stress response.
    d. immunoglobulin levels.

25. Fine motor development is evaluated in the 10-month-old infant by observing the:
    a. ability to stack blocks.
    b. pincer grasp.
    c. righting reflexes.
    d. tonic neck reflex.

26. Of the following characteristics, the one that disappears by about 3 months of age is the:
    a. ability to stack blocks.
    b. pincer grasp.
    c. righting reflexes.
    d. tonic neck reflex.

27. Which of the following assessment findings would be considered *most* abnormal?
    a. Infant displays head lag at 3 months of age.
    b. Infant starts to walk at 18 months of age.
    c. Infant begins to sit unsupported at 9 months of age.
    d. Infant begins to roll from front to back at 5 months of age.

28. If parents are concerned about the fact that their 14-month-old infant is not walking, the nurse should particularly evaluate whether the infant:
    a. pulls up on the furniture.
    b. uses a pincer grasp.
    c. transfers objects.
    d. has developed object permanence.

29. The factor that best determines the quality of the infant's formulation of trust is the:
    a. quality of the interpersonal relationship.
    b. degree of mothering skill.
    c. quantity of the mother's breast milk.
    d. length of suckling time.

30. According to Piaget's theory of cognitive development, the three crucial events of the sensorimotor phase are:
    a. trust, readjustment, and the regulation of frustration.
    b. separation, object permanence, and mental representation.
    c. imitation, personality development, and temperament.
    d. ordering, comfort, and satisfaction with his or her body.

31. The development of the sexual identity begins:
    a. after the first year.
    b. during the phallic stage.
    c. at birth.
    d. at puberty.

32. Parenting:
    a. is an instinctual ability.
    b. is a learned, acquired process.
    c. begins shortly after birth.
    d. shapes the infant's environment positively.

33. Separation anxiety and stranger fear normally begin to appear by:
    a. 4 weeks.
    b. 6 months.
    c. 14 months.
    d. 4 years.

34. A maltreated child who manifests behaviors such as limited eye contact and poor impulse control may be suffering from:
    a. separation anxiety.
    b. stranger fear.
    c. reactive attachment disorder.
    d. spoiled child syndrome.

35. Which of the following play activities would be *least* appropriate to suggest to parents for their 3-month-old infant?
    a. Playing music and singing along
    b. Using rattles
    c. Using an infant swing
    d. Placing toys a bit out of reach

36. Knowledge of the infant's temperament should *not* be used in helping parents to:
    a. see an organized view of the child's behavior.
    b. choose childrearing techniques.
    c. identify a difficult child.
    d. see their child in a better perspective.

37. If parents are concerned about "spoiling" their child, the nurse should encourage them to respond to the newborn's crying episodes with:
    a. a delayed response of holding the infant.
    b. a prompt response of holding the infant.
    c. letting the infant cry a little.
    d. maintaining a feeding schedule.

38. Which of the following examples provides the best evidence that the child is being spoiled by the parents?
    a. The child who has a difficult temperament and a short attention span
    b. The toddler who has a temper tantrum
    c. The infant who has colic
    d. The child who always cries if she doesn't get her way

39. Limit setting and discipline should begin in:
    a. middle childhood or adolescence.
    b. infancy, with voice tone and eye contact.
    c. early childhood, with voice tone and eye contact.
    d. infancy, with time-out in a chair for misbehavior.

40. In guiding parents who are choosing a daycare center, the nurse should stress that state licensure represents a program that maintains:
    a. optimal care.
    b. health features.
    c. minimum requirements.
    d. safety features.

41. To decrease dependence on non-nutritive sucking in young infants, the *best* strategy for the nurse to recommend would be to:
    a. provide a homemade pacifier.
    b. prolong the time the infant is fed.
    c. restrain the sucking fingers.
    d. prohibit the use of a pacifier.

42. A 12-month-old infant would be likely to have:
    a. 2 teeth.
    b. 4 teeth.
    c. 6 teeth.
    d. 12 teeth.

43. The main reason infants should wear shoes when they begin to walk is to:
    a. protect feet from injury.
    b. support foot muscles.
    c. support the ankles.
    d. protect the arches.

44. When the infant reaches 6 months of age, the breast-feeding mother may need to supplement the breast milk with:
    a. formula.
    b. nothing.
    c. water.
    d. vitamin D.

45. The greatest threat to successful breast-feeding for the employed mother is:
    a. lack of feeding options.
    b. danger of bacterial contamination.
    c. fatigue.
    d. inefficient breast pumping.

46. Which one of the following formula feeding patterns would warrant further evaluation for a 1-year-old infant?
    a. Four feedings of 5 oz each
    b. Five feedings of 8 oz each
    c. Three feedings of 6 oz each
    d. Four feedings of 6 oz each

47. The primary reason for introducing solid food to infants is to:
    a. increase their overall caloric intake.
    b. provide a substitute for the milk source.
    c. introduce a taste and chewing experience.
    d. increase their weight.

48. If sweetening of the infant's home-prepared foods is performed, the risk for botulism can be avoided by using:
    a. honey.
    b. corn syrup.
    c. refined sugar.
    d. none of the above.

49. Studies have shown that excessive fruit juice consumption increases the likelihood of:
    a. short stature.
    b. scurvy.
    c. rickets.
    d. nursing caries.

50. When introducing new food, the parents should *not*:
    a. decrease the quantity of the infant's milk.
    b. mix food with formula to feed through a nipple.
    c. introduce new foods in small amounts.
    d. offer the new food by itself at first.

51. Which one of the following techniques is recommended to assist in weaning an infant?
    a. Eliminate the nighttime feeding first.
    b. Always wean to a bottle first.
    c. Always wean directly to a cup.
    d. Gradually replace one bottle-feeding or breast-feeding at a time.

52. Describe the considerations that should be included in a culturally sensitive approach to weaning.

53. Co-sleeping with the parents is commonly associated with:
    a. sudden infant death syndrome.
    b. colicky infants.
    c. bottle-fed infants.
    d. breast-fed infants.

54. Match each sleep disturbance with its management technique.

    a. Nighttime feeding   d. Refusal to go to sleep
    b. Developmental night crying   e. Nighttime fears
    c. Trained night crying

    _____ Check at progressively longer intervals each night.
    _____ Keep a night-light on.
    _____ Reassure parents that this is a temporary phase.
    _____ Establish a consistent pre-bedtime routine.
    _____ Put infant to bed awake.

55. Which of the following side effects of immunization would *most* likely be considered severe?
    a. A febrile episode
    b. Malaise
    c. Encephalitis
    d. Behavioral changes

56. The nurse should withhold measles, mumps, and rubella (MMR) immunization if:
    a. the mother of the child is pregnant.
    b. a family member is immunodeficient.
    c. the child is receiving long-term immunosuppressive therapy.
    d. the child is infected with HIV.

57. Which one of the following techniques has been demonstrated by research to minimize local reactions when administering immunizations to infants?
    a. Select a 1-inch needle to deposit vaccine deep into the thigh muscle mass.
    b. Use an air bubble to clear the needle after the injection.
    c. Change the needle in the syringe after drawing up the vaccine.
    d. Apply a topical anaesthetic to the site for a minimum of 1 hour.

58. To prevent aspiration in the infant, the nurse should avoid using:
    a. baby powder made from cornstarch.
    b. pacifiers made from padded nipples.
    c. syringes to dispense oral medication.
    d. pacifiers with one-piece construction.

59. Which one of the following hazards causes the majority of deaths in young children?
    a. Plastic garment bags
    b. Ill-fitting crib slats
    c. Latex balloons
    d. Ill-fitting crib mattresses

60. Which one of the following situations involving cords would be considered *least* hazardous?
    a. A bib that is not removed at bedtime
    b. A pacifier that is hung around the infant's neck with a 10-inch string
    c. A play telephone with a 10-inch cord
    d. A toy tied to the playpen with a 15-inch ribbon

61. The *best* place for the infant car restraint is in the:
    a. back seat of the car, facing back.
    b. back seat of the car, facing front.
    c. front passenger seat of the car, with an air bag, facing front.
    d. front passenger seat of the car without an air bag, facing back.

62. Which of the following is *not* acceptable because of the risk for falls?
    a. Never leave the child on a changing table unattended.
    b. Keep necessary articles within easy reach.
    c. Change the infant's diaper on the floor.
    d. Use an infant walker to strengthen walking muscles.

63. Which of the following is *not* recommended as a way to distract an infant while changing his or her diaper?
    a. Give the infant a bottle of talc baby powder to hold.
    b. Sing and play with the infant.
    c. Play the same game each time.
    d. None of the above ideas are recommended.

Critical Thinking—Case Study

Jennifer Klein, a 6-month-old infant, is admitted to the pediatric unit with bronchiolitis. Both of the parents work, and Jennifer attends daycare. Jennifer is the first child, and the parents seem anxious about the admission, as well as about her care at home and her normal development. It is clear that the parents need information about general health promotion for their infant.

64. Place a check next to each of the following areas that should be assessed to determine the status of the parents' current health promotion practices? (Check all that apply.)

_____ Respiratory status (lung sounds)

_____ Nutrition

_____ Fever patterns

_____ Sleep and activity

_____ Number and condition of teeth

_____ Fluid and hydration status

_____ Condition of the mucous membranes of the mouth

_____ Immunization status

_____ Safety precautions used in the home

65. Which of the following nursing diagnoses would be used *most* often for health promotion related to development in an infant Jennifer's age?
    a. Activity intolerance
    b. Ineffective thermoregulation
    c. High risk for injury
    d. Altered parenting

66. Of the following strategies, the one used *most* often to help new parents like Jennifer's adjust to the parenting role is:
    a. parenting classes.
    b. anticipatory guidance.
    c. first aid courses.
    d. cardiopulmonary resuscitation courses.

67. By the time Jennifer is ready for discharge, the nurse evaluates that her parents have achieved improved parenting skills. Which one of the following would *best* confirm the plan's success?
    a. Jennifer is afebrile.
    b. Reports from the other staff are positive.
    c. Verbalizations from the parents indicate that they understand.
    d. A home visit demonstrates that positive changes have occurred.

CHAPTER 13

Health Problems During Infancy

1. The following terms are related to nutritional disturbances and feeding difficulties. Match each term with its description.

a. Coenzymes
b. Apoenzyme
c. Holoenzyme
d. Microminerals
e. Lacto-ovovegetarians
f. Vegans
g. Zen macrobiotics
h. Recommended Dietary Allowances (RDAs)
i. Dietary Reference Intake (DRIs)

j. Dietary Guidelines for Americans
k. Food Guide Pyramid
l. Diarrhea
m. Aflatoxin
n. Food allergy
o. Food intolerance
p. Allergens
q. Sensitization
r. Atopy

s. Lactase
t. Congenital lactase deficiency
u. Late onset lactase deficiency
v. Secondary lactase deficiency
w. Regurgitation
x. Spitting up
y. The Feeding Checklist

_____ More restrictive than pure vegetarians in that cereals, especially brown rice, are the mainstay of the diet

_____ Forms when vitamin coenzymes enter the body and combine with a protein apoenzyme

_____ Pure vegetarians who eliminate any food of animal origin, including milk and eggs

_____ Substances that regulate specific metabolic activity; e.g., vitamins

_____ Trace elements; have daily requirements of less than 100 mg

_____ A protein enzyme that has been synthesized with the cell

_____ Dietary advice for the public that replaces the basic four food groups; used to convey nutrition information to the public and applies to children as young as 2 years of age

_____ A mycotoxin mold that has been implicated in the etiology of kwashiorkor; present in large numbers in the intestines of children with the disease

_____ The standard developed by the National Academy of Sciences, Food and Nutrition Board; the most widely used standard that identifies areas of nutritional concern

_____ Those who exclude meat from their diet but eat milk and eggs and sometimes fish

_____ Guidelines for nutritional intake that encompass the RDAs yet extend their scope to include additional parameters related to nutritional intake; include estimated average nutrient requirements for age and gender categories, tolerable upper-limit nutrient intakes that are associated with a low risk for adverse effects and the standard RDAs

_____ A major factor in malnutrition in many developing and underdeveloped nations

_____ Dietary advice for the public that encourages eating a variety of foods, maintaining ideal body weight, consuming adequate starch and fiber and limiting intake of fat, cholesterol, sugar, salt, and alcohol

_____ Allergy with a hereditary tendency

_____ Hypersensitivity; refers to those reactions to food that involve immunologic mechanisms, usually immunoglobulin E

_____ Lactose intolerance that occurs when the intestinal lumen is damaged, causing a decrease or destruction of the enzyme lactase

_____ Refers to those reactions to food that involve known or unknown nonimmunologic mechanisms; e.g., the inability to properly digest lactose

_____ An enzyme that is needed for the digestion of lactose

_____ Return of undigested food from the stomach, usually accompanied by burping

_____ Usually proteins that are capable of inducing IgE antibody formation

_____ Dribbling of unswallowed formula from the infant's mouth immediately after a feeding

_____ The initial exposure of an individual to an allergen, resulting in an immune response, after which subsequent exposure induces a much stronger response that is clinically apparent

_____ A rare disorder that appears soon after the infant has consumed lactose-containing milk; an inborn error of metabolism that involves the complete absence or severely reduced presence of lactase

_____ A 25-item observational scale developed specifically for the purpose of observing mother-infant dyads with nonorganic failure to thrive

_____ Also referred to as _primary lactase deficiency_—the most common type of lactose intolerance; manifested at around 3 to 7 years of age; not a disease; more common in Asians, southern Europeans, Arabs, Israelis, and African Americans; characterized by abdominal pain, bloating, flatulence, and diarrhea that occur 30 minutes to several hours after lactose consumption

2. Match each term with its description.

   a. Example/demonstration
   b. Apparent life-threatening events (ALTEs)
   c. Plagiocephaly
   d. Infantile eczema
   e. Nursing Child Assessment Satellite Training (NCAST) Feeding Scale

   _____ Flattening of the skull that occurs when the infant's head position is not varied
   _____ A tool designed to assess the feeding interaction of infants up to 12 months of age
   _____ Teaching technique to use with parents of infants with nonorganic failure to thrive
   _____ Atopic dermatitis that begins at age 2 to 6 months, with spontaneous remission often occurring at age 3 years
   _____ Previously referred to by the expression "near-miss SIDS"; includes a combination of apnea, color change, and change in muscle tone that is frightening to the observer

3. In the United States, vitamin D deficiency is most likely to occur in an infant who:
   a. belongs to a low socioeconomic group.
   b. consumes yogurt as the primary milk source.
   c. had measles in the neonatal period.
   d. has the diagnosis of rheumatoid arthritis.

4. When hypervitaminosis is suspected, the vitamin that could cause the most harm is:
   a. folate.
   b. retinol.
   c. biotin.
   d. ascorbic acid.

5. To avoid problems associated with vitamin A deficiency, the American Academy of Pediatrics recommends that health care providers:
   a. screen all children between the ages of 6 month and 2 years for vitamin A deficiency.
   b. recommend supplementation of vitamin A (4000 mg) to breast-feeding mothers.
   c. consider vitamin A administration to children hospitalized for complicated measles.
   d. advise breast-feeding mothers to avoid highly pigmented fruits and vegetables.

6. The greatest concern with minerals is:
   a. deficiency.
   b. excess, causing toxicity.
   c. nervous system disturbances from excess.
   d. hemochromatosis.

7. Match each type of vegetarianism with its description.

   a. Lacto-ovovegetarianism
   b. Lactovegetarianism
   c. Pure vegetarianism (veganism)
   d. Zen macrobiotics
   e. Semi-vegetarianism

   _____ This group eliminates any food of animal origin, including milk and eggs.
   _____ This group is the most restrictive of all. Only small amounts of fruits, vegetables, and legumes are consumed.
   _____ This group excludes meat from their diet but eats milk, eggs, and sometimes fish.
   _____ This group excludes meat and eggs but drinks milk.
   _____ This group consumes a lacto-ovovegetarian diet with some fish and poultry

8. Nutritional assessment of any vegetarian family should focus on the amount of which nutrient?

9. List the four categories of the Dietary Reference Intakes (DRIs)

10. The source of nutrition information that replaces the basic four food groups and applies to children as young as 2 years of age is called:
    a. Recommended Dietary Allowances (RDAs).
    b. Dietary Reference Intakes.
    c. Food Guide Pyramid.
    d. Dietary Guidelines for Americans.

11. To ensure the most complete protein, a strictly vegetarian family should combine:
    a. milk and chicken.
    b. sunflower seeds and rice.
    c. rice and red beans.
    d. eggs and cheese.

12. In the United States, protein and energy malnutrition (PEM) occurs where:
    a. the food supply is inadequate.
    b. the food supply may be adequate.
    c. the adults eat first, leaving insufficient food for children.
    d. the diet consists mainly of starch grains.

13. Kwashiorkor occurs in populations where:
    a. the food supply is inadequate.
    b. the food supply is adequate for protein.
    c. the adults eat first, leaving insufficient food for children.
    d. the diet consists mainly of starch grains.

14. Childhood nutritional marasmus usually results in populations where:
    a. the food supply is inadequate.
    b. the food supply is adequate for protein.
    c. the adults eat first, leaving insufficient food for children.
    d. the diet consists mainly of starch grains.

15. It would be *inappropriate* to therapeutically manage PEM, kwashiorkor, or marasmus by:
    a. providing a high-protein, high-carbohydrate diet.
    b. replacing fluids and electrolytes.
    c. providing a high-fiber, high-fat diet.
    d. providing a structured play program.

16. Which of the following foods would be considered the least allergenic?
    a. Orange juice
    b. Eggs
    c. Bread
    d. Rice

17. A sensitivity to cow's milk in an infant may be manifested clinically by:
    a. irritability.
    b. colic.
    c. vomiting and diarrhea.
    d. all of the above.

18. Which one of the following diagnostic strategies is the *most* definitive for identifying a milk allergy?
    a. Stool analysis for blood
    b. Serum IgE levels
    c. Challenge testing with milk
    d. Skin testing

19. The American Academy of Pediatrics recommends treating cow's milk allergy in infants by changing the formula to:
    a. soy formula.
    b. goat's milk.
    c. casein hydrolysate formula.
    d. milk pretreated with microbial-derived lactase.

20. An acceptable substitute for the hydrolyzed formulas that the American Academy of Pediatrics recommends to avoid milk allergy is:
    a. yogurt.
    b. soy formula.
    c. cow's milk.
    d. goat's milk.

21. Congenital lactase deficiency is:
    a. a rare form of lactose intolerance.
    b. the form of lactose intolerance associated with giardiasis.
    c. an intolerance that is manifested later in life.
    d. a form of lactose intolerance caused by intestinal damage.

22. Late-onset lactase deficiency is also known as:
    a. congenital lactase deficiency.
    b. secondary lactose deficiency.
    c. primary lactase deficiency.
    d. congenital lactose intolerance.

23. One strategy for parents of infants with primary lactase deficiency would be to:
    a. substitute human milk for cow's milk.
    b. substitute soy-based formula for human milk.
    c. drink milk alone without other food or drink.
    d. substitute frozen yogurt for fresh yogurt.

24. If a sensitivity to cow's milk is suspected as the cause of an infant's colic, the parents should:
    a. try substituting casein hydrolysate formula.
    b. try substituting soy formula.
    c. be reassured that the symptoms will disappear spontaneously at about 3 months of age.
    d. be assessed for areas of improper feeding techniques.

25. The commonly accepted etiology for colic is:
    a. carbohydrate malabsorption.
    b. excessive air swallowing.
    c. colonic fermentation.
    d. infant temperament.

26. Which of the following phrases *best* defines rumination?
    a. It is the involuntary return of undigested food from the stomach, usually accompanied by burping.
    b. It is the dribbling of unswallowed formula from the infant's mouth immediately after a feeding.
    c. It is the active, voluntary return of swallowed food into the mouth.
    d. It is the same as vomiting.

27. Match each category of failure to thrive with its description.

    a. Organic failure to thrive (OFTT)
    b. Nonorganic failure to thrive (NFTT)
    c. Idiopathic failure to thrive

    _____ Has a definable cause that is unrelated to any physiologic disease process, such as disturbance in maternal-child attachment
    _____ Results from a physical cause, such as a congenital heart defect
    _____ Is unexplained by the usual organic and environmental etiologies and may also be classified as NFTT

28. List five factors other than parent-child interaction that can lead to inadequate feeding of the infant.

29. A term that health care workers may use to avoid the social stigma of *nonorganic failure to thrive* is

    _____.

30. If failure to thrive has been a long-standing problem, the infant will show evidence of:
    a. weight and height depression.
    b. weight depression only.
    c. height depression only.
    d. neither height nor weight depression.

31. Which one of the following characteristics in an infant with failure to thrive is *most* significant?
    a. Difficult feeding pattern with vomiting and aversion behavior
    b. Crying, excessive irritability and sleep pattern disturbances
    c. Lack of fit between the child's temperament and that of the parents
    d. Irregularity in activities of daily living and difficult temperament pattern

32. To increase the caloric intake of an infant with failure to thrive, the nurse might recommend:
    a. using developmental stimulation by a specialist during feedings.
    b. avoiding solids until after the bottle is well accepted.
    c. being persistent through 10 to 15 minutes of food refusal.
    d. varying the schedule for routine activities on a daily basis.

33. The incidence of diaper dermatitis is generally reported as greater in bottle-fed infants than in breast-fed infants, because in breast-fed infants there is a lower:
    a. ammonia content in the urine.
    b. pH content of the feces.
    c. microbial content of the feces.
    d. number of stools per day.

34. Parents of an infant with diaper dermatitis should be encouraged to:
    a. apply a petrolatum-based cream.
    b. mix zinc oxide thoroughly with antifungal cream.
    c. use a hand-held dryer on the open lesions.
    d. use diapers with super-absorbent gel.

35. Seborrhagic dermatitis is usually *not* manifested as:
    a. eczema.
    b. cradle cap.
    c. blepharitis.
    d. otitis externa.

36. Which one of the following recommendations for the care of atopic dermatitis is controversial?
    a. Apply emollient within the first few minutes after bathing.
    b. Apply cool wet compresses to sooth the skin.
    c. Limit the infant's exposure to allergens.
    d. Administer antihistamines to control pruritis.

37. Identify the following statements as either true or false.

    _____ The incidence of sudden infant death syndrome (SIDS) is associated with diphtheria, tetanus, and pertussis vaccines.

    _____ Maternal smoking during and after pregnancy has been implicated as a contributor to SIDS.

    _____ Parents should be advised to position their infants on their abdomen to prevent SIDS.

    _____ The nurse should encourage the parents to sleep in the same bed as the infant who is being monitored for apnea of infancy in order to detect subtle clinical changes.

    _____ Parents should avoid using soft, moldable mattresses and pillows in the bed to prevent SIDS.

Critical Thinking—Case Study

Six-month-old Jason Fitch has come to the office today for his routine immunizations. His mother says she thinks everything is just fine, except that Jason seems to have a lot of food intolerances. The nurse continues the assessment and finds that Jason is eating many of the food items the rest of the family eats, including milk products in very small amounts. There is no particular pattern to the way the new foods are being introduced. Jason exhibits a variety of symptoms related to skin irritations. He is developing rashes around his mouth, rectum, and elsewhere on his body when he eats certain foods.

38. Based on the prevalence of the common health problems of infancy, what areas should the nurse include in an initial assessment of a 6-month-old?
    a. Nutrition
    b. Temperament
    c. Sleep patterns
    d. All of the above

39. Based on the data from the assessment interview, which one of the following goals is *best* for the nurse to establish?
    a. To prevent outbreaks of food allergy
    b. To prevent death from anaphylaxis
    c. To prevent genetic transmission
    d. All of the above

40. Which one of the following recommendations would be *most* appropriate for Jason's mother?
    a. Reconsider breast-feeding.
    b. Eliminate cow's milk.
    c. Add only one new food at each 5-day interval.
    d. Eliminate solids until 9 months of age.

41. At an earlier visit, the nurse had determined that there was altered parenting related to lack of knowledge in Jason's family. Which one of the following outcome criteria would help the nurse to evaluate the ability of the mother to provide a constructive environment for Jason?
    a. Jason's mother is able to identify eating patterns that contribute to symptoms.
    b. Jason's mother is able to share her feelings regarding her parenting skills.
    c. Jason's mother is able to practice appropriate precautions to prevent infection.
    d. Jason's mother is able to identify the rationale for prevention of the skin rashes.

CHAPTER 14

Health Promotion of the Toddler and Family

1. Match each term with its description.

a. Terrible twos
b. Weight
c. Height
d. Head circumference
e. Chest circumference
f. Autonomy vs. doubt and shame
g. Negativism
h. Ritualism
i. Ego
j. Id
k. Superego

l. Tertiary circular reactions
m. New means through mental combinations
n. Domestic mimicry
o. Egocentrism
p. Preoperational phase
q. Egocentric speech
r. Collective monologue
s. Socialized speech
t. Preoperational thinking
u. Operations

v. Punishment and obedience orientation
w. Separation
x. Individuation
y. Parallel play
z. Toddler Temperament Scale and TBAQ
aa. Sibling rivalry
bb. Regression
cc. Fears
dd. Touch points

_____ Imitation of household activity

_____ The average at 2 years of age is 86.6 cm (34 in)

_____ Refers to the toddler years; period from 12 to 36 months of age

_____ Increases in size during the toddler years; also changes shape

_____ The persistent negative response to requests; characteristic of the toddler's behavior

_____ The average at 2 years of age is 12 kg (27 lb)

_____ The developmental task of the toddler years

_____ The toddler's need to maintain sameness and reliability; provides a sense of comfort

_____ The impulsive part of the psyche

_____ The fifth stage of the sensorimotor phase of development, when the child uses active experimentation to achieve previously unattainable goals; period during which object permanence is one of the most dramatic achievements

_____ May be thought of as reason or common sense during the toddler phase of psychosocial development

_____ The conscience

_____ Slows somewhat at the end of infancy; total increase during the second year is 2.5 cm.

_____ The final sensorimotor stage that occurs during ages 19 to 24 months

_____ The ability to envision situations from perspectives other than one's own

_____ Consists of repeating words and sounds for the pleasure of hearing oneself and is not intended to communicate

_____ The inability to manipulate objects in relation to each other in a logical fashion

_____ Spans ages 2 to 7 years; bridges the self-satisfying behavior of infancy and social behavior of latency; uses egocentric language dependent of perception

_____ Those achievements that mark children's assumption of their individual characteristics in the environment

_____ The child's emergence from a symbiotic fusion with the mother

_____ Playing alongside, not with, other children

_____ Egocentric speech that reflects the child's lingering self-centeredness

_____ The natural jealousy and resentment of children to a new child in the family

_____ Common during the toddler stage; includes problems with sleep, animals, engines, strangers, and separation

_____ Implies that children think primarily based on their own perception of an event; phase in which problem solving is based on what children see or hear directly, rather than on what they recall about objects and events

_____ A retreat from a present pattern of functioning to past levels of behavior; usually occurs in instances of stress, when the child attempts to cope by reverting to patterns of behavior that were successful in earlier stages of development; common in toddlers

_____ One of the two types of speech used by children in the toddler years; used for communication; egocentric in that children communicate about themselves to others

_____ Tools that assist in identifying temperamental characteristics; reliable instruments used to assess toddler temperament and other behaviors

_____ The most basic level of moral judgment, in which an action is judged good or bad depending on whether it results in reward or punishment

_____ Predictable times of regression

2. Match each term with its description.

a. Pedodontist
b. Plaque
c. Dental caries
d. Periodontal disease
e. Scrub method
f. Gingivitis
g. Swish-and-swallow method
h. Fluorosis
i. Nursing caries
j. Convertible restraint
k. Five-point harness
l. Padded shield
m. T-shield
n. Booster
o. Low-shield model
p. Belt-positioning model

_____ A booster that uses a lap/shoulder belt; the preferred type of booster

_____ A harness system that consists of retracting shoulder straps attached to a flat chest shield with a rigid stalk that attaches to a restraint between the legs

_____ A booster that primarily uses a lap belt

_____ Device that depends on the vehicle belts to hold the child in place

_____ Baby bottle caries (BBC); early childhood caries (ECC); occurs when the child is placed in the crib or bed with a bottle of milk, juice, soda pop, or sweetened water at nap or bedtime or uses the bottle as a pacifier while awake

_____ A harness system that consists of a strap over each shoulder, one on each side of the pelvis and one between the legs

_____ May be used to clean teeth when brushing is impractical

_____ A car seat that is suitable for infants in the rearward-facing position and for toddlers in the forward-facing position

_____ A condition characterized by an increase in the degree and extent of the enamel's porosity as a result of excessive fluoride ingestion by young children

_____ A brushing technique in which the tips of the bristles are place firmly at a 45-degree angle against the teeth and gums and are moved back and forth in a vibratory motion; suitable for cleaning primary teeth

_____ A harness system that uses shoulder straps attached to a shield held in place by a crotch strap

_____ Tooth decay

_____ Inflammation of the gums

_____ Gum disease

_____ A pediatric dentist who should examine toddlers soon after their first teeth erupt, usually around 1 year of age

_____ Soft bacterial deposits that adhere to the teeth and cause decay

3. If the chest circumference of a toddler is currently 50 cm, what would you expect the head circumference to be?
   a. 25 cm
   b. 35 cm
   c. 50 cm
   d. 60 cm

4. Which of the following characteristics *most* predispose toddlers to frequent infections?
   a. Short straight internal ear canal and large lymph tissue
   b. Slower pulse and respiratory rate and higher blood pressure
   c. Abdominal respirations
   d. Less efficient defense mechanisms

5. One of the most important digestive system changes completed during the toddler period is the:
   a. increased acidity of the gastric contents.
   b. voluntary control of the sphincters.
   c. protective function of the gastric contents.
   d. increased capacity of the stomach.

6. Which one of the following statements is *most* characteristic of a 24-month-old child?
   a. Motor skills are fully developed but occur in isolation from the environment.
   b. The toddler walks alone, but falls easily.
   c. The toddler's activities begin to produce purposeful results.
   d. The toddler is able to grasp small objects, but cannot release them at will.

7. Using Erikson's theory as a foundation, the primary developmental task of the toddler period is to:
   a. satisfy the need for basic trust.
   b. achieve a sense of accomplishment.
   c. learn to give up dependence for independence.
   d. acquire language or mental symbolism.

8. Piaget's theory of cognitive development depicts the toddler as a child who:
   a. continuously explores the same object each time it appears in a new place.
   b. is able to transfer information from one situation to another.
   c. has a persistent negative response to any request.
   d. has the rudimentary beginning of a superego.

9. The principal characteristics of Piaget's preoperational phase are:
   i.   dependence on perception in problem solving.
   ii. egocentric use of language.
   iii. the ability to manipulate objects in relation to one another in a logical way.
   iv. the ability to problem-solve based on what is recalled about objects and events.

   a. i, ii, and iii
   b. i and ii
   c. ii and iii
   d. ii, iii, and iv

10. Match each characteristic of preoperational thought with its description.

    a. Egocentrism   e. Animism
    b. Transductive reasoning   f. Irreversibility
    c. Global organization   g. Magical thinking
    d. Centration   h. Inability to conserve

    _____ Focusing on one aspect rather than considering all possible alternatives
    _____ Inability to envision situations from perspectives other than one's own
    _____ Inability to undo the actions initiated physically
    _____ Attributing lifelike qualities to inanimate objects
    _____ Thinking from the particular to the particular
    _____ Lack of understanding that a mass can be changed in size shape, volume, or length without
             losing or adding to the original mass
    _____ Believing that thoughts are all-powerful and can cause events
    _____ Changing any one part of the whole changes the entire whole

11. According to Kohlberg, the *best* way to discipline children is to:
    a. use a punishment and obedience orientation.
    b. withhold privileges.
    c. use power to control behavior.
    d. give explanations and help the child to change.

12. By the age of 2, the toddler generally:
    a. has clear body boundaries.
    b. participates willingly in most procedures.
    c. recognizes sexual differences.
    d. is unable to learn correct terms for body parts.

13. Which of the following skills is *not* necessary for the toddler to acquire before separation and individuation can be achieved?
    a. Object permanence
    b. Lack of anxiety during separations from parents
    c. Delayed gratification
    d. Ability to tolerate a moderate amount of frustration

14. The usual number of words acquired by the age of 2 years is:
    a. 50.
    b. 100.
    c. 300.
    d. 500.

15. The 2-year-old child living in a bilingual environment will generally have:
    a. advanced speaking ability without adequate comprehension.
    b. advanced speaking ability along with advanced comprehension.
    c. delayed speaking ability with adequate comprehension.
    d. delayed speaking without adequate comprehension.

16. As the child moves through the toddler period, there is a decrease in the frequency of:
    a. solitary play.
    b. imitative play.
    c. tactile play.
    d. parallel play.

17. List at least five characteristics of an 18- to 24-month-old child that would indicate readiness for toilet training.

18. Of the following techniques, which is the *best* to use when toilet training a toddler?
    a. Limit sessions to 5 or 10 minutes of practice.
    b. Remove child from the bathroom to flush the toilet.
    c. Ensure the toddler's privacy during the sessions.
    d. Place potty chair near a television to help distract the child during the sessions.

19. Which one of the following statements is *false* in regard to toilet training?
    a. Bowel training is usually accomplished after bladder training.
    b. Nighttime bladder training is usually accomplished after bowel training.
    c. The toddler who is impatient with soiled diapers is demonstrating readiness for toilet training.
    d. Fewer wet diapers signals that the toddler is physically ready for toilet training.

20. Of the following strategies, which is *most* appropriate for parents to use to prepare a toddler for the birth of a sibling?
    a. Explain the upcoming birth as early in the pregnancy as possible.
    b. Move the toddler to his or her own new room.
    c. Provide a doll for the toddler to imitate parenting.
    d. Tell the toddler that a new playmate will come home soon.

21. The *best* approach to stop a toddler's attention-seeking behavior of a tantrum with head banging is to:
    a. ignore the behavior.
    b. provide time-out.
    c. offer a toy to calm the child.
    d. protect the child from injury.

22. Of the following techniques, which is the *best* one to deal with the negativism of the toddler?
    a. Quietly and calmly ask the child to comply.
    b. Provide few or no choices for the child.
    c. Challenge the child with a game.
    d. Remain serious and intent.

23. Which of the following statements about stress in toddlers is true?
    a. Toddlers are rarely exposed to stress or the results of stress.
    b. Any stress is destructive because toddlers have a limited ability to cope.
    c. Most children are exposed to a stress-free environment.
    d. Small amounts of stress help toddlers develop effective coping skills.

24. List three sources of increased stress in toddlers.

25. Regression in toddlers occurs when there is:
    a. stress.
    b. a threat to their autonomy.
    c. a need to revert to dependency.
    d. all the above.

26. Which of the following statements is true in regard to nutritional changes from the infant to the toddler years?
    a. Caloric requirements increase from 102 kcal/kg to 108 kcal/kg.
    b. Caloric requirements decrease from 108 kcal/kg to 102 kcal/kg.
    c. Protein requirements decrease from 2.2 kcal/kg to 1.5 kcal/kg.
    d. Protein requirements increase from 1.2 kcal/kg to 2.2 kcal/kg.

27. Reduced fluid requirement in toddlers represents a decrease in total body fluid with:
    a. an increase in intracellular fluid.
    b. an increase in extracellular fluid.
    c. a decrease in intracellular fluid.
    d. a decrease in extracellular fluid.

28. Which nutritional requirement increases during the toddler years?
    a. Calories
    b. Proteins
    c. Minerals
    d. Fluids

29. Physiologic anorexia in toddlers is characterized by:
    a. strong taste preferences.
    b. extreme changes in appetite from day to day.
    c. heightened awareness of social aspects of meals.
    d. all of the above.

30. Healthy ways of serving food to toddlers include:
    a. establishing a pattern of sitting at a table for meals.
    b. permitting nutritious nibbling in lieu of meals.
    c. discouraging between-meal snacking.
    d. all of the above.

31. Developmentally, most children at 12 months:
    a. use a spoon adeptly.
    b. relinquish the bottle voluntarily.
    c. eat the same food as the rest of the family.
    d. reject all solid food in preference for the bottle.

32. The *best* approach to use for the toddler who prefers the bottle to all solid food is to:
    a. require the toddler to eat something.
    b. dilute the milk with water.
    c. withhold all food and water until the child takes solids.
    d. puree the solids and feed them through the bottle.

33. For a toddler with sleep problems, the nurse should suggest:
    a. using a transitional object.
    b. varying the bedtime ritual.
    c. restricting stimulating activities.
    d. all of the above.

34. Which of the following would be an *inappropriate* method to help a toddler adjust to the initial dental checkup?
    a. Explain to the child that a checkup won't hurt.
    b. Have the child observe his or her sibling's examination.
    c. Have the child perform a checkup on a doll.
    d. Ask the dentist to reserve a thorough exam for another visit.

35. The *most* effective way to clean a toddler's teeth is:
    a. for the child to brush regularly with a toothpaste of his or her choice.
    b. for the parent to stabilize the chin with one hand and brush with the other.
    c. for the parent to brush the mandibular occlusive surfaces leaving the rest for the child.
    d. for the child to brush all except the mandibular occlusive surfaces.

36. Flossing is necessary:
    a. only after the permanent teeth erupt.
    b. to prevent fluorosis.
    c. for the toddler to learn.
    d. even if teeth are widely spaced.

37. Adequate fluoride ingestion:
    a. prevents gingivitis.
    b. prevents fluorosis.
    c. alters the anatomy of the tooth.
    d. reduces the amount of plaque.

38. To prevent fluorosis, parents of toddlers should use all of the following strategies *except*:
    a. supervise the use of toothpaste.
    b. use fluoride rinses.
    c. store fluoride products out of reach.
    d. administer fluoride on an empty stomach.

39. One example of a treat that may damage the teeth is:
    a. aged cheese.
    b. celery sticks.
    c. sugarless gum.
    d. a handful of raisins.

40. Nursing bottle caries can result from:
    a. using a pacifier.
    b. feeding the last bottle just before bedtime.
    c. long, frequent nocturnal breast-feeding.
    d. all of the above.

41. Match each example of developmental status in a young child with its associated safety precaution that could be used to prevent injury.

    a. Has unrefined depth perception
    b. Is able to open most containers
    c. Has a great curiosity
    d. Walks, runs, and moves quickly
    e. Puts things in mouth
    f. Pulls on objects

    _____ Do not allow child to play near curb or parked cars.
    _____ Choose large toys without sharp edges.
    _____ Supervise closely at all times, especially near water.
    _____ Turn pot handles toward back of stove

_____ Remove unsecured or scatter rugs.

_____ Know the number of the poison control center.

42. _____ _____ injuries cause more accidental deaths in all pediatric age groups.

43. Children should use convertible car restraints until they:
    a. weigh 40 pounds.
    b. reach the age of 1 year.
    c. reach the age of 8 years.
    d. weigh 60 pounds.

44. The car restraint that consists of a standardized anchorage system uses a:
    a. five-point harness.
    b. convertible safety seat.
    c. universal child safety seat.
    d. belt-positioning model.

45. One of the *best* ways to prevent drowning in the toddler group is for parents to:
    a. learn cardiopulmonary resuscitation (CPR).
    b. supervise children whenever they are near any source of water.
    c. enroll the toddler in a swimming program.
    d. all of the above.

46. Prevention strategies have removed near-drowning as one of the leading causes of "vegetative" state in children.
    a. True
    b. False

47. Burn injuries in the toddler age group are most often the result of:
    a. flame burns from playing with matches.
    b. scald burn from hot liquids.
    c. hot object burns·from cigarettes or irons.
    d. electric burns from electrical outlets.

48. The *most* fatal type of burn in the toddler age group is:
    a. flame burn from playing with matches.
    b. scald burn from hot liquids.
    c. hot object burn from cigarettes or irons.
    d. electric burn from electrical outlets.

49. Poisonings in toddlers can be *best* prevented by:
    a. consistently using safety caps.
    b. storing poisonous substances in a locked cabinet.
    c. keeping ipecac syrup in the home.
    d. storing poisonous substances out of reach.

50. The parents should consider moving the toddler from the crib to a bed after the toddler:
    a. reaches the age of 2 years.
    b. will stay in the bed all night.
    c. reaches a height of 35 inches.
    d. is able to sleep through the night.

51. For each of the following potentially hazardous categories, give an example of an item that could cause aspiration or suffocation in the toddler (e.g., Foods: hard candy).

    Foods:

    Play objects:

    Common household objects:

    Electrical items:

Critical Thinking—Case Study

Tasha Jackson is a 12-month-old infant who is visiting the clinic for her well-baby checkup. Tasha's mother Dora is expecting her second child in 3 months. Dora works full-time and will be home for 6 weeks with the new baby. Tasha has been in daycare since she was a baby. Her husband also works full-time during the day.

52. List four areas that the nurse should assess to obtain the information necessary to adequately provide anticipatory guidance for a toddler at Tasha's age.

53. The *most* appropriate initial nursing intervention would be to:
    a. allow Mrs. Jackson to express her feelings.
    b. give Mrs. Jackson advice about daycare.
    c. give Mrs. Jackson advice about sibling rivalry
    d. all of the above.

54. Dora Jackson shares with the nurse that she is concerned about her daycare arrangements and is thinking about keeping Tasha at home for the 6 weeks after the baby is born. The highest priority intervention in this situation is to:
    a. stress the importance of preparing Tasha for the new sibling.
    b. recommend that Mrs. Jackson begin making plans to keep Tasha at home for the 6 weeks.
    c. recommend that any change in daycare should take place well before the new baby's arrival.
    d. explore Mrs. Jackson's concerns about her daycare arrangements.

55. The *best* way to evaluate and delineate whether Mrs. Jackson's daycare concerns are warranted would be to:
    a. make a home visit after the baby is born.
    b. visit the daycare center.
    c. observe a return demonstration of baby care.
    d. solicit feedback from Mrs. Jackson that she is comfortable with her postpartum arrangements.

CHAPTER 15

Health Promotion of the Preschooler and Family

1. Match each term with its description.

a. Preschool period
b. Placement stage
c. Shape stage
d. Design stage
e. Combine
f. Aggregate

g. Pictorial stage
h. Initiative
i. Guilt
j. Superego
k. Oedipal stage
l. Castration complex

m. Oedipus/Electra complex
n. Penis envy
o. Preoperational phase
p. Preconceptual phase
q. Intuitive thought phase

_____ Guilt that develops from a son's wish to marry his mother and kill his father or from a daughter's wish to marry her father and kill her mother

_____ Occurs in the preschool years, resulting in conflict when children overstep the limits of their ability and inquiry

_____ Time during which the child is 3 to 5 years of age

_____ Phallic stage

_____ The second stage of drawing development, in which the 3-year-old draws a single-line outline form such as a rectangle, circle, oval, cross, or other odd shape

_____ Period that occurs from ages 4 to 7 years, when the child begins to shift from totally egocentric thought to social awareness and the ability to consider other viewpoints

_____ The conscience

_____ The first stage of drawing development, in which a pattern of placing scribbles on paper appears by age 2 years and once developed, is never lost

_____ To create two united diagrams in a drawing

_____ The desire to have a penis

_____ To create three or more united diagrams in a drawing

_____ Guilt that develops regarding a son's feelings toward his father, making him fear the punishment of mutilation

_____ The fourth stage of drawing development, in which designs are recognizable as familiar objects

_____ Period that occurs from ages 2 to 4 years; the first phase of Piaget's preoperational phase

_____ The chief psychosocial task of the preschool period

_____ Period that spans the ages from 2 to 7 years; the stage of Piaget's cognitive theory that involves the preschooler

_____ The third stage of drawing development, in which simple forms are drawn together to make structured designs

123

2. Match each term with its description.

a. Play
b. Right and left concepts
c. Causality
d. Time concepts
e. Magical thinking
f. Punishment and obedience orientation
g. Naive instrumental orientation
h. Sex typing
i. Individuation-separation process
j. Telegraphic speech

k. Associative play
l. Imitative play
m. Imaginary playmates
n. Behavioral Style Questionnaire
o. Sexuality
p. Masturbation
q. Gifted/talented
r. Aggression
s. Frustration
t. modeling
u. Reinforcement

v. Quantity
w. Severity
x. Distribution
y. Onset
z. Duration
aa. Stuttering
bb. Animism
cc. Desensitization
dd. Dyslalia
ee. Mutual play
ff. DASE

_____ Play that occurs between the child and an adult (often the parent); fosters development and enriched opportunities

_____ The process by which an individual develops the behavior, personality, attitudes, and beliefs appropriate for his or her culture and sex

_____ Different manifestations of the behaviors that are used to differentiate between "normal" and "problematic" behavior

_____ Group play in similar or identical activities but without rigid organization or rules

_____ Actions directed toward satisfying the child's own needs and less commonly toward the needs of others

_____ Resembles logical thought superficially; the ability of preschoolers to explain a concept as they have heard it described by others, but with limited understanding

_____ The preschooler's belief that his or her own thoughts are all-powerful

_____ The child's way of understanding, adjusting to, and working out life's experiences

_____ The way that children from age 2 to 4 years judge whether an action is good or bad; based on whether the action results in reward or punishment

_____ Ideas that a preschooler does not have the ability to understand

_____ Complete by the preschool years; marked by preschoolers being able to relate to unfamiliar people easily and to tolerate brief separations from parents with little or no protest

_____ Imaginative play; dramatic play; self-expression

_____ Idea that is completely misunderstood by preschoolers, who interpret it according to their own frame of reference

_____ Behavior that attempts to hurt a person or destroy property

_____ Can shape aggressive behavior; closely associated with modeling of "masculine" behavior

_____ Usually occurs between the ages of 2½ and 3½ years; usually relinquished when child enters school

_____ The number of occurrences

_____ Used to identify temperamental characteristics in children who are in the age range of 3 to 7 years

_____ Occurs when the child is exposed to a feared object in a safe situation

_____ Self-stimulation of the genitals

_____ When a behavior starts, sudden changes in behavior being most significant

_____ The degree to which behavior interferes with social or cognitive functioning

_____ Stammering; a normal speech pattern in the preschooler

_____ A broad concept; the act of two people uniting intimately because of the special relationship they have

_____ Formation of sentences of about three to four words; includes only the most essential words to convey meaning

_____ The continual thwarting of self-satisfaction by parental disapproval, humiliation, punishment, and insults

_____ The amount of time a behavior lasts, significant periods being greater than 4 weeks

_____ Ascribing lifelike qualities to inanimate objects

_____ Used to refer to specific academic aptitude, creative or productive thinking, leadership ability, ability in the visual or performing arts, and/or psychomotor ability, either singly or in combination

_____ Imitating behavior of significant others; a powerful influencing force in preschoolers

_____ The Denver Articulation Screening Examination; a tool for assessing articulation skills in the child and for explaining to parents the expected progression of sounds

_____ Articulation problems

3. The approximate age range for the preschool period begins at age _____ years and ends at age

_____ years.

4. The average annual weight gain during the preschool years is _____ pounds.

5. Which one the following statements about the preschooler's physical proportions is true?
   a. Preschoolers have a squat and potbellied frame.
   b. Preschoolers have a slender, but sturdy frame.
   c. The muscle and bones of the preschooler have matured.
   d. Sexual characteristics can be differentiated in the preschooler.

6. Uninhibited scribbling and drawing can help to develop:
   a. symbolic language.
   b. fine muscle skills.
   c. eye-hand coordination.
   d. all of the above.

7. As preschool children begin to develop their own sense of morality, they primarily rely on:
   a. their association with other children.
   b. whether they are accepted for their attitudes.
   c. parental principles.
   d. all of the above.

8. The resolution of the Oedipus/Electra complex occurs when the child:
   a. identifies with the same-sex parent.
   b. realizes that the same-sex parent is more powerful.
   c. wishes that the same-sex parent were dead.
   d. notices physical sexual differences.

9. Because of the preschooler's egocentric thought, the *best* approach for effective communication is through:
   a. speech.
   b. play.
   c. drawing.
   d. actions.

10. Magical thinking, according to Piaget, is the belief that:
    a. events have cause and effect.
    b. God is an imaginary friend.
    c. thoughts are all-powerful.
    d. if the skin is broken, the child's insides will come out.

11. The moral and spiritual development of the preschooler is characterized by:
    a. concern for why something is wrong.
    b. actions that are directed toward satisfying the needs of others.
    c. thoughts of loyalty and gratitude.
    d. a very concrete sense of justice.

12. The preschooler's body image has developed to include:
    a. a well-defined body boundary.
    b. knowledge about his or her internal anatomy.
    c. fear of intrusive experiences.
    d. anxiety and fear of separation.

13. Sex typing involves the process by which the preschooler:
    a. forms a strong attachment to the same-sex parent.
    b. identifies with the opposite-sex parent.
    c. develops sexual identification.
    d. all of the above.

14. Language during the preschool years:
    a. includes telegraphic speech.
    b. is simple and concrete.
    c. uses phrases not sentences.
    d. includes the ability to follow complex commands.

15. According to Winsler and others, bilingual children would be most likely to experience:
    a. adverse affects to their receptive language development.
    b. adverse affects to performance in the majority language.
    c. proficiency in the majority language.
    d. adverse affects to areas in addition to language.

16. Which one of the following statements about social development of the preschooler is *false*?
    a. Imaginary playmates are a normal part of the preschooler's play.
    b. Preschoolers have overcome much of their anxiety regarding strangers.
    c. Preschoolers use telegraphic speech between the ages of 3 and 4 years.
    d. Preschoolers particularly enjoy parallel play.

17. Television and videotapes:
    a. hinder the preschooler's development.
    b. should be only a part of the preschooler's social and recreational activities.
    c. are not an interactive activity.
    d. do not provide learning for the preschooler.

18. In regard to the development of temperament in the preschool years:
    a. temperamental characteristics change considerably during the preschool years.
    b. the effect of temperament on adjustment in a group becomes important during the preschool years.
    c. children need to be treated the same regardless of differences in temperament.
    d. there really is no tool that will adequately identify temperamental characteristics during the preschool years.

19. List at least two strategies parents may use to help their child prepare for the preschool or kindergarten experience.

20. To guide parents in their quest to find a school with comprehensive services, the nurse should advise the parent to:
    a. find a school that focuses primarily on skill acquisition.
    b. visit the schools to observe their services personally
    c. select a licensed program to ensure the highest standard.
    d. all of the above.

21. The *best* way for parents to respond to a child's questions about sexuality is to give the child:
    a. an honest answer and find out what the child thinks.
    b. one or two sentences that answer the specific question only.
    c. an honest, short, and to-the-point answer.
    d. an honest answer but a little less information than the child expects.

22. Which of the following characteristics is *not* typically seen in a gifted/talented child?
    a. Asynchrony across developmental domains
    b. Insatiable curiosity
    c. Less need for attention than other children
    d. Intensity of feelings and emotions

23. Which one of the following factors influences aggressive behavior?
    a. Frustration
    b. Modeling
    c. Gender
    d. All of the above

24. Which one of the following dysfunctional speech patterns is a normal characteristic of the language development of a preschooler?
    a. Lisp
    b. Stammering
    c. Nystagmus
    d. Echolalia

25. Which one of the following sources of stress in the preschooler is typical of a three-year-old?
    a. Insecurity
    b. Masturbation
    c. Jealousy
    d. Sexuality

26. Which one of the following approaches is recommended to help prevent stress in children?
    a. Allow time for rest.
    b. Prepare the child for changes.
    c. Monitor the amount of stress.
    d. All of the above are recommended.

27. Which one of the following examples would *best* help a preschooler dispel his or her fear of the water when learning to swim?
    a. Fear of the water is a healthy fear. It should not be dispelled.
    b. Allow the child to sit by the water with other children, play with water toys, and get splashed lightly with the water.
    c. Reassure the child as he or she is brought slowly into the water with an adult who knows how to swim.
    d. Throw the child in the water and have an adult keep the child's head above water.

28. Identify the following statements as either true or false.

    _____ Sleep terrors can be described as a partial arousal from a very deep nondreaming sleep.

    _____ Nightmares usually occur in the second half of the night.

    _____ With sleep terrors, crying and fright persist even after the child is awake.

    _____ With nightmares the child is not very aware of another's presence.

29. When educating the preschool child about injury prevention, the parents should:
    a. set a good example.
    b. help children establish good habits.
    c. be aware that pedestrian/motor vehicle injuries increase in this age group.
    d. all of the above.

Critical Thinking—Case Study

Sheila Roth arrives at the office for a routine preschool physical. Her son Jacob, who is not quite 3 years old, will attend the 3-year-old preschool program at a local private school this year. Since he was a baby, Jacob has attended a home daycare program, while his mother managed her own interior decorating business. The daycare is run by an older woman who treats the 12 children in her program as if they were family. The helper at the daycare is also very loving. The program is very structured in regard to schedule and usual routines. Ms. Roth tells the nurse that she is looking forward to Jacob's new environment. His teacher is very creative and approaches the classroom from the perspective of the child's development. There will be a lot of choices for activities during the day.

30. Based on the information provided, which of the following is the *best* analysis?
    a. Jacob needs some preparation for this new preschool experience.
    b. Jacob will have less trouble adjusting than a child who has never attended daycare.
    c. Jacob is too young for such a drastic change.
    d. Jacob needs the individual attention he is getting at the daycare.

31. Which one of the following expected outcomes would be *most* reasonable to establish?
    a. The nurse will help Ms. Roth assess Jacob's readiness for preschool.
    b. Jacob will attend preschool without any behavioral indications of stress.
    c. Ms. Roth will verbalize at least five strategies that can be used to help prepare Jacob for his preschool experience.
    d. Jacob will demonstrate behavior that indicates that he is adjusting to his preschool experience.

32. Which one of the following interventions would be *inappropriate* for the nurse to suggest?
    a. Introduce Jacob to the teacher.
    b. Leave quickly the first day.
    c. Talk about the new school as exciting.
    d. Be confident the first day.

33. Which one of the following of Jacob's characteristics would indicate that he is ready for preschool?
    a. Social maturity
    b. Good attention span
    c. Academic readiness
    d. All of the above

CHAPTER 16

Health Problems of Early Childhood

1. Match each term with its description.

a. Communicable disease	g. Carrier	m. Pandemic
b. Epidemic	h. Contact	n. Prodromal period
c. Endemic	i. Direct	o. Control measures
d. Infectious agent	j. Vehicle	p. Isolation
e. Reservoir	k. Incubation period	q. Quarantine
f. Host	l. Period of communicability	

_____ Provides subsistence or lodging to infectious agent

_____ Harbors infectious agent without apparent disease

_____ Person or animal that has been in association with source that could provide the infected agent

_____ Illness caused by specific infectious agent through some transmission of agent

_____ Refers to disease occurring regularly within a geographic location

_____ Refers to disease occurring in greater-than-expected numbers within a community

_____ Environment in which infectious agent lives and multiplies

_____ Organism that is capable of producing infection

_____ Type of contact that results in immediate transfer of infectious agent (transfer by kissing)

_____ An object serving as intermediate means for transportation of infectious agent

_____ Time period in which infection may be directly or indirectly transported

_____ Time between exposure and appearance of symptoms

_____ Restriction of activities of exposed person until incubation period is completed

_____ Methods used to prevent spread of organism, including immunizations and health education

_____ Refers to disease affecting large portions of the populations throughout the world

_____ Separation of infected persons from noninfected persons for the period of communicability

_____ Interval between the time when early signs of disease appear and the time when overt clinical syndrome is evident

2. Janie, age 6 years, has been diagnosed with a communicable disease. The nurse, in preparing the plan of care, recognizes four goals. List them.

3. Match each communicable disease with its description or characteristics.

a. Varicella   e. Rubeola   h. Rubella
b. Diphtheria   f. Mumps   i. Scarlet fever
c. Fifth disease   g. Pertussis   j. Poliomyelitis
d. Roseola

_____ Rash appears in three stages; stage I is erythema on face, chiefly on cheeks.

_____ This condition begins as macule rash, rapidly progressing to papule rash and then to vesicles, eventually breaking and forming crusts.

_____ Tonsillar pharyngeal areas are covered with white or gray membrane; complications include myocarditis and neuritis.

_____ Rash is rose-pink macules or maculopapules, appearing first on trunk, then spreading to neck, face, and extremities; rash is nonpruriti.

_____ Cough occurs at night, and inspirations sound like crowing.

_____ This condition results in earache that is aggravated by chewing.

_____ Rash appears 3 to 4 days after onset and maculopapular eruption on face with gradual spread downward; koplik spots present before rash.

_____ Discrete pinkish red maculopapular rash appears on face and then spreads downward to neck, arms, trunk, and legs; greatest danger is teratogenic effect on fetus.

_____ Permanent paralysis may occur.

_____ Tonsils are enlarged, edematous, reddened, and covered with patches of exudate; rash is absent on face; desquamation occurs.

4. Assessment of which of the following is *not* helpful in identifying potentially communicable diseases?
   a. Recent travel to foreign country
   b. Immunization history
   c. Past medical history
   d. Family history

5. Primary prevention of communicable disease is *best* accomplished by:
   a. immunization.
   b. control of the disease spread.
   c. adequate water supply.
   d. implementing good handwashing among hospital personnel.

6. Certain groups of children are at risk for serious complications from communicable diseases. These children do *not* include which of the following groups?
   a. Children with an immunodeficiency or immunologic disorder
   b. Children receiving steroid therapy
   c. Children with leukemia
   d. Children who have recently undergone a surgical procedure

7. What antiviral agent is used to treat varicella infections in children at increased risk for complications associated with varicella?
   a. Varicella-zoster immune globulin
   b. Acyclovir
   c. Salicylates
   d. Steroids

8. Name the two diseases causes by the varicella zoster virus.

9. Identify a major responsibility of the school nurse working with children at high risk for communicable disease.

10. The American Academy of Pediatrics has recommended vitamin A supplements for certain pediatric patients with measles. Correct dosage of vitamin A and instructions to parents of these children include:
    i.   single oral dose of 200,000 IU in children 1 year old.
    ii. single oral dose of 100,000 IU in children 6 to 12 months old.
    iii. dosage may be associated with vomiting and headache for a few hours.
    iv. safe storage of the drug to prevent accidental overdose.

    a. i, ii, iii, and iv
    b. i, ii, and iv
    c. i, iii, and iv
    d. ii and iv

11. The nurse is conducting an educational session for the parents of a child diagnosed with varicella. Which one of the following is *not* an appropriate comfort measure to include in this session?
    a. Use Aveeno bath or oatmeal in bath water for added skin comfort.
    b. Use Caladryl lotion on rash to decrease itching.
    c. Use hot bath water to promote skin rash healing.
    d. Keep nails short and smooth to decrease infection from scratching.

12. Which one of the following does the nurse recognize as *contraindicated* in providing comfort measures to children with communicable diseases?
    a. Use of acetaminophen for control of elevated temperature in child with varicella
    b. Use of imposed bed rest in child with pertussis
    c. Use of aspirin to control elevated temperature and/or symptoms in child with varicella
    d. Use of lozenges and saline rinses in an 8-year-old child with sore throat

13. The nurse knows the child with chicken pox can return to school:
    a. 2 weeks after onset of rash.
    b. when all lesions have progressed to the vesicle stage.
    c. after administration of acyclovir.
    d. 5 days after onset of rash or when all lesions are crusted.

14. Clinical manifestations differentiate bacterial conjunctivitis from viral conjunctivitis. Which one of the following is present with bacterial conjunctivitis but *not* usually found with viral conjunctivitis?
    a. Child awakens with crusting of eyelids.
    b. Child has increase in watery drainage from eyes.
    c. Child has inflamed conjunctiva.
    d. Child has swollen eyelids.

15. When instructing the parents caring for an infant with conjunctivitis, the nurse will include which one of the following in the plan?
    a. Accumulated secretions are removed by wiping from outer canthus inward.
    b. Hydrogen peroxide placed on Q-tips is helpful in removing crusts from eyelids.
    c. Compresses of warm tap water are kept in place on the eye to prevent formation of crusting.
    d. Washcloth and towel used by the infant are kept separate and not used by others.

16. Identify the following statements about stomatitis as true or false.

_____ Aphthous stomatitis may be associated with mild traumatic injury, allergy, and emotional stress.

_____ Aphthous stomatitis is characterized by painful, small, whitish ulcerations that heal without complication in 4 to 12 days.

_____ Herpetic gingivostomatitis is caused by herpes simplex virus, usually type 1.

_____ Herpetic gingivostomatitis is commonly called "cold sores" or "fever blisters" and may appear in groups or singly.

_____ Treatment for stomatitis is aimed at relief of complications.

_____ When examining herpetic lesions, the nurse uses her uncovered index finger to check for cracks in the skin surface.

_____ Herpetic gingivostomatitis is associated with sexual transmission.

17. Anne, an 8-year-old, has been diagnosed with giardiasis. The nurse would expect Anne to have *most* likely presented with which of the following signs and symptoms?
    a. Diarrhea with blood in the stools
    b. Nausea and vomiting with a mild fever
    c. Abdominal cramps with intermittent loose stools
    d. Weight loss of 5 lb in the last month

18. The drug of choice for children diagnosed with giardiasis is:
    a. metronidazole (Flagyl).
    b. mebendazole (Vermox).
    c. erythromycin.
    d. tetracycline.

19. The nurse is instructing parents on the test-tape diagnostic procedure for enterobiasis. Which one of the following is included in the explanation?
    a. Use a flashlight to inspect the anal area while the child sleeps.
    b. Perform the test 2 days after the child has received the first dose of mebendazole.
    c. Test all members of the family at the same time using frosted tape.
    d. Collect the tape in the morning before the child has a bowel movement or bath.

20. Children with pinworm infections present with the principal symptom of:
    a. perianal itching.
    b. diarrhea with blood.
    c. evidence of small rice-like worms in their stool and urine.
    d. abdominal pain.

21. The nurse has an order to administer 100 mg of mebendazole (Vermox) to 5-year-old Megan for a positive pinworm test. The nurse recognizes which one of the following as an appropriate action when administering this medication?
    a. Vermox should be withheld in all children under 6 years of age.
    b. Treatment is limited to Megan until other family members have tested positive.
    c. Vermox will also effectively treat giardiasis.
    d. Treatment should be repeated in 2 weeks to prevent reinfection.

22. Reduction of poisonings in children and infants can be accomplished by:
    a. use of child-resistant containers.
    b. educating parents and grandparents to place products out of reach of small children.
    c. educating parents to relocate plants out of reach of infants, toddlers, and small children.
    d. all of the above.

23. The most common accidentally ingested medications in children under 6 years of age are:
    a. cold and cough preparations.
    b. analgesics such as acetaminophen and ibuprofen.
    c. hormones such as oral contraception.
    d. antibiotics.

24. The first action parents should be taught to initiate in a poisoning is to:
    a. induce vomiting.
    b. take the child to the family physician's office or emergency center.
    c. call the Poison Control Center.
    d. follow the instructions on the label of the product.

25. Each toxic ingestion is treated individually. Gastric decontamination and neutralization is aimed at removing the ingested toxic product by what five measures?

26. Identify the major principles of emergency treatment for poisoning.

27. When giving parents the proper instructions for administering ipecac syrup, the nurse includes which one of the following?
    a. Have full doses of emetic in the household for each child.
    b. Administer the emetic within 3 hours of toxic ingestion.
    c. Never administer out-of-date emetic.
    d. Force fluids and encourage activity after the emetic is administered to facilitate its effectiveness.

28. The nurse does *not* expect to assist in gastric lavage for the treatment of poisoning in which one of the following pediatric patients?
    a. The 8-month-old child admitted to the emergency center after eating 8 or 10 holly berries
    b. The 8-year-old child who has ingested three of his mother's birth control pills
    c. The 6-year-old child who has ingested an overdose of a noncorrosive substance and is convulsing
    d. The 13-year-old girl who has ingested an overdose of Valium and is comatose

29. Potential causes of heavy metal poisoning in children include _____,

    _____, and _____.

30. On routine physical exam, 2-year-old Zach is found to have an elevated blood lead level. The *most* likely cause for this finding is:
    a. Zach is allowed to play in the local sand box at the park.
    b. Zach lives in a house built after 1980.
    c. Zach's crib is positioned near windows with chipping, flaking paint.
    d. Zach's father is an artist and works at home.

31. Identify the following statements as true or false.

   _____ The neurologic system is of most concern when young children are exposed to lead, because the developing brain is very vulnerable.

   _____ Young children will absorb more of the lead to which they are exposed than will adults.

   _____ Lead-based paint in structures built before 1950 remains the most frequent source of lead poisoning in children.

   _____ Lead-containing pottery or leaded dishes do not contribute to lead poisoning, because food does not absorb lead.

   _____ If the venous blood value is below 10 µg/dl of lead, the child is considered to have a safe blood lead value.

   _____ The exposure risk for children living in leaded environments is lower if their diet is deficient in iron and calcium and high in fats, because the diet slows the absorption of lead.

   _____ Pica is the habitual, purposeful, and compulsive ingestion of nonfood substances.

   _____ Universal screening guidelines for BLL testing include all children between 1 and 2 years of age.

32. The nurse is to give a second injection of the chelation drug calcium disodium edetate. Which of the following does the nurse recognize as *most* helpful in preparing the young patient for the injection?
   a. Inspect intake and output records before administration to verify kidney function.
   b. Mix the drug with procaine to lessen the pain associated with the injection.
   c. Maintain seizure precautions at the bedside.
   d. Explanation of the treatment and medical play.

33. Diagnostic evaluations for lead poisoning include:
   a. blood levels for lead concentration, including screening by finger and heel sticks, with blood collected by venipuncture to confirm diagnosis.
   b. recommended universal screening for all children, with those ages 6 years or older given priority.
   c. identifying children at high risk for anemia, since these children will most likely have higher lead levels.
   d. understanding that a blood level for lead in the 10 to 14 µg/dl range is normal and needs no follow-up.

34. Therapeutic interventions for lead poisoning do *not* include:
   a. removal of the source of lead.
   b. improving nutrition.
   c. using chelation therapy.
   d. intravenous administration of dimercaprol.

35. Match each term with its description.

   a. Child neglect   d. Emotional abuse
   b. Physical neglect   e. Physical abuse
   c. Emotional neglect   f. Munchausen syndrome by proxy

   _____ Deliberate attempt to destroy a child's self-esteem
   _____ Failure to meet the child's needs for affection
   _____ Deprivation of necessities such as food and clothing
   _____ Failure to provide for the child's basic needs and adequate level of care
   _____ Deliberate infliction of physical injury on a child
   _____ An illness that one person fabricates or induces in another person

36. Which one of the following parental characteristics does *not* correctly describe abusive parent families?
    a. Teenage mothers are less likely to release frustration by striking out at their child.
    b. Abusive parents have difficulty controlling aggressive impulses.
    c. Free expression of violence is a consistent quality of abusive families.
    d. Abusive families are often more socially isolated and have fewer supportive relationships than nonabusive families.

37. A child who unintentionally contributes to the abusive situation *most* likely:
    a. fits into the "easy-child pattern."
    b. has a temperament that is incompatible with the parent's ability to deal with the behavioral style.
    c. has low self-esteem.
    d. comes from a low socioeconomic background.

38. Which one of the following statements is *false*?
    a. The position of the child in the family has little effect on the abusive situation.
    b. One child is usually the victim in an abusive family; removal of this child often places the other sibling at risk.
    c. The abusive family environment is one of chronic stress, including problems of divorce, poverty, unemployment, and poor housing.
    d. Child abuse is a problem of all social groups.

39. Match each term with its description.

    a. Incest   d. Pedophilia
    b. Molestation   e. Sexual abuse
    c. Exhibitionism   f. Shaken baby syndrome

    _____ The use, persuasion, or coercion of any child to engage in sexually explicit conduct
    _____ Preference for a prepubertal child by an adult as a means of achieving sexual excitement
    _____ Any physical sexual activity between family members
    _____ "Indecent liberties" such as touching or fondling
    _____ Violent shaking of infant that can cause fatal intracranial trauma
    _____ Indecent exposure

40. The nurse is talking with 13-year-old Amy, who has revealed that she is being sexually abused. Which one of the following is a *correct* guideline for the nurse to follow?
    a. Promise Amy not to tell what she tells you.
    b. Assure Amy that she will not need to report the abuse.
    c. Avoid using leading statements that can distort Amy's reporting of the problem.
    d. It is okay for the nurse to express anger and shock and to criticize Amy's family.

41. In identification of the abused child, the nurse knows:
    a. physical abuse can be readily identified during the physical exam.
    b. specific behavioral problems can be seen in the abused child.
    c. maltreated children easily admit to the abuse they received from their parents.
    d. incompatibility between the history and the injury is probably the most important criterion on which to base the decision to report suspected abuse.

Critical Thinking—Case Study

Jimmy is a 4-year-old preschool student who is brought to the school nurse's office by his teacher. She is concerned because Jimmy has purulent discharge in the corner of both eyes, with inflamed conjunctiva. The nurse observes Jimmy wiping his eyes frequently with his hands.

42. Based on the information provided, the nurse suspects that Jimmy has:
    a. bacterial conjunctivitis.
    b. viral conjunctivitis.
    c. allergic conjunctivitis.
    d. conjunctivitis caused by a foreign body.

43. Based on knowledge of communicable diseases, the nurse identifies which one of the following as the priority goal for Jimmy's plan of care?
    a. Will not become infected
    b. Will not spread disease
    c. Will experience minimal discomfort
    d. Will maintain skin integrity

44. The nurse calls Jimmy's parents to request that they come and pick Jimmy up from school. What is the *best* rationale for this action?
    a. Jimmy is tired and needs additional rest because of the infection.
    b. Jimmy is at high risk for spreading the disease because of his age and his inability to wash his hands after touching his eyes.
    c. Jimmy needs immediate medical attention to prevent complications.
    d. The nurse needs to discuss causes of this disease with Jimmy's mother so that its recurrence can be prevented.

45. It is important to include what information in the teaching plan for Jimmy's parents?
    a. Jimmy needs to have his own face cloth and towel.
    b. Eye medication will need to be administered before the eyes are cleaned.
    c. Jimmy cannot return to school until all symptoms have stopped.
    d. Jimmy will need his own eating utensils.

46. The nurse can expect treatment for Jimmy's condition to include:
    a. use of continuous warm compresses held in place on each infected eye.
    b. application of broad-spectrum topical ophthalmic agents.
    c. oral broad-spectrum antibiotics.
    d. all of the above.

47. The effectiveness of nursing interventions for Jimmy's condition is *best* demonstrated by which one of the following evaluations?
    a. There is no spread of the disease within the school and family.
    b. Parents are able to demonstrate appropriate eye care.
    c. Jimmy reports no eye discomfort.
    d. Child engages in normal activities.

48. Albert, age 7, has been diagnosed with pinworms, and Vermox has been ordered. The nurse knows that this drug should probably also be administered to:
    a. only Albert's siblings.
    b. only family members who test positive.
    c. all family members who are not pregnant or under 2 years of age.
    d. everyone who uses the same toilet facilities as Albert.

CHAPTER 17

Health Promotion of the School-Age Child and Family

1. Middle childhood is also referred to as the *middle years*, the *school years*, or the *school-age years*. What ages does this period represent?
   a. Ages 5 to 13 years
   b. Ages 4 to 14 years
   c. Ages 6 to 12 years
   d. Ages 6 to 16 years

2. Identify when the middle childhood years physiologically begin and end.

3. Which finding should the nurse expect when assessing physical growth in the school-age child?
   a. Weight increase of 2 to 3 kg per year
   b. Height increase of 3 cm per year
   c. Little change in refined coordination
   d. Decrease in body fat and muscle tissue

4. Identify the following statements about the school-age child as either true or false.

   _____ In middle childhood there are fewer stomach upsets, better maintenance of blood glucose levels, and an increased stomach capacity.

   _____ Caloric needs are higher in relation to stomach size when compared with the needs of preschool years.

   _____ The heart is smaller in relation to the rest of the body during the middle years.

   _____ During the middle years, the immune system develops little immunity to pathogenic microorganisms.

   _____ Backpacks are preferred to other book totes during middle years.

   _____ Physical maturity correlates well with emotional and social maturity during the middle years.

   _____ School-age children's muscles are still functionally immature as compared with those of the adolescent and are more easily damaged by muscular injury and overuse.

   _____ Physical maturity is correlated with emotional and social maturity for the school-age child.

   _____ There is no universal age at which the child assumes the characteristics of preadolescence.

   _____ Early appearance of physical sexual characteristics in girls and late appearance in boys has been linked to participation in risk-taking behaviors.

5. What period begins toward the end of middle childhood and ends at age 13?
   a. Puberty
   b. Preadolescence
   c. Early maturation
   d. All of the above

6. According to Freud, middle childhood is described as which one of the following periods?
   a. Anal
   b. Latency
   c. Oral
   d. Oedipal

7. According to Erikson, what is the developmental goal of middle childhood?
   a. Autonomy
   b. Trust
   c. Initiative
   d. Industry

8. Which of the following descriptions of school-age children is most closely linked to Erikson's theory?
   a. During this time, children experience relationships with same-sex peers.
   b. During this time, there is an overlapping of developmental characteristics between childhood and adolescence.
   c. During this time, temperamental traits from infancy continue to influence behavior.
   d. During this time, interests expand and children with a growing sense of independence engage in tasks that can be carried through to completion.

9. Accord to Piaget, what is the stage of development for middle childhood?
   a. Concrete operational
   b. Preoperational
   c. Formal operational
   d. Sensorimotor

10. Early appearance of secondary sex characteristics of girls during preadolescence may be associated with which of the following feelings?
    a. Satisfaction with physical appearance and higher self-esteem
    b. Increase in self-confidence and a more outgoing personality
    c. Dissatisfaction with physical appearance and lower self-esteem
    d. Increased substance use and reckless vehicle use

11. Generally, the earliest age at which puberty begins in girls is age _____; in boys, age _____.

12. Middle childhood is the time when children:
    i. learn the value of doing things with others.
    ii. learn the benefits derived from division of labor in accomplishing goals.
    iii. achieve a sense of industry and accomplishment.
    iv. expand interests and engage in tasks that can be carried to completion.

    a. i, ii, iii, and iv
    b. i, iii, and iv
    c. i and iv
    d. ii and iii

13. Dillon is a 6-year-old starting in a new neighborhood school. On the first day of school, he complains of a headache and tearfully tells his mother he does not want to go to school. Dillon's mother takes him to school, and the nurse is consulted. The nurse recognizes that Dillon is a slow-to-warm-up child and suggests which one of the following?
    a. Put Dillon in the classroom with the other children and leave him alone.
    b. Insist that Dillon join and lead the class song.
    c. Include Dillon in activities without assigning him tasks until he willingly participates in activities.
    d. Send Dillon home with his mom since he has a headache.

14. Which of the following accurately describes the expected cognitive development during the concrete-operational period of middle childhood?
    a. Children are able to follow directions but unable to verbalize the actions involved in the process.
    b. Children are able to use their thought processes to experience events and actions and make judgments based on what they reason.
    c. Children are able to view from an egocentric outlook that is rigidly developed around the action to be completed.
    d. Children progress from conceptual thinking to perceptual thinking when making judgments.

15. Easily distracted children:
    a. rarely pose a problem.
    b. usually exhibit discomfort when introduced to new situations.
    c. benefit from practice sessions before an event.
    d. should not be told when to stop activities, because this can trigger a reaction event.

16. The following terms relate to the accomplishment of cognitive tasks of middle childhood. Match each term with its description.

    a. Conservation   e. Classification skills   h. Metalinguistic awareness
    b. Identity   f. Serialize   i. Perceptual thinking
    c. Reversibility   g. Combinational skills   j. Conceptual thinking
    d. Reciprocity

    _____ Ability to arrange objects according to some ordinal scale
    _____ Ability to manipulate numbers and to learn the skills of addition, subtraction, multiplication, and division
    _____ Ability to group objects according to the attributes they share in common
    _____ Ability to think through an action sequence, anticipate the consequences, and return and rethink the action in a different direction
    _____ Ability to deal with two dimensions at one time and to comprehend that a change in one dimension compensates for a change in another
    _____ Ability to distinguish a shape change when nothing has been added or subtracted
    _____ Ability to comprehend that physical matter does not appear and disappear by magic
    _____ Ability to think about language and to comment on its properties
    _____ Ability to make decisions based on what one reasons
    _____ Ability to make decisions based on what one sees

17. A major difference in moral development between young school-age children and older school-age children is *best* described by which one of the following?
    a. Younger children believe that standards of behavior come from within themselves.
    b. Children 6 to 7 years of age know the rules and understand the reasons behind the rules.
    c. Older school-age children are able to judge an act by the intentions that prompted it and not only by the consequences.
    d. Rewards and punishments guide older school-age children's behavior.

18. Which one of the following *best* identifies the spiritual development of school-age children?
    a. They have little fear of "going to hell" for misbehavior.
    b. They begin to learn the difference between the natural and the supernatural.
    c. They petition to God for less tangible rewards.
    d. They view God as a deity with few human traits.

19. Which one of the following would the nurse *not* expect to observe as characteristic of peer group relationships of 8-year-old Mark?
    a. Mark demonstrates loyalty to the group by adhering to the secret code rules.
    b. Mark demonstrates a greater individual egocentric outlook as compared with other peer group members.
    c. Mark is willing to conform to the group's rule of "not talking to girls."
    d. Mark has a best friend within the peer group with whom he shares his secrets.

20. During the school-age years, children learn valuable lessons from age-mates. How is this accomplished?
    a. The child learns to appreciate the varied points of view within the peer group.
    b. The child becomes sensitive to the social norms and pressures of the group.
    c. The child's interactions among peers lead to the formation of intimate friendships between same-sex peers.
    d. All of the above

21. Which of the following is most characteristic of the relationship between school-age children and their family?
    a. Children desire to spend equal time with family and peers.
    b. Children are prepared to reject parental controls.
    c. The group replaces the family as the primary influence in setting standards of behavior and rules.
    d. Children need and want restrictions placed on their behavior by the family.

22. Ms. Jones is a single mother caring for her 10-year-old son James. At an office appointment for James, his mother asks the nurse how to prevent her son from becoming involved in gang violence. The *best* response is which one of the following?
    a. "Try to be more of a 'pal' to James so that he won't seek outside approval."
    b. "Relax restrictions on James. He needs to increase his independence, and this will show that you trust him."
    c. "Become aware of any gang-related activities in your community."
    d. "Don't allow James to join 'boys only' groups."

23. Children's self-concepts are developed by:

24. The nurse plans to conduct a sex education class for 10-year-olds. Which one of the following does the nurse recognize as *most* appropriate for this age group?
    a. Present sex information as a normal part of growth and development.
    b. Discourage question-and-answer sessions.
    c. Since sexual information supplied by parents usually produces feelings of guilt and anxiety in children, avoid parental assistance in conducting the program.
    d. Segregate boys from girls and include information related only to same sex in the discussion.

25. The school nurse is preparing information concerning acquired immunodeficiency syndrome (AIDS) for a group of school-age children. What should be included?

26. List three team membership characteristics that promote child development during the middle years.

27. School-age children:
    a. have little interest in complex board, card, or computer games.
    b. rarely collect items.
    c. tire of having stories read aloud.
    d. participate in hero worship.

28. Identify the following as true or false.
    _____ Successful adjustment to school entrance has little relationship to the child's physical and emotional maturity.
    _____ Children's attitudes toward school are influenced by the attitudes of their parents.
    _____ Television can increase the child's vocabulary, extend the child's horizon, and enrich the school experience.
    _____ Television can encourage children to believe that violence is an effective solution to conflict.
    _____ Children respond poorly to teachers who have attributes of caring parents.
    _____ The teacher's primary goal is guiding the child's intellectual development.
    _____ The reward and punishment administered by the teacher has little effect on the self-concept of the child.
    _____ Interaction between teacher and individual pupil affects the pupil's acceptance by the other children.
    _____ Being responsible for school work helps children learn to keep promises, meet deadlines, and succeed at jobs as adults.
    _____ Punitive interactions and corporal punishment are associated with decreasing disruptive behaviors in children.
    _____ Exposure to violence affects children's ability to concentrate and function.

29. A factor that *most* influences the amount and manner of discipline and limit-setting imposed on school-age children is:
    a. the age of the parent.
    b. the education of the parent.
    c. the response of the child to rewards and punishments.
    d. the ability of the parent to communicate with the school system.

30. List the purposes of discipline.

31. Seven-year-old Andy was caught taking a playmate's toy. Which of the following is an important understanding of this behavior?
    a. At this age, Andy's sense of property rights is limited, and he took the item simply because he was attracted to it.
    b. If Andy is caught and punished and promises "not to do it again," he will keep his promise.
    c. This stealing act is an indication that something is seriously lacking in Andy's life.
    d. Andy will learn the importance of respecting other's property if the parents unexpectedly give away an item of Andy's.

32. To assist school-age children in coping with stress in their lives, the nurse should:
    i.   be able to recognize signs that indicate the child is undergoing stress.
    ii. teach the child how to recognize signs of stress in herself or himself.
    iii. help the child plan a means for dealing with any stress through problem solving.
    iv. reassure the child that the stress is only temporary.

    a. ii, iii, and iv
    b. i, ii, and iii
    c. ii and iv
    d. i and iii

33. Identify which one of the following statements describing fears in the school-age child is true.
    a. School-age children are increasingly fearful of body safety.
    b. Most of the new fears that trouble school-age children are related to school and family.
    c. School-age children should be encouraged to hide their fears to prevent ridicule by their peers.
    d. School-age children with numerous fears need continuous protective behavior by parents to eliminate these fears.

34. The term *latchkey children* refers to whom?

35. By the end of middle childhood, children should be able to assume personal responsibility for self-

    care in the areas of _____, _____, _____,

    _____, _____, and _____.

36. What are the current dietary guidelines for healthy children between 2 and 11 years of age, as suggested by the ADA?

37. Sleep problems in the school-age child are often demonstrated by:
    a. delaying tactics, because the child does not wish to go to bed.
    b. the occurrence of night terrors that awaken the child during the night.
    c. the development of somatic illness that awakens the child during the night.
    d. the increasing need for larger amounts of sleep time as compared with preschool and adolescent children.

38. The nurse is planning to advise a school-age child's parents about appropriate physical activity for their child. Which fact does the nurse include?
    a. School-age children have the same stamina and control as 15-year-old teens.
    b. School-age children are prepared for participation in strenuous competitive athletics.
    c. Activities that promote coordination in the school-age child include running and skipping rope.
    d. Most children need continued encouragement to engage in physical activity.

39. Identify the following as true or false.

    _____ Sleepwalking occurs in the first 3 to 4 hours of sleep.

    _____ Children remember sleepwalking in the morning.

    _____ The best approach to sleepwalking is to awaken the child and put him or her back to bed.

    _____ Sleeptalking is purposeful and usually comprehensible.

    _____ Sleepwalking is usually self-limiting and requires no treatment.

    _____ Eruption of permanent teeth begins with the first or 6-year molar.

    _____ Children under 10 years of age often need parental assistance to brush back teeth.

    _____ Tooth brushes for school-age children should be soft nylon brushes with an overall length of about 6 inches.

40. List four components that should be included in the content of school health services.

41. The nurse is planning an educational session for a group of 9-year-olds and their parents aimed at decreasing injuries and accidents among this group. The nurse would *best* accomplish this goal by reviewing:
    a. safety rules to prevent burns when dealing with fire
    b. safety rules to prevent poisonings when dealing with toxic substances
    c. pedestrian safety rules and skills training programs to prevent motor vehicle accidents
    d. safety rules for the use of all-terrain vehicles, encouraging their use only with supervision

Critical Thinking—Case Study

Allen Thomas, age 9, is taken to the clinic by his mother for a school physical examination. Allen's mother is concerned because Allen wants to join the school soccer team this year. On physical examination, the nurse discovers that Allen has grown 2 inches in height and has gained 12 pounds since last year. His health history is unchanged from the previous year. Allen tells the nurse that he rides his bike more now than last year because he has a new best friend to go riding with.

42. Based on the information given, the nurse should expand assessment with Allen in which of the following areas at this visit?
    i.   His diet
    ii. His knowledge and use of safety precautions when riding his bike
    iii. His hygiene habits
    iv. His reasons for wanting to play soccer

    a. i, ii, and iii
    b. ii and iv
    c. i and ii
    d. i and iv

43. Which of the following would be the nurse's *best* response to the mother's concern about Allen playing soccer?
    a. "Allen is healthy, and playing soccer will allow him to increase strength and develop motor skill performance."
    b. "Allen is overweight for his age and should be encouraged to ride his bike less. Soccer is a better activity for him since it will help decrease his weight."
    c. "Allen is still too young to participate in strenuous sports like soccer. He should be able to participate in another year."
    d. "Let Allen play what he wants to. You worry too much about his activities."

44. Based on the information provided, the nurse plans an educational session for Allen and his mother. Which knowledge deficit would the nurse most likely identify for this family?
    a. Modified nutrition because of improper dietary habits.
    b. Improper nutrition related to less daily intake than the body needs.
    c. Lack of proper physical activity related to bike riding.
    d. Improper parenting skills related to overprotective mother.

45. Mrs. Thomas asks the nurse how she can foster Allen's development. What would be the *best* response by the nurse?
    a. "Don't interfere with Allen as long as he is doing well in school."
    b. "Give Allen recognition and positive feedback for his accomplishments."
    c. "Always point out to Allen how he incorrectly performs tasks so he can improve his accomplishments."
    d. "Try not to set rules for Allen. He needs to set his own limits during this period of development."

46. The nurse realizes that Allen's weight gain:
    a. is normal during this growth period.
    b. is probably related to a high-fat diet, rich in junk food intake.
    c. will be corrected by the increase in exercise of soccer and bike riding.
    d. is not influenced by the mass media.

CHAPTER 18

Health Problems of Middle Childhood

1. Functions performed by the skin include all of the following *except*:
   a. protection.
   b. heat regulation.
   c. sensation.
   d. nutrition.

2. The three layers of the skin are the _____, _____, and

   _____ _____.

3. Match each term related to assessment of the skin with its description.

   a. Pruritis
   b. Anesthesia
   c. Hyperesthesia
   d. Paresthesia

   e. Erythema
   f. Ecchymoses
   g. Petechiae
   h. Primary lesions

   i. Secondary lesions
   j. Distribution
   k. Configuration

   _____ Reddened area caused by increased amounts of blood
   _____ Localized purple discolorations
   _____ Pinpoint, circumscribed hemorrhagic spots
   _____ Skin changes caused by some causative factor to produce macules, papules, or vesicles
   _____ Changes related to rubbing, scratching, or medication
   _____ Used to describe whether the pattern of a skin condition is localized or generalized
   _____ The size and shape of the lesions or the group of lesions
   _____ Itching
   _____ Excessive sensitiveness
   _____ Absence of sensation
   _____ Abnormal sensation

4. Match each wound-related term with its description.

   a. Acute
   b. Chronic
   c. Pressure ulcer

   d. Abrasion
   e. Evulsion
   f. Laceration

   g. Incision
   h. Penetrating
   i. Puncture

   _____ Accidental cut, with either torn or jagged edges
   _____ Disruption of the skin that extends into the underlying tissue or into a body cavity
   _____ Heals uneventfully within the usual time frame
   _____ Does not heal in the expected time frame and can be associated with complications
   _____ Removal of the superficial layers of skin by scraping
   _____ Localized area of cellular necrosis that often becomes a chronic skin injury
   _____ Forcible pulling out or extraction of tissue
   _____ Wound with an opening that is small compared with its depth
   _____ Division of the skin made with a sharp object

145

5. Cindy, age 8 years, is brought to the clinic with a rash. On examination, the rash is found to consist of irregularly shaped areas of cutaneous edema with a pale pink appearance and a lighter center. Cindy says that the rash itches. Which of the following lesions should the nurse suspect?
   a. Macule
   b. Patch
   c. Plaque
   d. Wheal

6. Match each skin lesion with its description.

a.	Papule	e.	Pustule	i.	Lichenification
b.	Vesicle	f.	Cyst	j.	Scale
c.	Bulla	g.	Patch	k.	Crust
d.	Nodule	h.	Macule	l.	Keloid

   _____ Elevated, palpable, encapsulated
   _____ Flat, nonpalpable, irregular; greater than 1 cm in diameter
   _____ Caused by rubbing or irritation; rough, thickened epidermis
   _____ Dried serum, blood or purulent exudate; scab
   _____ Elevated, palpable, firm; less than 1 cm in diameter
   _____ Vesicle greater than 1 cm in diameter
   _____ Elevated, circumscribed; filled with serous fluid; less than 1 cm in diameter
   _____ Progressively enlarging scar caused by excess collagen formation
   _____ Heaped-up keratinized cells
   _____ Flat, nonpalpable, circumscribed; less than 1 cm in diameter
   _____ Elevated, superficial; filled with purulent fluid
   _____ Elevated, firm, palpable; 1 to 2 cm in diameter

7. Match each secondary skin lesion with its example.

a.	Scar	d.	Erosion
b.	Excoriation	e.	Ulcer
c.	Fissure		

   _____ Athlete's foot
   _____ Decubiti
   _____ Healed surgical incision
   _____ Abrasion, scratch
   _____ Variola following rupture

8. During wound healing, immature connective tissue cells migrate to the healing site and begin to secrete collagen into the meshwork spaces. What is this phase called?
   a. Scar contracture
   b. Inflammation
   c. Fibroplasia
   d. Scar maturation

9. Mary, age 7 years, fell and sustained a deep laceration to her chin. She was taken to the emergency center, where the laceration was sutured with the edges well approximated. The nurse expects the repair healing to take place by:
   a. primary intention.
   b. secondary intention.
   c. tertiary intention.

10. The nurse recognizes that which of the following is *not* indicated for use in promoting wound healing?
    a. Nutrition with sufficient protein, calories, vitamin C, and zinc
    b. Irrigation of wounds with normal saline
    c. Application of povidone-iodine daily
    d. Application of an occlusive dressing

11. Jimmy, age 9 years, has fallen and scraped his knee at school. He is brought to the school nurse for treatment. After cleaning the area and applying an over-the-counter first aid ointment, the nurse applies a gauze dressing. This type of dressing is considered to be:
    a. occlusive.
    b. semiocclusive.
    c. nonocclusive.
    d. impermeable.

12. Which one of the following does the nurse include in the educational plan when instructing parents about the use of topical corticosteroids?
    a. Do not use this cream on a fungal infection.
    b. Apply a thick layer of the cream and rub into the skin well.
    c. Do not use for longer than 3 days in chronic conditions.
    d. All of the above should be included.

13. Which of the following is true about topical therapy for acute treatment of dermatologic problems?
    a. Application of heat to the area will relieve itching.
    b. Children's broken or inflamed skin is more absorbent than their intact skin.
    c. Chemicals that are nonirritating to intact skin will be nonirritating to inflamed skin.
    d. Emollient action of soaks, baths, or lotions increases skin irritation.

14. Skin disorder assessment includes the objective data collected by inspection and palpation. Which one of the following is *not* an example of objective data?
    a. The lesion has an increased erythema margin edge.
    b. The rash appears as macules and papules.
    c. The lesion is painful and itches.
    d. The lesion is moist.

15. List the objective signs of wound infection.

16. The nurse is applying wet compresses of Burow's solution to Johnny's wound. Which one of the following does the nurse recognize as correct information about this type of topical therapy?
    a. After application of the compresses, the wound is washed with soap and water and rubbed dry.
    b. Compresses will loosen and remove crusts and debris.
    c. Burow's solution is applied directly onto the wound and then covered with a dry, soft gauze.
    d. All of the above are correct.

17. Care of bacterial skin infections in children may include all of the following *except*:
    a. good handwashing.
    b. keeping the fingernails short.
    c. puncturing the surface of the pustule.
    d. application of topical antibiotics.

18. Lisa, age 7, has been diagnosed with impetigo. Which one of the following does the nurse recognize as being a manifestation of this bacterial infection?
    a. Inflammation of skin and subcutaneous tissues with intense redness
    b. Honey-colored, crusty exudate
    c. Lymphangitis
    d. All of the above

19. Which one of the following is a fungal infection that lives on the skin?
    a. Tinea corporis
    b. Herpes simplex type 1
    c. Scabies
    d. Warts

20. Steve, age 8, has been diagnosed with tinea capitis. Which one of the following does the nurse include in the teaching plan for educating Steve and his parents?
    a. No animal-to-person transmission is associated with this infection.
    b. Steve can continue to share hair grooming articles with his younger brother.
    c. Griseofulvin should be administered with high-fat foods.
    d. Cleanliness is the best way to prevent this disease.

21. Johnny has been diagnosed with tinea capitis. His mother asks how he got this infection. The *best* response would be which of the following?
    a. "Transmission is from person-to-person or from animal-to-person contact."
    b. "Transmission is from person-to-person contact only."
    c. "Transmission is from animal-to-person contact only."
    d. "It is more important to talk about treatment than how Johnny got the disease."

22. Which one of the following statements about scabies is *incorrect*?
    a. Clinical manifestations include intense pruritus, especially at night, and papules, burrows, or vesicles on interdigital surfaces.
    b. Treatment is the application of 5% Elimite for all family members.
    c. After treatment, all previously worn clothing is washed in very hot water and dried at the high setting in the dryer.
    d. The rash and itching will be eliminated immediately after treatment.

23. What would the nurse look for in assessing whether a child has pediculosis?

24. In assisting parents to cope with pediculosis, the nurse should emphasize that:
    a. anyone can get pediculosis.
    b. lice will fly and jump from one person to another.
    c. cutting the child's hair short will prevent reinfestation.
    d. the condition can be transmitted by pets.

25. The nurse is instructing Angie's parents about using a pyrethrin shampoo for pediculosis. Which one of the following should be included in these instructions?
    a. Only one application is needed.
    b. The shampoo is avoided in children with contact allergy to ragweed or turpentine.
    c. The shampoo kills the lice and nits on contact.
    d. The shampoo will kill all the nits.

26. The treatment of choice for pediculosis capitis in a 2-year-old child is:
    a. 5% permethrin cream (Elimite).
    b. 1% lindane shampoo (Kwell).
    c. selenium sulfide shampoos.
    d. permethrin 1% cream rinse (Nix).

27. Children with lyme disease do *not* present with:
    a. a small erythematous papule that has a circumferential ring with a raised, edematous doughnut-like border.
    b. multiple, small secondary annular lesions with indurated centers on the palms and soles.
    c. flulike symptoms of headache, malaise, and lymphadenopathy.
    d. abdominal pain, splenomegaly, fatigue, and anorexia.

28. Susan, age 10 years, has been diagnosed with lyme disease. The nurse can expect the treatment to be:
    a. erythromycin.
    b. penicillin.
    c. ciprofloxin.
    d. doxycycline.

29. Match each term with its description.

    a. Histoplasmosis   d. Epidemic typhus

    b. Coccidiodomycosis   e. Endemic typhus

    c. Rocky Mountain spotted fever   f. Rickettsialpox

    _____ Transmitted by flea bite or by inhaling or ingesting flea excreta
    _____ transmitted from human to human by the body louse; requires that patient be isolated until deloused
    _____ Marked by maculopapular rash following primary lesion and eschar at site of bite; transmitted from house mouse to humans by infected mite
    _____ Infection caused by organism cultured from soil, especially where contaminated with fowl droppings
    _____ Transmitted by tick; maculopapular or petechial rash on palms and soles
    _____ Primary lung disease; endemic in southwestern United States

30. Children with cat scratch fever usually present with:
    a. headache, diarrhea, and fever.
    b. regional lymphadenopathy.
    c. maculopapular rash over the entire body.
    d. painful, pruritic papules at the site of inoculation.

31. Which of the following statements about cat scratch fever is true?
    a. It is caused by the scratch or bite of an animal, usually a cat or kitten.
    b. The animal will have a history of illness before transmission of the disease.
    c. Antibiotics shorten the duration of the illness.
    d. Analgesics are avoided during the disease process.

32. Billy has come in contact with poison ivy on a school picnic. The *best* intervention for the nurse to implement at this time is to:
    a. wash the area with a strong soap and water solution.
    b. apply Calamine lotion to the area.
    c. prevent spread by instructing Billy not to scratch the lesions.
    d. flush the area immediately with cold water.

33. When advising parents about the use of sunscreen for children, the nurse should tell them that:
    a. a waterproof sunscreen with a minimum 15 SPF is recommended for children.
    b. the lower the number of SPF, the higher the protection.
    c. sunscreens are not as effective as sunblockers.
    d. the sunscreen should be applied 1 hour before the child is allowed in the sun.

34. Which of the following information about sunscreen containing PABA is *false*?
    a. It may stain clothes.
    b. It can cause an allergic reaction.
    c. It provides little protection when the child is swimming or sweating.
    d. It is an effective sunscreen against UVB.

35. Match each term with its description.

    a. Chilblain
    b. Frostbite
    c. Sunscreen
    d. Sunblocker
    e. Ultraviolet A (UVA)
    f. Ultraviolet B (UVB)
    g. Hypothermia

    _____ Blocks out UV rays by reflecting sunlight
    _____ Partially absorbs UV light
    _____ Shorter light waves, responsible for tanning, burning, and most of the harmful effects attributed to sunlight
    _____ Longest light waves, causing only minimum burning but playing a significant role in photosensitive and photoallergic reactions
    _____ Condition in which ice crystals form in tissues
    _____ Redness and swelling of the skin from cold exposure
    _____ Cooling of the body's core temperature below 95° F

36. In caring for the child with frostbite, the nurse remembers that:
    a. slow thawing is associated with less tissue necrosis.
    b. the frostbitten part appears white or blanched, feels solid, and is without sensation.
    c. rewarming produces a small return of sensation with a small amount of pain.
    d. rewarming is accomplished by rubbing the injured tissue.

37. Skin disorders related to drug sensitivity include:
    a. impetigo.
    b. Stevens-Johnson syndrome.
    c. neurofibromatosis.
    d. all of the above.

38. Neurofibromatosis is:
    a. an autosomal dominant genetic disorder.
    b. suspected when the 5-year-old child presents with six or more cafe-au-lait spots larger than 5 mm in diameter.
    c. suspected when the infant develops axillary or inguinal freckling.
    d. all of the above.

39. Johnny's mother is calling the clinic because Johnny has developed a rash over his entire body. Two days ago he was prescribed amoxicillin for an ear infection, and now his mother tells the nurse she thinks Johnny may have gotten a small rash with this medication when he took it before. Which one of the following would be the *best* intervention by the nurse at this time?
    a. Question the mother about other symptoms that Johnny may have developed.
    b. Continue the medication and have Johnny come in tomorrow to see the practitioner.
    c. Stop the medication and inform the practitioner.
    d. Tell the mother to give only half the prescribed dose of the medication until Johnny can return to the clinic to see the practitioner.

40. Cindy is 12 years old and presents to the clinic because of a bald spot developing on her head. Cindy wears her hair tightly braided with beads. Which one of the following should the nurse suspect?
    a. Alopecia from trauma
    b. Tinea capitis
    c. Psoriasis
    d. Urticaria

41. Billy has been stung by a bee. A small reaction has occurred at the site. What is the *most* appropriate action at this time?
    a. Wait until Billy is at home to completely remove the stinger with forceps.
    b. Remove the stinger as soon as possible by scraping it off the skin.
    c. Wash the area with hot water and soap.
    d. Arrange for Billy to undergo skin testing.

42. The most effective method for tick removal in a child is to:
    a. use a curved forcep and grasp close to the point of attachment, then pull straight up with a steady, even pressure.
    b. apply mineral oil to the back of the tick and wait for it to back out.
    c. use the fingers to pull the tick out with a straight, steady, even pressure.
    d. place a hot match on the back of the tick and pick it up with gloved hands when the tick falls off.

43. Dog bites in children occur most often:
    a. in girls over 4 years of age.
    b. in children under 4 years of age.
    c. from stray dogs.
    d. in school yards and neighborhood parks.

44. Nora has been brought to the emergency department by her father after having been bitten by the family dog. Exam reveals three puncture wounds of the hand. Expected therapeutic management for these wounds includes:
    a. suturing the wounds.
    b. administering prophylactic antibiotics.
    c. irrigating with hydrogen peroxide.
    d. administering a tetanus toxoid booster since Nora's last booster was given 13 months ago.

45. On a field trip to a remote area with his boy scout troop, Peter is bitten by a snake. Which one of the following actions would be *contraindicated*?
    a. Remove Peter from the area and have him rest.
    b. Feel for a pulse distal to the bite area.
    c. Place ice from the ice cooler on the bite area.
    d. Apply a loose tourniquet above the bite area.

46. Human bites:
    a. are treatable at home.
    b. do not require tetanus immunization.
    c. should not have ice applied to the area.
    d. should receive medical attention if greater than ¼ inch.

47. The *most* common cause of malocclusion is:
    a. thumb sucking.
    b. tongue thrusting.
    c. hereditary factors.
    d. abnormal growth patterns.

48. Emergency care for tooth evulsion includes:
    a. replanting the tooth after bleeding has stopped.
    b. storing the tooth in tap water until it and the child can be transported to the dentist.
    c. holding the tooth by the root.
    d. rinsing the dirty tooth gently under running water before replanting.

49. The major nursing consideration in assisting the family of a child with nocturnal enuresis is to prevent the child from developing alterations in:
    a. body image.
    b. self-esteem.
    c. autonomy.
    d. peer acceptance.

50. The nurse is assisting the family of a child with a history of encopresis. Which one of the following should be included in the nurse's discussion with this family?
    a. Instructing the parents to sit the child on the toilet at two daily routine intervals
    b. Instructing the parents that the child will probably need to have daily enemas for the next year
    c. Suggesting the use of stimulant cathartics weekly
    d. Reassuring the family that most problems resolve successfully with some relapses during periods of stress

51. Barbara has been diagnosed with attention-deficit/hyperactivity disorder and placed on methylphenidate (Ritalin) by her physician. Which one of the following statements, if made by the nurse to Barbara's parents, is correct?
    a. "This drug will ultimately lead to stimulation of the inhibitory system of the central nervous system by increasing dopamine and norepinephrine levels in the body."
    b. "Dosage is usually unchanged until adolescence."
    c. "This medication takes 2 to 3 weeks to achieve an effect."
    d. "Barbara's appetite will be increased with this drug."

52. Identify the following as true or false.
    _____ Dyslexia is a learning disability characterized by reading letters in reverse.
    _____ Children with learning disabilities have below-average intelligence.
    _____ Children with learning disorders grow up to be adults with learning disabilities.
    _____ Learning disabilities include learning problems that result from visual, hearing, or motor disabilities.

53. Therapeutic management for a child with a tic disorder primarily consists of:
    a. behavioral modification to teach the child to suppress the tic disorder.
    b. administration of haloperidol to suppress the tic disorder.
    c. education and support for the child and family with reassurance about the prognosis.
    d. genetic counseling for the parents.

54. Which of the following statements about Tourette's syndrome (TS) is true?
    a. Manifestations are stable in intensity and rarely change once developed.
    b. Children with TS have no associated obsessive-compulsive symptoms.
    c. Tics lead to physical deterioration and affect life expectancy.
    d. Behaviors are involuntary.

55. Identify the following statements as true or false.

    _____ Posttraumatic stress disorder typically involves life-threatening events.

    _____ School phobia is more common in boys than in girls.

    _____ Children with school phobia are correctly viewed as delinquent children.

    _____ A frequent source of fear in school phobia is separation anxiety based on a strong dependent relationship between the mother and the child.

    _____ The primary goal for the child with school phobia is to return the child to school.

    _____ Prevention of dependency problems in childhood is based on encouraging independence at appropriate times during infancy and early childhood.

    _____ Recurrent abdominal pain of childhood is defined as three or more separate episodes of abdominal pain during a 3-month period.

    _____ Children at risk for recurrent abdominal pain tend to be high achievers with great personal goals or whose parents have unusually high expectations.

    _____ Parents of children with conversion reaction seldom display problems in communication or depression.

    _____ Depressed children usually exhibit low-esteem, think of themselves as hopeless, and explain negative events in terms of their personal shortcomings.

    _____ Three risk factors identified for childhood schizophrenia are genetic characteristics, gestational and birth complications, and winter birth.

Critical Thinking—Case Study

Carol, age 9, went on a picnic yesterday with her family. Today she returns to school and is showing her classmates several leaves that she collected yesterday on her picnic. The teacher notes that three of the leaves are from a poison ivy plant. The teacher takes Carol to the school nurse because of a rash that has developed on her arms and legs. Carol tells the nurse that the rash is "very itchy."

56. The nurse completes a diagnostic assessment of the skin rash to include a complete history and physical examination. The nurse knows that this history should include:
    a. inspection of the rash, including size and shape of lesions.
    b. symptoms, past and recent exposure to causative agents, medications taken, and history of previous similar rashes.
    c. palpation of the rash for increased heat, edema, and tenderness.
    d. skin scrapings from the site for microscopic examination.

57. The primary action the school nurse should take at this time is to:
    a. call Carol's parents to pick her up at school. Isolate Carol from other classmates until her parents arrive.
    b. give the poison ivy leaves to the school janitor to be destroyed in the school incinerator.
    c. instruct the teacher to make sure all classmates who had contact with the poison ivy plant wash these areas with mild soap and water.
    d. reassure Carol that everything is going to be fine, apply Calamine lotion to her rash, and instruct Carol not to scratch the rash.

58. What is the *best* nursing diagnosis for Carol at this time?
    a. Impaired skin integrity related to environmental factors
    b. High risk for infection related to presence of infectious organisms
    c. Pain related to skin lesions
    d. Body image disturbance related to presence of rash

59. Goals for Carol will include which of the following?
    a. Carol will not experience secondary damage, as infection, from scratching.
    b. Carol will demonstrate acceptable levels of comfort from itching.
    c. Carol will be able to recognize and avoid precipitating agent in the future.
    d. All of the above should be included.

60. In educating Carol and her parents about caring for the rash, the nurse should tell them to:
    i.   bath in tepid or cool water.
    ii.   bath in hot water.
    iii. apply hydrogen peroxide to the rash daily.
    iv.   apply calamine lotion to the rash.
    v.   administer over-the-counter diphenhydramine orally to decrease itching.
    vi.   keep fingernails short.
    vii. wear heavy clothing to prevent contamination.
    viii. understand that the rash is contagious and will weep.

    a. i, iii, iv, vi, and vii
    b. i, iv, v, and vi
    c. ii, v, vi, and vii
    d. iii, iv, v, and viii

CHAPTER 19

Health Promotion of the Adolescent and Family

1. In the female adolescent who has reached puberty, the luteinizing hormone (LH) initiates which of the following actions?
   a. Production of estrogen
   b. Growth of ovarian follicles
   c. Production of gonadotropin-releasing hormone
   d. Ovulation

2. The hormone in the female that causes growth and development of the vagina, uterus, fallopian tubes, and breasts is:
   a. estrogen.
   b. progesterone.
   c. follicle-stimulating hormone.
   d. luteinizing hormone.

3. Identify the following statements regarding adolescence as either true or false.

   _____ The adolescent is considered potentially fertile from the first menstrual period or first ejaculation.

   _____ Development of secondary sexual characteristics occurs in a predictable sequence.

   _____ The Tanner developmental stages are based on maturity of secondary sex characteristics and can be used when assessing adolescent growth.

   _____ The hypothalamic-pituitary-gonadal system is maintained in an active state throughout childhood because of the low secretion of gonadotropin-releasing hormone.

   _____ The development of a small bud of breast tissue is the earliest, most easily visible change of puberty.

   _____ The average age for beginning menstruation is 13 years.

   _____ In girls, physical maturation leads to greater satisfaction with their appearance.

   _____ Genetic endowment is the most important determinant of the onset, rate, and duration of pubertal growth.

4. Match each term with its description.

   a. Thelarche
   b. Adrenarche
   c. Physiologic leukorrhea
   d. Menarche
   e. Gynecomastia
   f. Puberty
   g. Ovulation

   _____ Biologic changes of adolescence
   _____ Onset of menstrual periods
   _____ Development of breast tissue
   _____ Male breast enlargement and tenderness
   _____ Development of pubic hair
   _____ Normal vaginal discharge
   _____ Release of an ovum by a follicle

155

5. Julie, 12 years old, is brought to the nurse practitioner's office by her mother. Julie has started to develop breast tissue and some pubic hair. Both the mother and daughter are concerned because Julie has been having increased vaginal discharge. Julie tells the nurse, "I wash my private area every day, but I still have fluid that comes out." What is the nurse's *best* response?
   a. "It sounds like you have an infection. We'll have the nurse practitioner check you to see what is causing this discharge."
   b. "Have you been using soap when you wash?"
   c. "This sounds like a normal discharge that happens to all girls as they start to mature. It is a sign your body is preparing for your periods to begin."
   d. "This is probably not related to hygiene. Are you concerned that this discharge might be causing an odor?"

6. Girls may be considered to have _____ _____ if breast development has not occurred by age 13 or if menarche has not occurred within 4 years of the onset of breast development.

7. The first pubescent change in boys is:
   a. appearance of pubic hair.
   b. testicular enlargement with thinning, reddening, and increased looseness of the scrotum.
   c. penile enlargement.
   d. temporary breast enlargement and tenderness.

8. Tommy is brought in by his father for his yearly physical. On examination, the nurse notes that since last year Tommy has developed pubic hair, testicular enlargement, and related scrotal changes. In planning anticipatory guidance, the nurse recognizes that which one of the following subjects would *best* be discussed with Tommy as soon as possible?
   a. Nocturnal emission
   b. Sexually transmitted disease prevention
   c. Pregnancy prevention
   d. Hygiene needs

9. The _____ _____ refers to the increased development of muscles, skeleton, and internal organs that peaks during puberty.

10. During assessment, the nurse observes that Gail has sparse growth of downy hair extending along the labia. Which of the following Tanner stages would be suspected?
    a. Stage 1
    b. Stage 2
    c. Stage 4
    d. Stage 5

11. Ben has just turned 16 years of age and is in for his routine physical. The nurse notes that Ben has pubescent changes and determines that Ben is in Tanner stage 3. What findings would *best* describe this Tanner stage?
    a. Testes, scrotum, and penis are adult in size and shape.
    b. No pubic hair is present.
    c. There is initial enlargement of scrotum and testes; reddening and texture changes of the scrotal skin; long, straight, downy hair at base of penis.
    d. There is initial enlargement of penis in length; testes and scrotum are enlarged; hair is darker, coarser, and curly over entire pubis.

12. Which one of the following statements about pattern of growth during adolescence is true?
    a. Knowing the correct sequence of the growth pattern is useful only when assessing abnormal growth patterns versus normal growth patterns.
    b. Girls usually begin puberty and reach maturity about 2 years earlier than boys do.
    c. Girls and boys experience an increase of muscle mass that begins during early puberty and lasts throughout adolescence.
    d. Girls and boys experience an increase in linear growth that begins for both during midpuberty.

13. On the average, girls gain _____ to _____ inches in height and _____ to _____ pounds during

    adolescence, while boys gain _____ to _____ inches and _____ to _____ pounds.

14. Which one of the following *best* describes the formal operational thinking that occurs between the ages of 11 and 14 years?
    a. Thought process includes thinking in concrete terms.
    b. Thought process includes information obtained from the environment and peers.
    c. Thought process includes thinking in abstract terms, possibilities, and hypotheses.
    d. Thought process is limited to what is observed.

15. Jimmy, a 13-year-old, is sent to the school nurse because he and some of his peers were caught chewing tobacco while playing baseball. The nurse knows that the *best* way to influence Jimmy's behavior for health promotion would be which of the following?
    a. Tell Jimmy that he will be suspended from school if he continues to chew the tobacco.
    b. Show Jimmy pictures of oral cancers from chewing tobacco.
    c. Tell Jimmy about the dangers of chewing tobacco and stress the fact that girls do not like boys who chew tobacco.
    d. Arrange for a local baseball hero to talk with Jimmy and his friends, stressing that he does not use chewing tobacco, his friends do not chew tobacco, and that chewing tobacco causes ugly teeth.

16. Adolescent egocentrism may lead to a pattern of personal fable. An example of a personal fable is:
    a. "Everyone is coming to the play just to see me."
    b. "Mary Sue got pregnant, but it won't happen to me."
    c. "I hate taking my clothes off for gym class because everyone stares at me."
    d. "Mary is very envious of how I dress."

17. Adolescents develop the social cognition change of mutual role-taking. Which one of the following is the *best* description of this ability?
    a. Heightened sense of self-consciousness
    b. Understanding the perspectives of others and that actions can influence others
    c. Beliefs that are more abstract and rooted in ideologic principles
    d. Realization that others have thoughts and feelings

18. The development of a personal value system or value autonomy during adolescence usually occurs by what age?
    a. 14 to 16 years of age
    b. 18 to 20 years of age
    c. 13 to 14 years of age
    d. 16 to 18 years of age

19. Elements of principled moral reasonings emerge during adolescence. Which of the following is the *best* description of this moral development?
    a. Moral guidelines are seen to emanate from authority figures.
    b. Moral standards are seen as objective and not to be questioned.
    c. Absolutes and rules are questioned and subject to disagreement.
    d. A personal value system is developed.

20. Spiritual development during adolescent years can *best* be described by which of the following?
    a. Places less emphasis on what a person believes
    b. Places more emphasis on whether a person attends religious services
    c. Becomes more focused on spiritual and ideologic matters and less towards observing religious customs
    d. Becomes more focused on observing religious customs and less on ideologic matters

21. According to Erikson, a key to identity achievement in adolescence is:
    a. related to the adolescent's interactions with others and serves as a mirror reflecting information back to the adolescent.
    b. linked to the role the adolescent plays within the family.
    c. related to the adolescent's acceptance of parental guidelines.
    d. related to the adolescent's ability to complete his or her plans for future accomplishments.

22. Expected characteristics of emotional autonomy during early adolescence include:
    a. increased independence from friends.
    b. increased need for parental approval.
    c. belief that parents are all-knowing and all-powerful.
    d. less emotional dependence on parents.

23. The formation of sexual identity development during adolescence usually involves which of the following?
    a. Forming close friendships with same-sex peers during early adolescence
    b. Developing intimate relationships with members of the opposite sex during later adolescence
    c. Developing emotional and social identities separate from those of families
    d. All of the above

24. Nationally, what percentage of boys and girls have had sexual intercourse by the twelfth grade?
    a. 67% of boys and 76% of girls
    b. 84% of boys and 58% of girls
    c. 66% of girls and 64% of boys
    d. 84% of girls and 58% of boys

25. The development of sexual orientation includes seven developmental milestones during late childhood and throughout adolescence. These milestones do not always occur in the same order or in the same time frame. List these milestones.

26. Intimate relationships are *not* necessarily characterized by:
    a. concern for each other's well-being.
    b. sharing of sexual intimacy.
    c. a willingness to disclose private, sensitive topics.
    d. sharing of common interests and activities.

27. Changes in family structure and parental employment result in changes for adolescents, including:
    a. adolescents having more time unsupervised by adults.
    b. adolescents having more time for communication and intimacy with parents.
    c. adolescents having less time to spend with peers.
    d. adolescents requiring more supervision by outside family members.

28. Adolescents who feel close to their parents show:
    i.   more positive psychosocial development.
    ii. greater behavioral competence.
    iii. less susceptibility to negative peer pressure.
    iv. less tendency to be involved in risk-taking behaviors.

    a. i, iii, and iv
    b. i and ii
    c. iii and iv
    d. i, ii, iii, and iv

29. Describe authoritative parenting and results related to this type of parenting.

30. Only about 10% of the variations found in risk behaviors of seventh- and eighth-grade adolescents can be explained by the effects of their ethnic group, income and family structure.
    a. True
    b. False

31. During adolescence, advances in cognitive development bring which one of the following changes?
    a. Beliefs become more concrete and less rooted in general ideologic principles.
    b. Adolescents show an increasing emotional understanding and acceptance of parents' beliefs as their own.
    c. Adolescents encounter few new opportunities for decisions based on their past experiences.
    d. Adolescents develop a personal value system distinct from that of significant adults in their lives.

32. As compared with childhood peer groups, adolescent peer groups are:
    a. more likely to include peers from the opposite sex.
    b. less autonomous.
    c. less likely to influence members' socialization roles.
    d. more likely to require parental supervision.

33. The timing of the transition from elementary school to junior high can be advantageous to the adolescent if it:
    a. occurs at the same time as the rapid physical changes of puberty.
    b. precedes the changes of puberty.

34. While Jenny, age 16, is in for her routine checkup, her mother tells the nurse that Jenny wants to get a job at a local fast-food restaurant, where she would work 30 hours a week to earn extra money for clothes. The mother wonders whether this is a good idea. Which one of the following is the nurse's best response?
    a. "Jenny is healthy and there is no reason she could not take the job."
    b. "All adolescents are preoccupied with clothes, so let her go ahead."
    c. "That sounds like a dead-end job. Why would Jenny want to work there?"
    d. "Working 30 hours a week may take time away from her studies and extracurricular activities and increase fatigue. Looking together at Jenny's future career goals may help identify alternatives."

35. List three primary causes of mortality accounting for 75% of all adolescent deaths.

36. To *best* effect adolescent health promotion activity, the nurse should incorporate which one of the following in the plan?
    a. The adolescent's definition of health
    b. The adolescent's past health promotion activities
    c. A complete assessment of the adolescent's past medical treatment
    d. A complete physical examination

37. Health concerns consistent with middle adolescents include:
    a. school performance.
    b. emotional health issues.
    c. physical appearance.
    d. future career or employment.

38. Adolescents are more likely to participate in health care services when:
    a. they understand the potentially negative consequences of their health behavior.
    b. they rank confidential care and respect higher than site cleanliness.
    c. they view their health problems as not organic in nature.
    d. they see the health care provider as caring and respectful.

39. Identify the following statements as true or false.

    _____ Routine exercise can reduce risk for depression and emotional distress in adolescents.

    _____ Nearly 20% of ninth- through twelfth-graders have reported considering suicide.

    _____ When used alone, media campaigns still have a substantial direct influence on changing health behaviors in adolescents.

    _____ Protective factors that characterize adolescents who cope successfully with adverse life situations include the ability to adapt to new persons and situations.

    _____ The nurse involved with adolescent health promotion should plan interventions that decrease exposures to stressful life events and increase sources of emotional support.

    _____ The most successful adolescent health promotion programs are aimed at single issues presented with a focused educational approach.

    _____ When interviewing adolescents, the nurse begins with questions of a less sensitive nature and ends with those of a more sensitive area.

    _____ For older African-American teens the most likely cause of death is homicide.

    _____ School-based clinics have not increased adolescents' access to preventive services.

    _____ All adolescents who participate in homosexual activity will become homosexual adults.

    _____ Gay, lesbian, and bisexual adolescents need specific sexuality education that is different from that provided to other adolescents.

    _____ Students with below-average grades are more likely to engage in health-compromising behaviors.

    _____ Students who are exposed to repeated teasing and harassment are more likely to skip school and to attempt suicide.

    _____ Students who are regularly harassed are more likely to bring weapons to school.

    _____ Dropout rates are highest among Hispanic and American Indian adolescents.

    _____ Parental involvement has not been shown to increase effectiveness of high schools.

    _____ African-American and Native American males have a higher risk for premature mortality than do other racial/ethnic groups.

    _____ Adolescents should be made aware of the reporting process before information about abuse is disclosed to local authorities.

    _____ Teenagers who drop out of school can expect to earn approximately one-third less income each year than those who graduate.

40. Effective health care services for adolescents must be _____ and

_____.

41. List three strategies that nurses can use in school and clinical settings to promote adolescent self-advocacy skills.

42. List three elements that are critical in establishing a trusting relationship with an adolescent during a health interview.

43. During the adolescent health screening interview, the nurse will focus on which of the following to *best* address injury prevention?
    a. Drownings
    b. Burns
    c. Motor vehicle crashes
    d. Drug use

44. The most appropriate way to prevent firearm injury among adolescents is:
    a. teaching the adolescent proper use of the firearm.
    b. counseling the adolescent on nonviolent ways to resolve conflict.
    c. passing laws to prevent parents from having guns.
    d. telling parents to keep the gun and the ammunition in separate locations within the house.

45. Adolescent girls of low socioeconomic status are particularly at risk for dietary deficiencies of:
    i.   calories.
    ii. sodium.
    iii. calcium.
    iv. folic acid.
    v.   iron.

    a. i, ii, and iii
    b. ii, iii, iv, and v
    c. iii, iv, and v
    d. i, iii, and v

46. When is a screening hemoglobin or hematocrit recommended for adolescents?
    a. At the first health provider encounter with an adolescent
    b. At the end of pubertal development
    c. At the end of puberty
    d. All of the above

47. A dietary and health assessment should be done to determine risk for morbidity in adolescents if:
    i.   the BMI has decreased in the last 12 months.
    ii.   there is a positive family history of diabetes, premature heart disease, hypertension, or obesity.
    iii. the adolescent is concerned about weight.
    iv.   the adolescent has an elevated serum cholesterol.
    v.   the adolescent has a history of sweating and breathing hard for at least 20 minutes.

    a. i, ii, and iii
    b. ii, iii, and iv
    c. i, ii, and v
    d. i, ii, iii, iv, and v

48. List four risk factors that should be targeted in the adolescent to prevent the development of adult cardiovascular disease.

49. Susan, age 15 years, comes to the school-based clinic and complains to the nurse practitioner about a vaginal discharge. After the nurse has established a trusting and confidential relationship, Susan confides that she has been sexually active with three different partners within the past 6 months. She thinks they used condoms every time, but she is not sure. Susan's last period was 3 weeks ago and she had a Pap test a little over 2 months ago. What tests would the nurse assisting the nurse practitioner expect to prepare for?
    i.   Pap test
    ii.   Gonorrhea test
    iii. Chlamydial test
    iv.   HIV test
    v.   Pregnancy test
    vi.   Syphilis test

    a. i, ii, iii, and iv
    b. ii, iii, iv, and vi
    c. ii, iii, and v
    d. i, ii, iii, and vi

50. The troubled adolescent thinking about suicide should be immediately referred for acute intervention

    when _____.

Critical Thinking—Case Study

Shawna, a 16 year old, visits the nurse practitioner for a routine checkup. Shawna is an A and B student in school and a member of the girls' drill team. She matured early and started to menstruate at the age of 10. Her menses are now regular. She has a boyfriend and has been dating since the age of 13. Shawna tells the nurse she has no specific concerns.

51. Based on risk factors associated with teens of Shawna's age, the nurse recognizes which one of the following as the *most* important to discuss with Shawna at this time?
    a. Shawna's perception and concerns about health
    b. Shawna's nutritional habits
    c. Shawna's sexual activity
    d. Shawna's relationship with her family

52. The nurse establishes a trusting relationship with Shawna, who admits to having been sexually active with five boys since she started dating. Besides educating her on the risks for sexually transmitted diseases and pregnancy, which one of the following is *most* important for the nurse to include in her plan of care for Shawna at this time?
    a. Discuss with Shawna how she can tell her parents about her sexual activity.
    b. Explore possible reasons for Shawna's behavior with her.
    c. Assess Shawna's immunization status for hepatitis B.
    d. Assess how Shawna feels about the possibility of getting pregnant.

53. Mrs. Smith complains to you that her 15-year-old son, Ben, has begun to drift away from the family and that he finds fault with everything she and her husband do. She is worried about the relationship between them and Ben and doesn't understand what she and her husband have done wrong. "Why does Ben seem to suddenly dislike us so much?" Based on your knowledge of adolescent behavior, which one of the following would be the *best* explanation?
    a. "Ben's behavioral standards are set by his peer group, and he is acting this way because of fear of rejection by this group."
    b. "Ben is defining his moral values, and you and your husband will need to have the same moral values as Ben if you want to continue to be close to him."
    c. "Ben is developing the capacity for abstract thinking and increasing his concern about social issues. He will return to share your views shortly."
    d. "Ben is defining independence-dependence boundaries and beginning to disengage from parents."

54. Christy, age 14, comes to the clinic for a physical exam. It has been longer than 2 years since her last exam. Upon review of Christy's immunization record, the nurse notes that Christy had a diphtheria-tetanus (DT) booster at age 4 years and a measles-mumps-rubella (MMR) vaccine at age 15 months. Christy has been healthy in the past with normal childhood diseases including varicella. Which of the following immunizations would you expect Christy to receive today?
    a. Influenza, pneumococcal, and chickenpox
    b. MMR, hepatitis B, and hepatitis A
    c. MMR, DT, and hepatitis B
    d. Mantoux tuberculin, hepatitis B, and hepatitis A

55. Carl, age 16 years, has been brought to the clinic after taking some drugs given to him by friends at school. He is now alert and, after talking to the nurse, confides that he is gay. Carl's parents do not know he is gay. Which one of the following *most* likely explains Carl's drug-taking behavior?
    a. Carl is suicidal.
    b. Carl is a chronic drug user.
    c. Carl used the drugs as an escape from anxieties and emotional distress related to keeping his gay sexuality secret.
    d. Carl took the drugs as an attempt to call attention to himself and his gay lifestyle.

CHAPTER 20

Physical Health Problems of Adolescence

1. Which one of the following current beliefs about acne formation is true?
   a. Cosmetics containing lanolin and lauryl alcohol are not known to contribute to acne formation.
   b. There is scientific research to support the theory that stress will cause an acne outbreak.
   c. Exposure to oils in cooking grease can be a precursor to acne in adolescents working over fast-food restaurant oils.
   d. Acne usually worsens with dietary intake of chocolates and other foods high in sugars.

2. Nancy, age 16 years, presents to the nurse because of acne on her face, shoulders, and neck areas. After talking with Nancy, the nurse makes a nursing diagnosis of knowledge deficit, related to proper skin care. Which one of the following would the nurse include in the instruction plan for Nancy?
   a. Wash the areas vigorously with antibacterial soaps.
   b. Brush the hair down on the forehead to conceal the acne areas.
   c. Avoid the use of all cosmetics.
   d. Gently wash the areas with a mild soap once or twice daily.

3. The practitioner has prescribed Retin-A for Nancy's acne, and Nancy returns for a follow-up visit after 2 weeks of treatment. During the nursing assessment, Nancy tells the nurse that she has "done everything" that she was told to do and asks, "Why is my acne no better?" The nurse's *best* reply is:
   a. "Since the medication prevents the formation of new comedones, it will take at least 6 weeks for improvement to be obvious."
   b. "You must not be using the medication right. Show me how you apply it to your face."
   c. "Acne is caused by dirt or oil on the surface of the skin. You will need to increase the number of times you wash these areas each day."
   d. "You will probably need to ask the practitioner about changing your medicine as soon as possible."

4. The nurse is conducting an educational session with Cindy and her parents on medications used for acne. Which one of the following is correct information?
   a. Tretinoin gel has a bleaching effect on bed coverings and towels.
   b. Topical clindamycin is applied only to the individual lesions.
   c. Oral contraceptive medications contain estrogen, which will increase acne formation and should be avoided.
   d. Tretinoin requires that Cindy protect herself from sun exposure.

5. The proper use of Accutane for adolescents includes:
   i. reserving its use to severe, cystic acne that has not responded to other treatments.
   ii. limiting treatment to 20 weeks.
   iii. watching for side effects, including mood changes, depression, and suicidal ideation.
   iv. watching for detrimental effects on bone mineralization.
   v. recognizing that it is contraindicated in pregnancy and in sexually active females not using an effective contraceptive method.
   vi. monitoring for elevated cholesterol and triglyceride levels before and during treatment.

   a. i, ii, iv, and v
   b. i, iii, v, and vi
   c. i, ii, iii, v, and vi
   d. i, ii, iii, iv, v, and vi

6. The most common solid tumor in males 15 to 34 years of age is:
   a. varicocele.
   b. testicular torsion.
   c. priapism.
   d. testicular cancer.

7. The adolescent with testicular cancer is *most* likely to present with which of the following signs and symptoms?
   a. Tender, painful swelling of the testes
   b. A mass in the posterior aspect of the scrotum that can be transilluminated
   c. A heavy, hard, painless, mass palpable on the anterior or lateral surface of the testicle
   d. An asymptomatic scrotal mass that aches, especially after exercise or penile erection

8. In teaching the adolescent male how to perform testicular self-examination, the nurse includes which of the following in the instructions?
   a. Perform the procedure once a month after a warm shower.
   b. A raised swelling palpated on the superior aspect of the testicle indicates an abnormality.
   c. Use the second and third fingers on each hand, holding each testicle between the fingers while palpating it with the other fingers.
   d. All of the above should be included.

9. The nurse knows that which of the following adolescent females should be scheduled for her first pelvic examination?
   i.   The 16-year-old who has not become sexually active
   ii.   The adolescent who has been menstruating for 2 years
   iii. The adolescent who wants to start taking birth control pills
   iv.   The 18-year-old who has not become sexually active
   v.   The sexually active adolescent

   a. i, iii, and v
   b. ii, iii, and v
   c. iii and v
   d. iii, iv, and v

10. Match each term with its definition. (Terms may be used more than once.)

   a. Varicocele   c. Testicular torsion
   b. Epididymitis   d. Gynecomastia

   _____ Breast enlargement that occurs during puberty
   _____ Wormlike mass that is palpated above the testicle and becomes smaller in size when the adolescent lies down
   _____ Benign and temporary disease that occurs in about 50% of adolescents
   _____ Inflammation that is a result of either infection or local trauma
   _____ Marked by the testis hanging free from its vascular structure; results in partial or complete venous occlusion
   _____ Characterized by unilateral scrotal pain, redness, and swelling; may include urethral discharge, dysuria, fever, and pyuria; treated with antibiotics
   _____ Presents with scrotum that is swollen, painful, red, and warm; presence of pain radiating to groin, accompanied by nausea, vomiting, and abdominal pain; generally, an absence of fever and urinary symptoms; immediate surgery required to treat

11. _____ _____ is defined as an absence of menses by age 17.

_____ _____ is defined as an absence of menses for 6 months in a previously menstruating female, when pregnancy has been excluded.

12. Linda, age 16, started her menses at age 13 years. She now presents at the school-based clinic with a history of secondary amenorrhea. Linda is an honor student and a long-distance runner who runs an average of 50 miles per week. The physical exam is normal, and Linda has been requested to decrease her running distance and to improve her nutrition. She is scheduled for a follow-up visit and told that if her menses are not more regulated, oral birth control pills will be prescribed. Linda wants to know why she would have to take the pills since she is not sexually active. How would you respond?

13. The treatment of choice for adolescents with dysmenorrhea is:
    a. acetaminophen.
    b. oral contraceptives.
    c. nonsteroidal antiinflammatory drugs.
    d. estrogen-suppression drugs.

14. Adverse effects of intensive physical exercise on an adolescent's reproductive cycle may include:
    a. delayed menarche.
    b. anovulation associated with dysfunctional uterine bleeding.
    c. amenorrhea.
    d. all of the above.

15. Match the term with its description.

    a. Dysmenorrhea
    b. Premenstrual syndrome
    c. Endometriosis
    d. Dysfunctional uterine bleeding

    e. Vaginitis candidiasis
    f. Pelvic inflammatory disease
    g. Trichomoniasis vaginalis

    h. Oligomenorrhea
    i. Leukorrhea
    j. Bacterial vaginosis (BV)

    _____ Condition that has more than 100 associated physical, psychologic, and behavioral symptoms
    _____ Condition that may be caused by the presence of endometrial tissue outside the uterine cavity
    _____ Abnormal vaginal bleeding, usually associated with anovulation
    _____ Symptoms that include thin, malodorous vaginal discharge; diagnosis confirmed by clue cells on microscopic exam
    _____ Painful menses
    _____ Abnormally light or infrequent menstruation
    _____ Infection of the upper genital tract, commonly caused by gonorrhea or chlamydia
    _____ Condition that may present with vaginal pruritus and dysuria and is not an STD; treated with over-the-counter topical antifungal creams
    _____ An STD caused by an anaerobic parasitic protozoa
    _____ Glutinous, gray-white vaginal discharge caused by physical, chemical, or infectious agents

16. Evidence suggests that effective treatments of premenstrual syndrome include:
    a. vitamin B_6, vitamin E, and magnesium.
    b. primrose oil combined with 1200 mg/dl of calcium.
    c. serotonin reuptake inhibitors.
    d. all of the above.

17. Gail has been diagnosed with vaginitis. The nurse is preparing to instruct her on prevention. Describe what information the nurse should include in her instructions.

18. Indicate whether the following statements are true or false.

    _____ Approximately 50% of high school students report having had sexual intercourse by their senior year in high school.

    _____ Adolescents who have at least one supportive parent engage in less risky behavior.

    _____ The pregnancies of adolescents under 15 years old are less frequently complicated by obstetric problems.

    _____ Adolescent mothers are just as likely to complete high school as are other adolescents.

    _____ During a second pregnancy for a teenager, obstetric risk and risk to the infant is lower.

    _____ Teens between 12 and 16 years are at high risk for prolonged labor related to fetopelvic incompatibility.

    _____ Pregnant adolescents often have diets deficient in iron, calcium, and folic acid.

    _____ Effective parent-child communication about sexuality topics can delay the onset of first sexual intercourse.

    _____ The teenage pregnancy rate continues to increase for all age groups.

    _____ The abortion rate has fallen more quickly than the drop in pregnancy rate for adolescents.

19. Lesley is a sexually active adolescent. She presents to the clinic with abdominal pain and vaginal bleeding. The nurse recognizes that which of the following must be ruled out immediately?
    a. Ectopic pregnancy
    b. Ovarian cyst
    c. STDs
    d. Endometriosis

20. The nurse knows that which of the following adolescents would be at high-risk for pregnancy?
    a. Those who have early initiation of sexual activity
    b. The adolescent who does not use a reliable method of contraception regularly
    c. The adolescent female who has poor school performance
    d. All of the above

21. Infants of adolescents are at risk because:
    a. teenage mothers often neglect their infants, leaving them for long periods with grandparents.
    b. teenage mothers supply excessive amounts of cognitive stimulation to their infants.
    c. adolescents often lack knowledge about normal infant growth and development.
    d. adolescents are less likely to treat their infant as love objects or playthings.

22. The first goal in nursing care of the pregnant teenager is:
    a. to arrange for the pregnant teen to register for food supplement programs to ensure proper nutrition.
    b. to assist the pregnant teen in obtaining prenatal care.
    c. to involve the boyfriend and parents in the pregnancy so that the pregnant teen will have support during her pregnancy.
    d. to educate the pregnant teen regarding child care.

23. Postpartum care of adolescents should be directed toward:
    a. preventing subsequent pregnancies.
    b. reestablishment with high school counselors for completion of education.
    c. arranging for childcare classes.
    d. increasing interaction among the father, the new mother, and the newborn.

24. A drug approved for medical abortion is mifepristone. Which of the following statements about this drug is true?
    a. The drug can be used to provide nonsurgical abortion at 49 days or less of pregnancy.
    b. The drug prevents receptor binding of endogenous or exogenous progesterone.
    c. The abortion completion rate is 92% to 95% in pregnancies if used correctly.
    d. All of the above.

25. Emily is an unmarried 17-year-old who is 6 weeks pregnant and has decided to have an abortion. One nursing action used to assist Emily would be:
    a. explaining to Emily that it is wrong for her to have an abortion and arranging for her to visit an adoption center.
    b. referring Emily to an appropriate abortion agency when she is 4 months pregnant.
    c. providing Emily with relaxation strategies to be used during the abortion procedure.
    d. calling Emily's parents so that they can be present for the abortion.

26. In discussing prevention of sexually transmitted diseases, the nurse tells the adolescent that which one of the following is *most* effective?
    a. Birth control pills
    b. Norplant
    c. Spermicides
    d. Condoms

27. Nancy, age 17, is brought to the family planning clinic by her mother for birth control. Which of the following is *most* important to include in a plan for Nancy at this time?
    a. Discussion of the effectiveness rates of various methods and importance of compliance
    b. Including Nancy's partner in the discussions
    c. Discussion of Nancy's perception of the likelihood of getting pregnant and her desire to prevent pregnancy versus her desire for pregnancy
    d. Cost of the various methods of contraception

28. Which of the following is *not* recommended as a birth control method for Nancy at age 17 years?
    a. Intrauterine device
    b. Sponge
    c. Depo-Provera
    d. Diaphragm

29. The nurse is conducting a sexual education program. What technique has been found helpful when dealing with the subject of sexual abstinence?

30. Rape victims display a variety of manifestations. Which of the following might the nurse see in 16-year-old Sally as she arrives at the emergency center for treatment after being raped?
    a. Hysterical crying or giggling
    b. Calm and controlled behavior
    c. Anger and rage alternating with helplessness and agitation
    d. All of the above

31. The primary goal of nursing care for the adolescent rape victim is:
    a. not to inflict further stress on the victim.
    b. obtaining a complete history of the incident.
    c. assisting in the physical examination.
    d. notifying the police and the parents of the victim before proceeding with assessment.

32. Identify the following statements about STDs in adolescence as true or false.

    _____ Adolescent females are at a lower risk for chlamydia and human papilloma virus because of the immature adolescent endocervix.

    _____ In the adolescent, the immune system provides excellent localized antibody response to infectious agents at the cervical level.

    _____ Research has demonstrated that as the use of hormonal contraception increases, the use of condoms declines among adolescents.

    _____ Adolescents ages 15 to 19 have the highest overall incidence of gonococcal infection.

    _____ Symptoms of gonorrhea can occur 1 day to 2 weeks after sexual contact, or there may be no symptoms.

    _____ Treatment for uncomplicated gonorrhea is with a single dose each of cefixime 400 mg PO plus azithromycin 1 g PO.

    _____ Conjunctiva gonorrhea is always sexually transmitted.

    _____ Treatment for gonorrhea includes both the partner and the patient and provides life-long immunity.

    _____ A major effect of untreated chlamydial infections among adolescent females is infertility.

    _____ Long-term effects of PID include infertility because of tubal scarring.

33. Therapeutic management for chlamydia includes:
    a. doxycycline, 100 mg bid for 7 days in the pregnant adolescent and her partner.
    b. intramuscular injection of ceftriaxone (rocephrin) 125 mg for the patient and partner.
    c. intramuscular injection of penicillin 2.4 million units for the patient and partner.
    d. azithromycin 1 g PO in a single dose for the patient and her partner.

34. Shirley, age 17, has been diagnosed with pelvic inflammatory disease caused by gonorrhea. The nurse can expect treatment to include which one of the following?
    a. Shirley will be admitted to the hospital immediately.
    b. Shirley will be given ceftriaxone (rocephrin) intramuscularly, with oral antibiotics as outpatient treatment for 14 days.
    c. No treatment of Shirley's partner will be necessary.
    d. Shirley will be prescribed oral contraceptives.

35. The most common STD in the United States is _____ _____,

    which causes _____ _____. Individuals with this infection are at

    risk for development of _____ _____ and

    _____.

36. Oncogenic risk categories for HVP include types _____, _____, _____, _____, and

    _____. The treatment for external warts can be either applied by the _____ or

    administered by the _____.

37. One STD for which there is an immunization recommended for all adolescents is:
    a. human immunodeficiency virus.
    b. hepatitis B virus.
    c. syphilis.
    d. herpes simplex type 2 virus.

38. Connie, age 15 years, has requested information about prevention of STDs. As the nurse begins to discuss HIV and AIDS, Connie tells the nurse to skip information on this topic. Based on knowledge about adolescents, which of the following is the *most* likely reason for Connie's response?
    a. Connie does not think she has at-risk behavior for AIDS.
    b. Connie already knows as much about AIDS as is necessary.
    c. Connie is not sexually active.
    d. Connie wants information about birth control but is afraid to ask.

Critical Thinking—Case Study

Bryan, age 14, has come to the clinic because he has started breaking out with acne on his face, chest, and shoulders. He says he is embarrassed to go out, because his friends stare at him and girls avoid him. The physician has started medical treatment and sent him to you for further guidance.

39. Based on the information provided, what is a priority nursing diagnosis for Bryan at this time?
    a. Altered family process related to the adolescent with a skin problem
    b. Body image disturbance related to perception of acne lesions
    c. Bathing/hygiene self-care deficient related to skin care
    d. Altered role performance related to perceived peer separation

40. The *best* goal for Bryan would be which of the following?
    a. Will have a positive body image
    b. Will receive appropriate education for hygiene
    c. Will have a reduction in dietary fat and calories
    d. Will receive appropriate referral to skin specialist

41. Subjective data collection on Bryan should include which of the following?
    a. Family history of acne
    b. Location and size description of visible lesions
    c. Culture and sensitivity for identifying organism
    d. All of the above

42. The nurse has established a plan of care with Bryan. Which one of the following would be an expected component of the plan to improve Bryan's body image?
    a. Help him find mechanisms to reduce emotional stress.
    b. Explain the disorder and therapy prescribed to increase family understanding.
    c. Emphasize the positive aspects, as well as the limited nature of the disorder, and assist Bryan with grooming to enhance appearance.
    d. Discourage peer relationships until Bryan's facial appearance has improved from medication.

Sixteen-year-old Jenny is pregnant and coming to the school-based clinic for prenatal care. Jenny and the baby's father, Doug, are still seeing each other, but their relationship has "cooled" since Jenny found out she was pregnant. Jenny is living at home. She is expecting her mother to help in the raising of the infant while Jenny continues school.

43. The nurse is planning for prenatal and childrearing classes that both Jenny and Doug could attend. Based on knowledge of adolescent fathers, the nurse would:
    a. realize that adolescent fathers have little association with their infants.
    b. understand that Doug will want to start breaking the contact with Jenny and will refuse to go.
    c. realize that Doug is still most influenced by his male peer friends and is embarrassed about getting Jenny pregnant and will not go.
    d. realize that active participation in the pregnancy by Doug will have positive effects on Jenny's self-esteem and will decrease her level of distress and depression.

44. Which of the following does the nurse recognize as the *best* plan for Jenny and her infant?
    a. Have Jenny move out of her mother's house and care for the infant on her own.
    b. Have Jenny leave the care of the infant completely to her mother and get on with her life.
    c. Have Jenny go along with whatever her mother says to avoid open conflicts around the infant.
    d. Have Jenny care for her child even when other adults are involved.

45. Which one of the following statements, if made by Jenny, would reflect the concept of a personal fable that could lead to risk-taking behaviors?
    a. "I don't want to get an STD, so it won't happen to me."
    b. "Only girls that are permissive get STDs."
    c. "Abstinence is the only way to prevent an STD."
    d. "All my friends have sex."

CHAPTER 21

Behavioral Health Problems of Adolescence

1. Identify the following statements as either true or false.

   _____ The number of fat cells may be established at an early age, and overfeeding during this time may have a significant influence on the development of obesity at a later age.

   _____ Obesity is the most common nutritional disturbance of children.

   _____ During the adolescent growth spurt, the distribution of fat in girls decreases sharply.

   _____ Obesity refers to the state of weighing more than average for height and body build and may or may not include an increased amount of fat.

   _____ Birth weight is an indicator of childhood obesity.

   _____ In Prader-Willi syndrome, children exhibit characteristics of slow intellectual development, short stature, and obesity and go to great lengths to obtain food.

   _____ Obesity in adolescents can be caused by overeating or low activity levels.

   _____ Obese persons eat more at a given sitting and tend to eat more rapidly than those who are not obese.

   _____ Obese adolescents are characteristically night eaters who skip meals, especially breakfast.

   _____ Obese children are often from families that emphasize large meals or scold children for leaving food on their plates.

   _____ Obesity in childhood and adolescence is a significant risk factor for adult obesity.

   _____ African Americans, Hispanics, and Filipinos engage in less physical activity than non-Hispanic whites.

   _____ Parents who use food as a positive reinforcer for desired behavior may be encouraging the child to continue to use food as a reward and a means to deal with feelings of depression. This may lead to weight problems.

2. Increased obesity among children is related to:
   a. decreased physical activity in elementary and secondary schools.
   b. parental obesity and low levels of physical activity within the family.
   c. increased television viewing.
   d. all of the above.

3. Gail, age 14, comes to the school nurse's office because she is obese and wants to lose weight. The nurse's assessment will include:
   a. Gail's physical activity.
   b. dietary intake and meal patterns for Gail.
   c. eating patterns of Gail's family.
   d. all of the above.

4. Adolescents with obesity have common emotional problems of:
   a. poor body image.
   b. low self-esteem.
   c. social isolation and feelings of rejection.
   d. all of the above.

5. List three factors that can contribute to the development of a disturbed body image in the obese adolescent.

6. A main difference with the new BMI growth charts is that they were designed to allow health care

   providers to _____.

7. Weight-reduction management in adolescents should include:
   a. significant caloric restriction.
   b. elimination of physical hunger cues.
   c. regular physical activity.
   d. appetite-suppressant drugs.

8. Janie, age 14, wants to discuss with the nurse how to modify her eating habits to reduce her weight. Which one of the following methods does the nurse recognize as *least* helpful in assisting Janie to meet her goals?
   a. Have Janie keep a list of everything she eats.
   b. Request that Janie's parents remind Janie not to eat junk foods.
   c. Establish a system of rewards for changes in eating habits.
   d. Discuss with Janie methods other than eating than can be used to deal with emotional stress.

9. Obesity and overweight nutritional counseling is aimed at preventing an increase in body fat during growth. List the three aspects of changing eating habits that can *best* accomplish this.

10. The age range for anorexia nervosa is _____ to _____ years. This disorder is characterized by

    _____.

11. Individuals with bulimia are divided into two different types. Identify and define each type.

12. Cindy, age 16, has been sent to the school nurse because her gym teacher has noticed a marked decrease in Cindy's weight since vacation. Which one of the following does the nurse recognize as a common finding among adolescent girls with anorexia nervosa?
    a. Wears form-fitting clothes like tank tops and jeans
    b. Has strong peer relationships with classmates and several best friends
    c. Has poor schoolwork performance because of little interest in school
    d. Is present at meals, selects foods, and appears to family and friends to be eating appropriately

13. Cindy has been diagnosed with anorexia nervosa. Her therapeutic management plan includes hospitalization. Which one of the following would the nurse recognize as a possible reaction of Cindy to the treatment plan?
    a. Exhibits high-energy-level activity participation, especially with marked preoccupation with food preparation
    b. Becomes dependent on her parents, especially her mother
    c. Attempts to control the situation and views the treatment plan as an attempt to remove her autonomy
    d. Regards her appearance as abnormal or ugly

14. Cindy is about to be discharged after treatment for anorexia nervosa. The nurse has formulated a nursing diagnosis related to family coping with a goal that the family will be prepared for home care. Which one of the following interventions would best help meet this goal?
    a. Make certain both patient and family understand the therapeutic plan.
    b. Observe family interaction for assessment of family coping patterns.
    c. Explore feelings and attitudes of family members.
    d. Convey an attitude of caring and acceptance to family and patient.

15. In treating anorexia nervosa:
    a. weight gain is a reliable sign of positive progress.
    b. when a therapeutic environment is removed, relapses seldom occur.
    c. antianxiety or antidepressant drug use has not been proven effective.
    d. psychotherapy is aimed at resolving adolescent identity crises and distorted body image.

16. Bulimia is observed most frequently in _____.

    _____ bulimics are uncommon.

17. Which one of the following does the nurse recognize as being an adolescent group at high risk for bulimia?
    a. Adolescents in the lower socioeconomic level
    b. Adolescents who want to be tough, muscular football players
    c. Adolescents who aspire to careers that require low weight
    d. Adolescents with good self-image

18. Karen is suspected of being bulimic. The nurse recognizes which of the following as clinically characteristic of this disease?
    a. Bulimia often begins with decreased dietary intake due to poor relationships with family members.
    b. Once started, the binges decrease in frequency to only about 2 to 3 times per day.
    c. Insulin production is decreased because of excessive self-induced vomiting.
    d. Caloric intake may range from 20,000 to 30,000 calories per day.

19. The patient with bulimia must be watched by the nurse for medical complications. Which one of the following findings does the nurse recognize as needing *immediate* intervention?
    a. Backs of the hands scarred and cut from self-induced vomiting
    b. Potassium depletion from diuretic abuse
    c. Erosion of teeth enamel from self-induced vomiting
    d. Chronic esophagitis from self-induced vomiting

20. Treating the adolescent with bulimia requires the integration of medical, psychologic, and nutritional approaches. What group of antidepressants has been shown to diminish the obsessive-compulsive urge to binge and vomit in some adolescent patients?

21. Nurses encountering young people with "fear of fat" syndrome should focus on assisting these patients:
    a. to reduce intake of cereal, breads, and pastas.
    b. to increase exercise level.
    c. to understand the fact that they are not overweight and demonstrate this with ideal body weight graphs.
    d. by providing education directed at normal body changes and hazards of dieting.

22. Identify the following statements about substance abuse as either true or false.

    _____   A person may be physically dependent on a narcotic without being addicted.

    _____   The adolescent abusing drugs has often adopted the use of a substance as a means of coping with feelings of depression, boredom, and emptiness.

    _____   Identification of the pattern of drug use in the adolescent is essential but offers little help in developing a successful approach to the problem.

    _____   The usual goal for the compulsive drug user is peer acceptance.

    _____   One of the hazards associated with drug use is the risk for injury while driving under the influence of the drug.

    _____   National surveys have shown a steady decrease in the incidence of adolescents between the ages of 12 and 18 using tobacco, alcohol, and marijuana.

    _____   The absence of aldehyde dehydrogenase (ALDH), an enzyme that assists with the breakdown of ethanol in the body, reduces the likelihood that alcoholism will develop.

23. Which one of the following adolescents does the nurse recognize as *least* likely to begin smoking?
    a. Johnny, age 16 years, whose father quit smoking 2 years ago
    b. Karen, age 13 years, whose older sister smokes
    c. Ted, age 17 years, who smoked a cigarette at home in front of his parents
    d. Lilly, age 12, who feels uncomfortable with her early maturing body

24. Johnny, age 16, has tried his first cigarette because of peer pressure to "look cool." The nurse correctly notes that Johnny is in what stage of becoming a smoker?
    a. Preparation
    b. Initiation
    c. Experimentation
    d. Regular smoking

25. The school nurse is planning an educational program centered on smoking prevention for junior high school adolescents. Which of the following methods does the nurse recognize as the *most* effective way to present this program?
    a. Ban smoking in the school.
    b. Teach methods of resistance to peer pressure.
    c. Use peer-led programs that emphasize social consequences.
    d. Use media, videotapes, and films on smoking prevention.

26. Which one of the following statements is true?
    a. Smokeless tobacco is a safe alternative to cigarette smoking.
    b. Smokeless tobacco is often linked to periodontal disease and lesions in the oral soft tissue.
    c. Smokeless tobacco is not addictive.
    d. Smokeless tobacco users are less likely to become cigarette smokers.

27. Adolescent alcoholics are often described as:
    a. hard to live with and indecisive.
    b. good students with a strong desire to complete school.
    c. rarely denying their problem.
    d. having poor role models but excellent peer relations.

28. Certain protective factors have been identified as helping at-risk adolescents to resist pressures to use drugs and alcohol. List five recognized protective factors.

29. The motivation phase of treatment and rehabilitation of young drug users is directed toward:
    a. assessment of the drug habits and amount of drugs used.
    b. exploring the factors that influence drug use.
    c. prevention of relapse into drug use.
    d. all of the above.

30. Complete the following statements about drug abuse.

    a. The form of cocaine known as the purer and more menacing form is _____.

    b. Cocaine taken by _____ is associated with the highest levels of dependence.

    c. Cocaine is a potent _____ _____, and the crash after a cocaine

       high usually consists of _____.

    d. Physical signs of narcotic abuse include _____

       _____.

    e. _____, also known as the "date rape drug," is 10 times more powerful than diazepam and produces short-term memory loss.

    f. _____, with the street names of "crank" and "crystal," produces more stimulation than cocaine, and the user can remain "up" for hours.

    g. Inhalant abuse usually gives the child an inexpensive euphoria but is extremely dangerous and can

       cause _____.

31. The increase in suicide and depression during adolescence may be due to:
    a. expected low self-esteem among this population.
    b. the importance of peer pressures among this group.
    c. cognitive development and the ability to observe one's self.
    d. higher substance abuse among this group.

32. Jim, who has no history of previous suicide attempt, is talking with the school nurse about his feelings of despair and hopelessness about the future. He tells the nurse he would be better off dead. The nurse's *best* response is which one of the following?
    a. Recognize that Jim is going through a common phase of adolescence.
    b. Recognize that Jim is at low risk for suicide since he has not previously attempted suicide.
    c. Explain to Jim that suicide never solved anything and that he will feel better tomorrow.
    d. Take Jim seriously, allow time for him to verbalize his feelings, and stay with him until referral.

33. The nurse has been asked to present an educational program on prevention of adolescent stress and suicide. In planning the program, the nurse should include:
    a. the importance of being supportive and establishing positive communication patterns between family and teens.
    b. the precipitating factors for suicide.
    c. effective coping mechanisms and problem-solving skills.
    d. all of the above.

34. Mark, age 14 years, has been rushed to the emergency department because of illegal drug ingestion at a party. Which of the following is *most* important for the nurse to collect to assist in the emergency treatment plan?
    i.   The type and amount of drug taken
    ii. The time the drug was taken and mode of administration
    iii. Number of times Mark has previously overdosed
    iv. Why the drug was taken

    a. i and ii
    b. i, ii, and iii
    c. i only
    d. i, ii, iii, and iv

35. Match the term with its description.

    a. Suicidal ideation   d. Suicide   g. Overweight
    b. Suicide attempt   e. Contagion suicide   h. Anorexia nervosa
    c. Parasuicide   f. Obesity   i. Bulimia

    _____   Behaviors ranging from gestures to serious attempts to kill oneself
    _____   Increase in body weight from excess fat
    _____   Deliberate act of self-injury with death as result
    _____   Deliberate but unsuccessful act of self-injury
    _____   Weighing more than average for height and body build
    _____   Thoughts about killing oneself
    _____   Phenomenon resulting from excessive media coverage after an adolescent suicide
    _____   Denial of the existence of hunger
    _____   Binge eating followed by purging

Critical Thinking—Case Study

Kenny, 16 years of age, visits the clinic for follow-up of a recent infection. While talking with the nurse, he tells her that he has recently broken up with his girlfriend after going steady for 11 months. Kenny has a history of having a difficult home situation. His recent school performance has declined, and this has further upset Kenny's parents and their expectations for him. Physical examination of Kenny reveals an expressionless face with a slight smell of alcohol on his breath and signs consistent with depression.

36. You suspect that Kenny might be suicidal. Which factors in the preceding data might support this assumption?
    i.   Alcohol consumption
    ii. Recent breakup with girlfriend
    iii. History of difficult home situation
    iv. Depression
    v.   Age and gender

    a. i, ii, iii, and iv
    b. ii, iii, and iv
    c. ii, iv, and v
    d. i, ii, iii, iv, and v

37. Upon questioning by the nurse, Kenny admits to suicidal ideation. What should the nurse first assess to determine risk?
    a. History of suicide attempts within the family
    b. Past methods of coping with stress by the individual
    c. Whether Kenny has a plan for suicide
    d. Whether Kenny has a gun available to him

38. Which one of the following nursing diagnoses would the nurse develop to *best* deal with Kenny's suicide thoughts?
    a. High risk for injury related to feelings of rejection
    b. Sleep pattern disturbance related to inability to sleep
    c. Social isolation related to withdrawal from friends
    d. High risk for self-directed violence related to excessive alcohol use

39. The *most* important goal in the nursing management for Kenny at this time should focus on:
    a. reestablishing Kenny's relationship with his girlfriend.
    b. teaching Kenny how to cope with the stress of being an adolescent.
    c. maintaining physical safety for Kenny.
    d. assisting Kenny to express his emotional pain and regain his ability to perform assigned tasks.

CHAPTER 22

Family-Centered Care of the Child with Chronic Illness or Disability

1. Match each term with its description.

   a. Chronic illness
   b. Congenital disability
   c. Developmental delay
   d. Developmental disability

   e. Disability
   f. Handicap
   g. Impairment
   h. Technology-dependent

   i. Home care
   j. Mainstreaming

   _____ A barrier imposed by society

   _____ A disability that has existed since birth but is not necessarily hereditary

   _____ Requiring the routine use of a medical device for support of a life-sustaining bodily function

   _____ A condition that interferes with daily functioning for more than three months

   _____ Any mental and/or physical disability that is manifested before age 22 years and is likely to continue indefinitely

   _____ A system of care with the goals to normalize the child's life, lessen disruption on the family, and maximize the child's growth and development

   _____ A maturational lag

   _____ The process of integrating children with special needs into regular classrooms and child care centers

   _____ A loss or abnormality of a structure or function

   _____ A long-term reduction in the child's ability to engage in day-to-day activities because of a chronic condition

2. Match each program with its description.

   a. Education for All Handicapped Children Act of 1975
   b. Individuals with Disabilities Education Act (IDEA)
   c. Individual Education Program (IEP)
   d. The Education of the Handicapped Act Amendments of 1986
   e. Individual Family Service Plan (IFSP)
   f. Americans with Disabilities Act (ADA)

   _____ The 1990 amendment to the Education of All Handicapped Children Act of 1975 that changed name of the program

   _____ A program that requires daycare providers to make "reasonable modifications" for equal access to program participation

   _____ The approach in which a multidisciplinary team writes a plan that includes special education and therapeutic strategies and goals for each eligible child

   _____ A program developed jointly by families and professionals; includes information about the infant/toddler's present level of development, family strengths and needs relating to enhancing development, major outcomes expected, services needed, identification of a case manager, and transition steps to preschool services

_____ The public law that is largely responsible for the development of a variety of supplemental programs in the school system to accommodate children with special needs

_____ The program that directs states to develop and implement statewide comprehensive, coordinated, multidisciplinary interagency programs of early intervention services for infants and toddlers with disabilities, as well as support services for their families

3. Match each term with its description.

   a. Special Olympics
   b. VSA arts
   c. Coping Health Inventory for Parents (CHIPS)
   d. Approach behaviors
   e. Avoidance behaviors
   f. Trajectory model

   g. Family management styles theory
   h. Guilt
   i. Anger/bitterness
   j. Overprotection
   k. Rejection
   l. Denial

   m. Gradual acceptance
   n. Chronic sorrow
   o. Functional burden
   p. Programs for Children with Special Health Needs

   _____ Offers disabled children an opportunity to celebrate and share their accomplishments in a variety of expressive activities such as art, music, poetry, dance, and drama

   _____ An emotional response of parents manifested throughout the life span of the disabled or chronically ill child; includes elements of permanence with episodic surges in the presence of developmental or situational crisis; may include resurgence of grief triggered by events that remind the parent of what could have been

   _____ An 80 item checklist providing self-report information about how parents perceive their overall response to the management of family life with a child with a chronic illness

   _____ A program that offers children with physical disabilities an opportunity to compete with their peers and to achieve athletic skill

   _____ Those coping mechanisms that result in movement toward adjustment and resolution of the crisis

   _____ A theory about chronic illness that acknowledges that the condition has a course that varies and changes over time

   _____ Self-accusation; a feeling that is often greatest when the cause of a disorder is directly traceable to the parent, as in cases of genetic disease

   _____ A concept that considers the issues associated with caring for and living with the chronically ill/disabled child in relation to the family's resources and ability to cope

   _____ Common and normal reactions of families to a chronic illness diagnosis; emotions that typically manifest in the parents, the ill child, and siblings; e.g., verbal self-degrading, arguments, withdrawal, and complaints about nursing care

   _____ Characterized by parents acting as if the child's disorder does not exist or attempting to have the child overcompensate for the disability

   _____ A theory about chronic illness that emphasizes the family's role in actively responding to a child's illness

   _____ Behavior in which parents fear allowing the child to achieve any new skill, avoid all discipline, and cater to the child's desires to impede frustration

   _____ Coping mechanism with the result of movement away from adjustment to the crisis

   _____ Behavior in which parents detach themselves emotionally from the child but usually provide adequate physical care or constantly nag and scold the child

   _____ Formerly called Crippled Children's Services; provides financial assistance for children with various disabling conditions

   _____ Behavior in which parents place necessary and realistic restrictions on the child, encourage self-care activities, and promote reasonable physical and social abilities

4. Which one of the following diseases is the most common chronic childhood illness?
   a. Asthma
   b. Congenital heart disease
   c. Cancer
   d. Spina bifida

5. Which of the following is an example of how chronic illness and disability affect children's health, functional status, and family functioning?
   a. Families do not bring the disabled child for health care often.
   b. Siblings' routines are completely separated from the disabled child's.
   c. Parents are usually not able to meet the child's normal developmental needs.
   d. Disabled children are absent from school often.

6. Emphasizing the characteristics that the disabled child has in common with other children rather than viewing the disabilities within a pathological framework *best* describes which one of the following approaches to care of the disabled child?
   a. Chronological
   b. Developmental

7. A goal that would be considered *inappropriate* for family-centered care would be to:
   a. maintain family routine in the hospital.
   b. empower the family members.
   c. support the family during stressful times.
   d. maintain a high level of professional control.

8. The individual family service plan (IFSP) is:
   a. developed jointly by families and professionals.
   b. a comprehensive insurance plan for families with a disabled child.
   c. developed by a team of professionals for the disabled child.
   d. a plan that finances direct services for the disabled child.

9. When working with people of other cultural backgrounds who are caring for a child with a disability, the nurse should plan care that:
   a. uses a family member to translate into the language of the family.
   b. incorporates the generalized culture of the United States.
   c. recognizes that culture fully defines how the child and family will react.
   d. remains consistent with the cultural practices of the family when possible.

10. Match each developmental stage with the particular area of development in which a disability poses a challenge or risk at this stage.

   a. Infant   d. School-age child
   b. Toddler   e. Adolescent
   c. Preschooler

   _____ Self-concept/body image
   _____ Social development
   _____ Attachment
   _____ Mobility
   _____ Participation

11. A strategy that is recommended to promote normalization in children with special needs would be to:
    a. avoid discussing issues of appearance in the adolescent.
    b. focus on the areas of ability and competence.
    c. establish special family rules for the child with a disability.
    d. allow children with special needs to make all decisions about their care.

12. The child who is disabled tends to develop appropriate independence and achievement when the parents:
    a. protect the child from all dangers.
    b. establish reasonable limits.
    c. emphasize their limits.
    d. isolate the child to avoid peer rejection.

13. Which one of the following strategies would be *inappropriate* for the nurse to use when teaching families with children who are disabled?
    a. Give information that meets the current needs of the child.
    b. Give as much information as possible at the time of diagnosis.
    c. Answer the child's questions openly.
    d. Repeat information as often as needed.

14. The adolescent patient with a disability or chronic illness should be transferred to an adult provider:
    a. when the patient reaches the age of 18 years.
    b. when the patient reaches the age of 16 years.
    c. when the patient knows about his/her condition and is prepared for the transition.
    d. none of the above; it is better not to change providers.

15. The purpose of the initial assessment of the coping mechanisms of a child who is disabled is for the nurse to:
    a. determine help that the family may want or need.
    b. establish a rapport with the child and family.
    c. provide care from stage to stage of development.
    d. provide care from phase to phase of the disorder.

16. Which one of the following statements is *false* about family members' perceptions of a child's illness or disability?
    a. Children may interpret the reason for the illness/disability as a punishment.
    b. Family members are usually shocked to learn that their child has a serious illness/disability.
    c. Parents may interpret illness/disability as a punishment.
    d. Family members usually have no knowledge about the disorder when they learn their child has it.

17. Which of the following statements about the time of diagnosis is *false*?
    a. Parents may not remember all that is said.
    b. Parents remember the tone of the communication.
    c. Parents cannot sense the tone of communication.
    d. Parents may not hear all that is said.

18. When initially informing the family of a child's serious condition, the nurse should:
    a. explain that with time, everything will be all right.
    b. accept any emotional reaction without judgment.
    c. decide when and how to tell the child about the diagnosis.
    d. use therapeutic touch to stimulate free expression of feelings.

19. Describe at least three guidelines for the nurse to use when providing ongoing information to the family with a disabled or chronically ill child.

20. Parents in thriving families:
    a. stress normalcy and feel confident.
    b. have an enduring management style.
    c. feel competent but burdened.
    d. feel dominated by the illness.

21. The two most important environments of the child who is disabled or chronically ill are:

    _____ and _____.

22. Which one of the following factors is more characteristic of a father than a mother in adjusting to a child's chronic illness? The father is more likely to:
    a. use a practical approach or withdraw.
    b. use an emotional release.
    c. perceive he is coping poorly.
    d. view the child's temperament as influential.

23. To help siblings prepare for the changes that will occur in the disabled child, the nurse should:
    a. wait until questions are asked, because siblings often desire little or no involvement.
    b. recognize that permitting sibling hospital visits will increase stress in the whole family.
    c. reassure siblings that they will continue to be involved in the care whenever possible.
    d. help the sibling realize that the disabled child needs more parental attention.

24. Research indicates that compared with their peers, siblings of a child with a disability exhibit:
    a. greater independence.
    b. more maturity.
    c. an increased sense of responsibility.
    d. all of the above.

25. Which one of the following characteristics would most likey indicate that a sibling of a child with a disability is having difficulty?
    a. Sharing
    b. Withdrawal
    c. Competing
    d. Compromising

26. Describe how an extended family member may be a source of stress to the parents of the disabled or chronically ill child.

27. Identify each of the following coping behaviors as an approach behavior or an avoidance behavior.

    a. _____ A father stops at a friend's house and talks about his child's poor prognosis.

    b. _____ A father's alcohol use increases to the point of being excessive.

    c. _____ A mother tells the nurse that she is afraid to tell her child about his or her poor prognosis.

    d. _____ A mother never carries a glucose source for her toddler who takes insulin for type 1 diabetes mellitus.

    e. _____ A mother begins to cry in the nurse's office at school, saying that she always gets depressed at the beginning of the new year.

    f. _____ A father asks the nurse to explain a diagnosis again.

    g. _____ A mother asks her neighbor to watch her older child for a few hours while she is at the clinic.

28. Corbin and Strauss's "chronic illness trajectory" model is based on the idea that the:
    a. family understands the meaning of the illness situation.
    b. course of the illness changes over time.
    c. family member roles do not change with illness.
    d. coping patterns for the illness can be learned.

29. The adaptive coping process includes:
    a. cognitive tasks.
    b. behavioral tasks.
    c. emotional tasks.
    d. all of the above.

30. If the reaction of a family member to the diagnosis of a chronic illness is denial, the nurse would recognize that denial is:
    a. an abnormal response to grieving this type of loss.
    b. preventing treatment and rehabilitation.
    c. necessary to prevent disintegration.
    d. necessary for the child's optimum development.

31. Health professionals frequently work with people in denial, but many health professionals typically do *not*:
    a. actively attempt to remove the denial behaviors.
    b. repeatedly give blunt explanations.
    c. label denial as maladaptive.
    d. understand the concept of denial.

32. Hope in the chronically ill child's family would be considered:
    a. a way to absorb stress in a manageable way.
    b. negative coping with a serious diagnosis.
    c. a maladaptive mechanism for dealing with the inevitable death.
    d. to have the same meaning for the nurse and the family.

33. Describe at least two effective methods of support that would help families manage their emotional response to the diagnosis of a disability or chronic illness in their child.

34. A strategy for the nurse to encourage parents to express their feelings about the diagnosis of a chronic illness in their child would be to:
    a. tell them that what they are going through is completely understandable.
    b. help them focus on their emotions.
    c. explain the policies and procedures regarding visiting hours.
    d. review the disease process with them.

35. Parents who provide adequate physical care but detach themselves emotionally from the child characterizes the type of parental reaction known as:
    a. overprotection.
    b. denial.
    c. gradual acceptance.
    d. rejection.

36. The nurse's response to anger in parents of the disabled child should be:
    a. reciprocal anger.
    b. disapproval.
    c. acceptance.
    d. avoidance.

37. List at least five characteristics of parental overprotection.

38. Nurses who provide support to parents of a child with a disability should develop an attitude that has all of the following characteristics *except* the belief that:
    a. every person has burdens to bear.
    b. trust is a foundation for good communication.
    c. parents are experts about their own child.
    d. parents and professionals are colleagues.

39. When the parents of a child with special needs experience chronic sorrow, the process:
    a. of grief is pronounced and self-limiting.
    b. involves social reintegration after grieving.
    c. is characterized by realistic expectations.
    d. is interspersed with periods of intensified grief.

40. Which one of the following stressors can usually be predicted for a child with special needs?
    a. The approximate cost of the yearly medical bills
    b. The future needs for residential care
    c. The types of schooling and vocational training that will be needed
    d. The stress of developmental milestones and the start of school

41. The adjustment of the family to caring for and living with the child with special needs is greatly influenced by the:
    a. functional burden.
    b. severity of the condition.
    c. complexity of the care.
    d. resources required for care.

42. The effectiveness of the family's support system depends on the:
    a. ability to match the best source of support for each need.
    b. diversity of the family's social network.
    c. extended family and their availability.
    d. extended family and their resources.

43. Which of the following is *not* necessarily a criterion to consider when selecting parents to offer support to *other* parents of children with disabilities?
    a. The parents should possess advocacy and problem-solving skills.
    b. The parents should have a child with the same diagnosis.
    c. The parents should have a nonjudgmental approach to problem solving.
    d. The parents should be good listeners.

44. Fill in the blanks in the following statements.

    a. _____ _____ _____ is the term used for the interaction style of parents who have a high level of trust in the nurse and usually comply with rules.

    b. Parents who fit in the _____ _____ _____ category usually are very uncertain and may visit on a limited or irregular basis.

    c. If the parent is able to coordinate the child's complex chronic care and uses the nurse for consultation and direct care, he or she can be said to follow the pattern of a _____ _____

    _____.

    d. Parents who keep track of the staff and seek detailed information are referred to as

    _____ _____ _____.

45. Out-of-home placement of a child with a disability:
    a. may be the best option if the integrity of the family unit is in jeopardy.
    b. occurs if coping strategies are not employed within the home.
    c. is becoming increasingly more difficult to accomplish.
    d. demonstrates that the family is maladjusted.

46. The Crippled Children's Services, which provides financial assistance for children with many disabling conditions, is now known as:
    a. Programs for Children with Special Health Needs.
    b. National Information Center for Children and Youth with Disabilities.
    c. Association for the Care of Children's Health.
    d. Alliance for Health, Physical Education, Recreation and Dance.

Critical Thinking—Case Study

Jerome Thomas is a 15-month-old infant who was born prematurely and was discharged from the hospital at age 3 months after multiple invasive procedures, including intubation, ventilation, and surgery. He is delayed in his motor development, but other areas of development are progressing as would be expected for a prematurely born infant of his age. Jerome has recently been diagnosed with cerebral palsy. He is at the physician's office for a routine health check. His mother is with him.

47. In order to assess the family's adjustment to the diagnosis, the nurse would gather more information. One area that could be deferred to a later date would be the assessment of the family's:
    a. goals for the future.
    b. available support system.
    c. coping mechanisms.
    d. perception of the disorder.

Jerome's mother has returned to work part-time as a partner in a computer consulting firm. Jerome's father is a marketing consultant in the food industry and travels frequently. The parents, who are in their late thirties, have hired a woman whom they trust with Jerome's many needs to come into the home. Jerome, who is an only child, goes out of the home several times a week for therapy.

48. Based on the information given, select the *best* nursing diagnosis for Jerome.
    a. High risk for injury
    b. Maladaptive family processes
    c. Delayed growth and development
    d. Disturbed body image

49. With the selected diagnosis in mind, what is the expected outcome with the highest priority for Jerome?
    a. Jerome will attain the physical development that is appropriate for any 15-month-old.
    b. Jerome will attain psychosocial and cognitive development that is appropriate for any 15-month-old.
    c. Jerome will attain physical, psychosocial, and cognitive development that is appropriate for his age and abilities.
    d. Jerome's parents will set realistic goals for themselves and Jerome.

50. An intervention that would address the issues involved with altered family process related to the birth of Jerome and the complexity of his care after birth would be to:
    a. teach safety precautions.
    b. help the family achieve a realistic view of Jerome's capabilities and limitations.
    c. stress the importance of sound health practices and frequent health supervision.
    d. encourage responsibility of use of equipment and appliances.

51. Between now and Jerome's next visit at 24 months of age, the nurse should provide anticipatory guidance to the parents about Jerome's growth toward developing:
    a. a sense of trust and attachment to his parents.
    b. mastery of self-care skills.
    c. a sense of body image.
    d. through sensorimotor experiences.

CHAPTER 23

Family-Centered End-of-Life Care

1. Match each term with its description.

   a. Euthanasia   e. Palliative care   i. Burnout
   b. Assisted suicide   f. Hospice   j. Detached concern
   c. Drug tolerance   g. DNR
   d. Addiction   h. The Compassionate Friends

   _____ Occurs when someone provides the patient with the means to end his or her life and the patient uses that means to do so

   _____ Psychological dependence on the side effects of a drug; usually not a factor in pain management of terminally ill children

   _____ Active total care of patients whose disease is not responsive to curative treatment

   _____ The act of ending the life of a person who is suffering from a terminal condition; carried out by a person other than the suffering person; commonly referred to as "mercy killing"

   _____ One of the reasons for administering high doses of opioids for pain control in order to maintain the same level of pain relief

   _____ The level of involvement that allows sensitive, understanding care as a result of being sufficiently neutral to make objective rational decisions

   _____ A community health care organization that specializes in the care of dying patients and their families; combines the philosophy of dying as a natural process with palliative care

   _____ A state of physical, emotional, and mental exhaustion that occurs as a result of prolonged involvement with individuals in situations that are emotionally demanding; an occupational hazard to which nurses are susceptible

   _____ An indication to withhold cardiopulmonary resuscitation in response to cardiac arrest; "do not resuscitate"; no code

   _____ An international organization for bereaved parents and siblings

2. In children 5 to 9 years of age, the most frequent causes of death are:
   a. accidents, trauma, infectious illness, and suicide.
   b. injuries/trauma, cancer, and congenital anomalies.
   c. accidents/trauma, homicide, suicide, and cancer.
   d. prematurity, congenital birth defects, and infectious illness.

3. According to the American Nurses Association Code for Nurses, when caring for a terminally ill child, nurses are permitted to provide interventions that:
   a. actively aim to end a suffering child's life.
   b. relieve symptoms in a suffering child's life only if doing so poses a low risk for hastening death.
   c. offer relief to the dying child even if there is risk that death will occur.
   d. present the family with the means to end the dying child's life.

4. Describe three strategies nurses can use to communicate with families of children with life-threatening illness.

5. A nurse is about to present facts to parents about the possible death of their child. In this case, which of the following techniques would most effectively provide a setting conducive to communication?
   a. Acknowledging denial in the parents whenever it occurs
   b. Using only medical terms for all explanations
   c. Using body language to communication caring
   d. Recognizing feelings and reactions but not acknowledging them

6. When communicating with dying children, the nurse should remember that:
   a. older children tend to be concrete thinkers.
   b. when children can recite facts, they understand the implications of those facts.
   c. if children's questions direct the conversation, the assessment will be incomplete.
   d. games, art, and play provide a good means of expression.

7. When assisting parents in supporting their dying child, the nurse should stress the importance of honesty, because if parents are honest and openly discuss their fears, the child is more likely to:
   a. discuss his or her fears.
   b. ask fewer distressing questions.
   c. lose his or her sense of hope.
   d. do all of the above.

8. Fear of the unknown is one of the greatest threats to seriously ill children of which age group?
   a. Toddlers
   b. Preschoolers
   c. School-age children
   d. Adolescents

9. Immobilization is one of the greatest threats to seriously ill children of which age group?
   a. Toddlers
   b. Preschoolers
   c. School-age children
   d. Adolescents

10. Fear of punishment is one of the greatest threats to seriously ill children of which age group?
    a. Toddlers
    b. Preschoolers
    c. School-age children
    d. Adolescents

11. Inability to use their parents for emotional support is one of the greatest threats to seriously ill children of which age group?
    a. Toddlers
    b. Preschoolers
    c. School-age children
    d. Adolescents

12. Which one of the following age groups is most likely to suffer negative reactions to an altered body image as a result of a life-threatening illness?
    a. Young children
    b. School-age children
    c. Adolescents
    d. All age groups affected equally

13. Describe at least three benefits of implementing the hospice concept in the child's home environment.

14. Which one of the following interventions is *most* important for the dying child?
    a. Emotional support
    b. Preparing parents to deal with fears
    c. Relief from pain
    d. Control of pain

15. When the parent of a child who is dying tells the nurse the child is in pain, even when the child appears comfortable, the nurse should be sure that:
    a. p.r.n. pain control measures are instituted.
    b. pain control is administered on a regular preventive schedule.
    c. parents understand that pain is a physical process.
    d. parents understand that the child is probably in less pain than the parents think.

16. Interventions to help the family prepare for the care of a terminally ill child include:
    a. educating the family about complications of overfeeding or overhydration.
    b. providing a supply of medications to alleviate discomfort.
    c. encouraging fun and memorable activities.
    d. all of the above.

17. The sibling of a dying child may feel:
    a. displaced.
    b. isolated.
    c. resentful.
    d. all of the above.

18. List at least five physical signs of approaching death.

19. Methods to support the grieving families at the time of death and in the grieving period after death include:
    a. encouraging family members to avoid upsetting each other by keeping their feelings to themselves.
    b. consoling with phrases such as "I know how you feel."
    c. emphasizing that the painful grieving usually lasts less than a year.
    d. allowing the family time to stay with the child after the death.

20. List at least three activities that are characteristic of a child's behavior as death approaches.

21. The extended phase of mourning:
    a. usually takes about a year.
    b. is accompanied by support of the family at the funeral.
    c. may extend over years.
    d. can be eliminated if the family is well prepared.

22. Which one of the following strategies would be *best* for the nurse to use to support the family's spiritual needs when their child's death is imminent and a clergy member is unavailable?
    a. Pray appropriately with the family.
    b. Implement relaxation techniques.
    c. Make an appointment for the family to speak with an expert.
    d. Review the physical signs of death with the family.

23. When a child dies suddenly, which one of the following interventions would be *least* beneficial?
    a. Avoid having the family view the body of a disfigured child.
    b. Inform the family of what to expect when they see the disfigured body of their child.
    c. Offer the parents the opportunity to see the child's body even after resuscitation was performed.
    d. Arrange to have a health care worker with bereavement training meet with the family

24. Identify each of the following statements as either true or false.

    _____ Children with cancer, chronic disease, or infection or who have suffered prolonged cardiac arrest are excellent candidates for organ donation.

    _____ The nurse should never inquire whether organ donation was discussed with the child but should allow the family to come forward with this information on their own.

    _____ If organs are donated, the family will most likely need to choose a closed-casket funeral service.

    _____ Most families choose not to donate organs because of the high cost.

    _____ Many body tissues and organs can be donated, but their removal may cause mutilation of the body.

25. In regard to whether a child should attend the funeral of a loved one, the nurse should consider:
    a. the age of the child.
    b. that it will be a frightening experience.
    c. their responsibility to protect the child from distressing events.
    d. that attending the funeral may be useful to the child.

26. Current research supports the notion that:
    a. involvement in the experiences of the dying sibling is beneficial.
    b. siblings of children who died in the hospital reported readiness for the death.
    c. protecting the sibling of the dying child from the death rituals is beneficial.
    d. it is better for the sibling to remember the dying child as he or she was when alive.

27. Which one of the following techniques would be considered an example of the *most* therapeutic communication to use with the bereaved family?
    a. Cheerfulness
    b. Interpretation
    c. Validating loss
    d. Reassurance

28. Which one of the following helping statements would be *least* therapeutic for the nurse to use with the bereaved family?
    a. "You can stay with him and hold him if you wish."
    b. "It must be painful for you to return to the doctor's office without her."
    c. "Fortunately his suffering is over now."
    d. "Will your husband return to be with you soon?"

29. Which one of the following symptoms would be considered normal grief behavior?
    a. Depression
    b. Obsessive-compulsive behavior
    c. Hearing the dead person's voice
    d. All of the above

30. The resolution of grief usually:
    a. occurs in sequential phases.
    b. is completed in about 2 years.
    c. is completed in about 3 years.
    d. may take years with periods of intensification of grief.

31. Reorganization after the death of a child means that the:
    a. loved one is forgotten.
    b. pain is gone.
    c. survivors have "let go."
    d. survivors have recovered from their loss.

32. List at least three of the reactions that nurses have when caring for children with fatal illnesses.

33. Intervening therapeutically with terminally ill children and their families requires:
    a. only self-awareness.
    b. nursing practice that is based on a theoretical foundation.
    c. years of experience.
    d. all of the above

Critical Thinking—Case Study

Julie is a 6-year-old child with leukemia. She has undergone a bone marrow transplant with associated complications and has had several remissions. After the last remission she deteriorated rapidly. Her parents tell the nurse that they believe Julie is now in the final stages of her illness. Her parents also express their feelings of discouragement and depression.

34. How should the nurse approach the parents in regard to their feelings about Julie's impending death?
    a. The nurse should begin by assessing the reason for the depression.
    b. The nurse should be sure that Julie's parents know that repeated relapses with remissions are associated with a better prognosis.
    c. The nurse should begin to help the parents work through their depression.
    d. The nurse should use heavy sedation to help Julie and her parents cope with this phase.

35. As Julie's parents express their concerns, it becomes very clear that pain control is a fear for Julie and her parents. What strategy should the nurse use to help them deal with this fear?
    a. The nurse should assure the parents that all of Julie's pain will be eliminated.
    b. The nurse should use heavy sedation to help Julie and her parents cope with this phase.
    c. A regular preventive medication schedule should be adopted as pain develops.
    d. The pain medications should be given only intravenously when Julie is near death.

36. After Julie's death in late December, which one of the following evaluation strategies is *most* likely to help support and guide the family through the resolution of their loss?
    a. A written questionnaire
    b. A telephone call placed in early January
    c. A meeting with the family at the time of death
    d. A telephone call placed in early February

37. Which one of the following would be the *best* expected outcome for the nursing diagnosis of fear/anxiety when planning care for Julie in this terminal stage?
    a. Julie will discuss her fears without evidence of stress.
    b. Julie will exhibit no evidence of loneliness.
    c. Julie's parents are actively involved in Julie's care.
    d. Julie's parents demonstrate ability to provide care for her.

CHAPTER 24

The Child with Cognitive, Sensory, or Communication Impairment

1. Match each cognitive impairment with its description.

a. Cognitive impairment
b. Educable mentally retarded
c. Trainable mentally retarded
d. Bayley Mental and Motor Scales
e. Wechsler Preschool and Primary Scales of Intelligence (WPPSI-R)
f. Vineland Adaptive Behavior Scale
g. Primary prevention strategies
h. Secondary prevention activities
i. Tertiary prevention strategies
j. Task analysis
k. Trisomy 21
l. Translocation of chromosome 21
m. Mosaicism
n. Atlantoaxial instability
o. Fragile site

_____ Identification and early treatment of conditions; including (in the case of mental retardation) prenatal diagnosis or carrier detection of disorders such as Down syndrome and newborn screening for treatable inborn errors of metabolism such as congenital hypothyroidism, phenylketonuria, and galactosemia

_____ A general term that encompasses any type of mental deficiency; mental retardation

_____ Comprises about 10% of the mentally retarded population; moderately mentally retarded

_____ Comprises about 85% of all people with mental retardation; mildly retarded

_____ Used during the preschool years to make the diagnosis of mental retardation

_____ One of the tests most commonly used to diagnose mental retardation in infants, along with the Cattell Infant Intelligence Scale

_____ Used, along with the AAMR Adaptive Behavior Scale, to assess adaptive behaviors

_____ Treatment to minimize long-term consequences, including (in the case of mental retardation) early identification of conditions and appropriate therapies and rehabilitation services; medical treatment of coexisting problems such as hearing and visual impairment in Down syndrome and programs for infant stimulation, parent treatment, preschool education, and counseling services to preserve the integration of the family unit

_____ Interventions designed to preclude the occurrence of the condition, including (in the case of mental retardation) rubella immunization, genetic counseling (especially in terms of Down or fragile X syndrome), and preventing neural tube defects by the use of folic acid supplements during pregnancy

_____ Refers to cells with both normal and abnormal chromosomes; associated with 1%–3% of persons with Down syndrome; degree of impairment related to the percentage of cells with the abnormal chromosome makeup

_____ The process used to delineate the components for each step so that each step can be taught completely before proceeding to the next activity

_____ A genetic aberration that is usually hereditary and associated with 3%–6% of Down syndrome cases

_____ An extra chromosome 21 (group G), 92%–95% of Down syndrome cases have this genetic pattern

_____ Occurs in 15%–20% of children with Down syndrome; includes symptoms of neck pain, weakness, and torticollis, although most affected children are asymptomatic

_____ A region on the chromosome that fails to condense during mitosis; characterized by a nonstaining gap or narrowing

2. Match each hearing impairment term with its description.

a. Deaf
b. Hard of hearing
c. Conductive hearing loss
d. Sensorineural hearing loss
e. Mixed conductive-sensorineural hearing loss
f. Central auditory imperception

g. Organic type of central auditory imperception
h. Aphasia
i. Agnosia
j. Dysacusis
k. Functional type of hearing loss
l. Decibel (dB)

m. Hearing-threshold level
n. Cochlear implants
o. Closed captioning
p. Acoustic feedback
q. ASL/SEE/BSL
r. Telecommunication devices for the deaf (TDD)

_____ Refers to a person whose hearing disability precludes successful processing of linguistic information through audition, with or without a hearing aid

_____ Middle-ear hearing loss; results from the interference of transmission of sound to the middle ear; most common of all types of hearing loss; frequently a result of recurrent serous otitis media; mainly involves interference with loudness of sound

_____ Refers to a person who, generally with the use of a hearing aid, has residual hearing sufficient to enable successful processing of linguistic information through audition

_____ Includes all hearing losses that do not demonstrate defects in the conductive or sensorineural structures; divided into organic and functional classifications

_____ Perceptive deafness; nerve deafness; involves damage to the inner ear structures and/or the auditory nerve; commonly caused by congenital defects or a consequence of an acquired condition such as kernicterus; results in distortion of sound and problems in discrimination

_____ Results from interference with transmission of sound in the middle ear and along neural pathways; frequently caused by recurrent otitis media and its complications

_____ Defect involving the reception of auditory stimuli along the central pathways and the expression of the message into meaningful communication; e.g., aphasia, agnosia, and dysacusis

_____ Hearing loss with no organic lesion; e.g., conversion hysteria, infantile autism, and childhood schizophrenia

_____ Inability to express ideas in any form, either written or verbal

_____ The measurement of an individual's hearing threshold by means of an audiometer

_____ Inability to interpret sound correctly

_____ Difficulty in processing details or in discrimination among sounds

_____ A unit of loudness measured in frequencies; cycles per second

_____ A surgically implanted prosthetic device that converts sound to electrical impulses and feeds them directly to the auditory nerve

_____ Visual-gestural languages that use hand signals and concepts in the English language that roughly correspond to specific word; commonly referred to as "signing"

_____ A special decoding device that translates the audio portion of a television program into subtitles that appear written on the television screen

_____ An annoying whistling sound usually caused by improper fit of the ear mold of the hearing aid

_____ Special teletypewriters that help deaf people communicate over the telephone

3. Match each visual impairment term with its description.

a. Legal blindness
b. Partially sighted
c. Visual impairment
d. Refraction
e. Myopia
f. Hyperopia
g. Penetrating wounds of the eye

h. Nonpenetrating wound of the eye
i. Tapping method
j. Guides
k. Blindisms
l. Braille
m. Braillewriter

n. Braille slate/stylus
o. Library of Congress
p. Finger spelling
q. Tadoma method
r. John Tracy Clinic

_____ Trauma to the eye that is most often a result of sharp instruments such as sticks, knives, or scissors

_____ Portable systems for written communication used by the blind person

_____ A human or dog used to help a person who is visually impaired move around in the environment and avoid obstacles

_____ A general term that includes both school vision and legal blindness

_____ Condition in which light rays enter the lens and, rather than falling directly on the retina, fall in front of it

_____ A system that uses six raised dots to represent each letter and number

_____ Condition in which light rays enter the lens and, rather than falling directly on the retina, fall beyond it

_____ May be a result of foreign objects in the eye, lacerations, a blow from a blunt object such as a baseball or fist, or thermal or chemical burns

_____ Communication technique in which the letters are spelled into the deaf-blind child's hand and the child spells out ideas to the other person

_____ School vision; defined as visual acuity better than 20/200 but worse than 20/70 in the better eye with correction

_____ Use of a cane to survey the environment for direction and avoid obstacles

_____ Refers to the bending of light rays as they pass through the lens of the eye

_____ Self-stimulatory activities such as body rocking, finger flicking, or arm twirling; usually discouraged because they tend to retard the child's social acceptance

_____ A small typewriter-like device that enables the blind child to write a message

_____ Offers a home correspondence course for parents of the deaf-blind child

_____ Has talking books, braille books, and a special record program available for no cost to the blind person

_____ Defined as visual acuity of 20/200 or less and/or a visual field of 20 degrees or less in the better eye

_____ A type of tactile communication that involves the child placing the hand over the speaker's face and neck to monitor facial movements associated with speech production

4. Match each communication impairment term with its description.

a. Language
b. Receptive language
c. Expressive language
d. Speech
e. Developmental language disorder
f. Articulation errors

g. Dysfluencies
h. Stuttering/stammering
i. Block
j. Voice disorders
k. Blissymbols
l. Direct observation
m. Indirect assessment

n. Denver Articulation Screening Examination
o. Early Language Milestone Scale (ELM)
p. Denver II
q. Peabody Picture Vocabulary Test III

_____ A standardized screening instrument for assessing language development in children less than 3 years of age

_____ A method of assessing speech and language development that uses spontaneous language interaction between the child and nurse for children less than 3 years of age

_____ Speaking verbal symbols

_____ A communication impairment that occurs without impairment in other developmental realms

_____ Understanding the spoken word

_____ Rhythm disorders; usually consist of repetitions of sounds, words, or phrases

_____ Primarily refers to the symbol system used to convey thoughts or feelings to others

_____ The oral production of language, including articulation of sounds, rhythm, and tone

_____ One of the most common and potentially serious dysfluencies, characterized by tense repetition of sounds or complete blockages of sound or words; a normal characteristic of language development during the preschool years

_____ Sounds that a child makes incorrectly or inappropriately

_____ A highly stylized communication system consisting of graphic symbols that represent words, ideas, and concepts

_____ A useful screening instrument for word comprehension used for children ages 2 1/2 to 18 years

_____ A reliable, effective screening test to measure speech development that takes about 10 minutes to administer

_____ A stutter that is characterized by no sound coming out when the person tries to speak

_____ A revision of the Denver Developmental Screening Test that includes an expanded section with language items

_____ Characterized by differences in pitch, loudness, and/or quality

_____ A method of evaluating speech and language development that relies on parental information obtained through a history

5. Match each level of retardation/IQ range with its appropriate example of maturation or development.

a. Mild (50–55 to about 70)
b. Moderate (35–40 to 50–55)

c. severe (20–25 to 35–40)
d. profound (below 20–25)

_____ A preschool-age child with noticeable delays in motor development and in speech

_____ An adolescent who may walk but needs complete custodial care

_____ A school-age child who is able to walk and who can profit from systematic habit training

_____ A preschool-age child who may not be noticed as retarded but is slow to walk, feed self, and talk

6. The American Association on Mental Retardation definition of *mental retardation* includes:
   a. an intelligence quotient that is lower than 50.
   b. an emphasis on function.
   c. only intelligence and no other criteria.
   d. an age limit of 12.

7. List at least four early behavioral signs that are suggestive of cognitive impairment.

8. When teaching a child with a cognitive impairment, the *best* strategy for the nurse to use to present symbols in an exaggerated concrete form is:
   a. singing.
   b. memorizing.
   c. verbal explanation.
   d. ignoring the child.

9. Define the term *fading*.

10. Define the term *shaping*.

11. Acquiring social skills for the child who is mentally retarded includes:
    a. learning acceptable sexual behavior.
    b. being exposed to strangers.
    c. learning to greet visitors appropriately.
    d. all of the above.

12. Describe the pros and cons involved in the advisability of a marriage between two individuals with significant cognitive impairment.

13. Which of the following strategies would best help the mentally retarded child acquire social skills?
    a. Use discipline and negative reinforcement.
    b. Provide information about the importance of socialization skills.
    c. Use active rehearsal with role-playing and practice sessions.
    d. Use all of the above.

14. For the child who is cognitively impaired, the contraceptive choice that requires little compliance, produces amenorrhea, and provides long-term protection from pregnancy is:
    a. the intrauterine device.
    b. Depo-Provera.
    c. the diaphragm.
    d. oral contraception.

15. Define *task analysis* and describe its use when teaching a child who is mentally retarded.

16. The primary purpose of record keeping for 7 days prior to toilet training a mentally retarded child is to:
    a. determine the child's patterns of behavior and parents' response.
    b. determine the amount of urinary output and usual times the child urinates.
    c. assess the child's physical and psychological readiness to use the toilet.
    d. determine all of the above.

17. Describe the conditions necessary for a child with cognitive impairment to begin learning how to dress.

18. The mutual participation model of care for the child who is cognitively impaired and needs hospitalization would include:
    a. isolating the child from others to avoid conflicts.
    b. encouraging the parents to room in.
    c. having the parents perform all activities of daily living.
    d. having the nurse perform all activities of daily living.

19. Another name for trisomy 21 is:
    a. phenylketonuria.
    b. Turner syndrome.
    c. Down syndrome.
    d. galactosemia.

20. Testing of the parents is necessary to identify the carrier and offer genetic counseling when Down syndrome is caused by:
    a. mosaicism.
    b. translocation.
    c. maternal age over 40.
    d. paternal age over 40.

21. List five physical features that are found in the infant with Down syndrome.

22. Some research has shown that families who keep the child with Down syndrome at home report having:
    a. negative feelings for the child.
    b. a more accepting attitude toward others.
    c. higher divorce rates.
    d. more sibling problems.

23. Decreased muscle tone in the infant with Down syndrome:
    a. indicates inadequate parenting.
    b. is a sign of infant detachment.
    c. compromises respiratory expansion.
    d. predisposes the infant to diarrhea.

24. Fragile X syndrome is:
    a. the most common inherited cause of mental retardation.
    b. the most common inherited cause of mental retardation next to Down syndrome.
    c. caused by an abnormal gene on chromosome 21.
    d. caused by a missing gene on the X chromosome.

25. In regard to fragile X syndrome, an individual who is a carrier would have 50 to 100 excess repeats of nucleotide base pairs in a specific DNA segment of the X chromosome. This characteristic is also called:
    a. fragile site.
    b. fragile X syndrome.
    c. full mutation.
    d. permutation.

26. The correct term to use for a person whose hearing disability precludes successful processing of linguistic information through audition is:
    a. deaf-mute.
    b. mute.
    c. deaf.
    d. deaf and dumb.

27. Conductive hearing loss in children is most often a result of:
    a. the use of tobramycin and gentamicin.
    b. the high noise levels from ventilators.
    c. congenital defects.
    d. recurrent serous otitis media.

28. At what decibel (dB) level would a hearing loss be considered profound?
    a. Less than 30 dB
    b. 55–70 dB
    c. 71–90 dB
    d. Greater than 91 dB

29. One behavior associated with hearing impairment in the infant is:
    a. a monotone voice.
    b. consistent lack of the startle reflex to sound.
    c. a louder than usual cry.
    d. inability to form the word "da-da" by 6 months.

30. In the assessment of the child to identify whether a hearing impairment has developed, the nurse would look for:
    a. a loud monotone voice.
    b. consistent lack of the startle reflex.
    c. a high level of social activity.
    d. attentiveness, especially when someone is talking.

31. All of the following strategies will enhance communication with a child who is hearing-impaired *except*:
    a. touching the child lightly to signal presence of a speaker.
    b. speaking at eye level or a 45-degree angle.
    c. using facial expressions to convey the message better.
    d. moving and using animated body language to communicate better.

32. In order to *best* promote socialization for the child with a hearing impairment, teachers should:
    a. discourage hearing-impaired children from playing together.
    b. use frequent group projects to promote communication.
    c. use audiovisual-assisted instruction as much as possible.
    d. minimize background noise.

33. Care for the hearing-impaired child who is hospitalized should include:
    a. supplementing verbal explanations with tactile and visual aids.
    b. communicating only with parents to ensure accuracy.
    c. discouraging parents from rooming in.
    d. sending nonvocal communication devices home to avoid loss.

34. Which of the following situations would be considered abnormal?
    a. A neonate who lacks binocularity
    b. A toddler whose mother says he looks cross-eyed
    c. A five-year-old who has hyperopia
    d. Presence of a red reflex in a 7-year-old

35. If a child has a penetrating injury to the eye, the nurse should:
    a. apply an eye patch.
    b. attempt to remove the object.
    c. irrigate the eye.
    d. use strict aseptic technique to examine the eye.

36. Match each type of visual impairment with its description or characteristics.

    a. Astigmatism   d. Strabismus
    b. Anisometropia   e. Cataract
    c. Amblyopia   f. Glaucoma

    _____ Increased intraocular pressure
    _____ Squint or cross-eye; malalignment of eyes
    _____ Different refractive strength in each eye
    _____ Unequal curvatures in refractive apparatus
    _____ Opacity of crystalline lens
    _____ Lazy eye; reduced visual acuity in one eye

37. List at least eight strategies the nurse can use during hospitalization of a child who has lost his sight.

38. Which of the following statements is correct about eye care and sports?
    a. Glasses may interfere with the child's ability in sports.
    b. Face mask and helmet should be required gear for softball.
    c. Contact lenses provide less visual acuity than glasses for sports.
    d. It is usually very difficult to convince children to wear their glasses to play sports.

39. The method of communication used with the deaf-blind child that involves spelling into the child's hand is called:
    a. finger spelling.
    b. the Tadoma method.
    c. blindism.
    d. the tapping method.

40. In order to help the deaf-blind child establish communication, parents should:
    a. always place the child in the same place in the room to help identify surroundings.
    b. select a cue that is always used to help the child discriminate one person from another.
    c. limit the cues that are sent and received.
    d. limit stimulation to allow the child to feel safe.

41. Which one of the following examples would be *most* indicative of a language disorder?
    a. A 22-month-old child who has not uttered his first word
    b. A 38-month-old who has not uttered his first sentence
    c. An 18-month-old who uses short "telegraphic" phrases
    d. A 4-year-old who stutters

42. Which of the following statements about stuttering is correct?
    a. Stuttering is normal in the school-age child.
    b. Stuttering occurs because children do not know what they want to say.
    c. Undue emphasis on a stutter may cause an abnormal speech pattern.
    d. Chances for reversal of stuttering are good until about age 3 years.

43. One of the clinical manifestations associated with the speech sounds known as *articulation errors* is the:
    a. omission of consonants at the beginning of words.
    b. deviation in pitch or quality of the voice.
    c. pauses within a word.
    d. frequent use of circumlocutions.

44. Diagnostic criteria for autism include symptoms related to:
    a. social interaction.
    b. qualitative communication.
    c. repetitive behavior patterns.
    d. all of the above.

45. Strategies to use when caring for the hospitalized child with autism include:
    a. maintaining eye contact when explaining procedures.
    b. using holding and touch to comfort the child.
    c. adhering to a strict diet consisting of hypoallergenic foods.
    d. all of the above.

46. The parents of a child who is stuttering should be encouraged to:
    a. have the child start again more slowly.
    b. give the child plenty of time.
    c. show concern for the hesitancy.
    d. reward the child for proper speech.

47. Define the term *situated approach*.

48. Detecting communication disorders during early childhood:
    a. adversely affects the child's social relationships.
    b. increases the child's difficulty with academic skills.
    c. increases the child's ability to correct deficit skills.
    d. adversely affects the child's emotional interactions.

49. Following assessment and detection of a language problem, the nurse should advise the family to:
    a. wait and see what happens.
    b. wait, because the child will grow out of it.
    c. obtain a specialized evaluation.
    d. repeat words so that the child will learn more language.

50. Which one of the following findings would indicate a need for referral regarding a communication impairment?
    a. A 5-year-old who stutters
    b. A 3-year-old who omits word endings
    c. A 2-year-old with unintelligible speech
    d. A 3-year-old who substitutes easier sounds for difficult ones

Critical Thinking—Case Study

Paula Larson, a 9-month-old infant with Down syndrome (DS) who is also blind and deaf, is admitted to the hospital with pneumonia. She holds her head steady but cannot sit without support or pull up on the furniture. Paula squeals and laughs but does not imitate speech sounds or have any words, not even "da-da" or "ma-ma." She can shake a rattle but cannot pass a block from one hand to the other. She smiles spontaneously and holds her own bottle, but she does not play "pattycake" or wave "bye-bye."

Along with the developmental deficits, Paula has congenital heart anomalies and has been hospitalized many times for pneumonia and bronchiolitis. Paula's parents knew that she would be born with DS. They have chosen to care for Paula at home. Paula's care has become increasingly more time-consuming. During the admission assessment interview, Mr. and Mrs. Larson state they are both exhausted.

51. The nurse determines that Paula's developmental lag is *least* pronounced in the area of:
    a. gross motor skills.
    b. language skills.
    c. fine motor skills.
    d. personal-social skills.

52. Paula's parents have cared for her at home since her birth. Mrs. Larson expresses concern that she is not doing a good enough job and that perhaps it is time to consider placement out of the home for Paula. The nurse responds based on the knowledge:
    a. that the potential for development varies greatly in DS.
    b. that every available source of assistance to help Mr. and Mrs. Larson with the care of Paula should be explored.
    c. that the nurse's responses may influence Mr. and Mrs. Larson's decisions.
    d. all of the above.

53. Which one of the common nursing diagnoses used in planning care for mentally retarded children should take priority in Paula's current situation?
    a. Altered growth and development
    b. Altered family processes
    c. Anxiety related to the hospitalization
    d. Impaired social interaction

54. Mr. and Mrs. Larson make the decision to explore residential care for Paula. The *best* expected outcome during this time for Paula Larson would be for the parents to:
    a. demonstrate acceptance of Paula.
    b. express feelings and concerns regarding the implications of Paula's birth.
    c. make a realistic decision based on Paula's needs and capabilities as well as their own.
    d. identify realistic goals for Paula's future home care.

CHAPTER 25

Family-Centered Home Care

1. Match each term with its description.

   a. Home care
   b. Hospice
   c. Home care implementation areas
   d. Cost of care
   e. Individualized home care plan (IHCP)
   f. Care coordination
   g. Nurse case manager
   h. American Nurses Credentialing Center
   i. The Hospice Nurses Association
   j. Collaborative caring

   _____ The approach to nursing practice that allows the nurse and family to work together and share outcomes in a deep and meaningful way

   _____ Offers certification in hospice nursing

   _____ A single person who works with the family to accomplish the many tasks and responsibilities involved; should have a minimum of a baccalaureate degree in nursing and 3 years of experience; needs to be knowledgeable about community resources

   _____ Care provided for children and families with complex health care needs in the place of residence; for the purpose of promoting, maintaining, or restoring health or for maximizing the level of independence while minimizing the effects of disability and illness, including terminal illness

   _____ Intermittent skilled nursing visits and private-duty nursing

   _____ A subsidiary of the American Nurses Association; offers generalist and clinical specialist certification in both home health and community health

   _____ A program of palliative and supportive care services that provides physical, psychological, social, and spiritual care for dying persons, their families, and their loved ones

   _____ A critical factor that influences the numbers of technology-dependent children that are returned home more quickly than ever

   _____ The coordination of care across hospital, home, educational, therapeutic, and other settings to ensure continuity for the child and family; general focus is cost control, attainment of desired clinical outcomes, and the monitoring and evaluation of care provided

   _____ A general plan developed before discharge that ideally is developed with multidisciplinary input; should address the range of needs identified as part of the comprehensive predischarge assessment

2. Name at least two major reasons why care for complex medical conditions has moved from the hospital to the home setting.

3. Private-duty nursing is the area of pediatric home care nursing most likely to be used to care for:
   a. a child at risk, such as one with nonorganic failure to thrive.
   b. a medically stable child with multiple skilled nursing needs.
   c. a technology-dependent child (e.g., ventilator-dependent).
   d. all of the above.

205

4. The cost of home care for children dependent on medical technology is usually more than the cost of hospital care for:
   a. third-party payers.
   b. the government.
   c. the family.
   d. all of the above.

5. Pediatric home care is planned based on assessment of:
   a. parental ability.
   b. the complexity of the family.
   c. the home environment.
   d. all of the above.

6. Which one of the following situations would be of *most* concern to the nurse who was evaluating a family for the possibility of a discharge with home care?
   a. The preterm infant who will be managed with home care is stable after surgery for his congenital heart anomaly.
   b. The family of a child who will be on a ventilator at home has no telephone.
   c. The parents are asking about the availability of respite care.
   d. The mother plans to stop working outside the home to be with the infant.

7. List four major areas of predischarge assessment for the child who is dependent on medical technology.

8. List the elements of a quality home care agency.

9. The *best* strategy to use when planning for transition from hospital to home for the child with complex home care requirements is to:
   a. give the parents a trial period at home during which the parents provide some of the care.
   b. teach a family member all aspects of the child's care.
   c. allow the parents to provide total care in the hospital with support from the staff as needed.
   d. arrange a predischarge visit during the hospitalization by the home care nurse.

10. Ideally, home care of the child who is technology-dependent should be based on the concept of:
    a. traditional case management.
    b. independent care.
    c. primary care management.
    d. case management with care coordination.

11. According to the American Nurses Association, the qualifications of the nurse case manager should include:
    a. a baccalaureate degree in nursing.
    b. 3 years of experience.
    c. knowledge about community resources.
    d. all of the above.

12. List the responsibilities involved in pediatric home care coordination.

13. The pediatric home care nurse's practice includes all of the following *except*:
    a. consultation with peers to make most daily decisions.
    b. a high level of technical clinical expertise.
    c. knowledge of child development.
    d. the ability to support family autonomy.

14. The pediatric nurse in home care practice is expected to adhere to standards of practice developed by:
    a. the World Health Organization.
    b. the American Nurses Association.
    c. the Society for Pediatric Nurses.
    d. the National League for Nursing.

15. Strategies that promote the central goal of family-centered home care would include all of the following *except*:
    a. emphasizing family strengths.
    b. identifying family coping mechanisms.
    c. developing unidirectional communication.
    d. promoting family empowerment.

16. List five characteristics of collaborative caring.

17. Basic principles used to communicate with the family include all of the following *except*:
    a. informing families who will have access to the information.
    b. assuring families that they have the right to confidentiality.
    c. collecting all information firsthand.
    d. restricting communications with other professionals to clinically relevant information.

18. The nurse should use all of the following guidelines for communication with family members *except*:
    a. giving information slowly and repeating it as necessary.
    b. answering questions honestly.
    c. using medical terminology.
    d. encouraging family members to ask questions.

19. When conflict occurs between the family and the treatment nurse about the child's treatment, the nurse should first:
    a. call the physician and negotiate a change.
    b. contact the home care supervisor.
    c. respect parental preferences if no danger is posed.
    d. explain the correct way and have the family return a demonstration.

20. The nursing process in home care nursing practice integrates:
    a. normalization.
    b. various disciplines.
    c. family priorities.
    d. all of the above.

21. In home nursing practice the nurse allows the family members to maintain control over:
    a. their home.
    b. their child's care.
    c. their personal lives.
    d. all of the above.

22. When a family chooses *not* to pursue developmental intervention, the nurse should:
    a. develop an individual family service plan.
    b. ensure that developmental needs have been explained in a meaningful way.
    c. notify child protective services.
    d. perform all of the above.

23. Describe at least three of the general guidelines a nurse should use when a disagreement among the nurse and the family members arises in regard to the care of the child at home.

24. The school-age child who is physically able may be expected to participate in his or her own care by:
    a. doing no more than holding equipment and discarding used supplies.
    b. administering his or her own medicines with supervision.
    c. assuming responsibility for scheduling home visits.
    d. none of the above; the school-age child is too young to participate in his or her own care.

25. When a child requiring special medical care enters an education setting, the school personnel should:
    a. develop parent advocacy skills.
    b. train staff and caregivers.
    c. coordinate the educational plan.
    d. carry out all of the above.

26. A safety issue, specific to the home care child who is dependent on electrical equipment is the need to:
    a. have a telephone on site.
    b. be cared for by trained individuals.
    c. notify the telephone and electric companies that the family needs to be placed on a priority service list.
    d. have someone in the house at all times who knows how to perform cardiopulmonary resuscitation.

27. At night, the care of the child dependent on medical technology poses what safety concern?
    a. The child may become frightened from the strange noises.
    b. Accidental strangulation on equipment wires can occur during sleep.
    c. The lights must be kept brightly lit all night so that procedures can be performed correctly.
    d. All of the above.

28. Family-to-family support:
    a. promotes family strength through shared experiences.
    b. often relieves the health professional from his or her role in the primary support system.
    c. meets the specific emotional needs of all families.
    d. accomplishes all of the above.

Critical Thinking—Case Study

William Patterson, who is now 18 months old, was born with Werdnig-Hoffmann disease, a congenital neuromuscular disorder. His disease has developed to the point that he is unable to breathe for more than a few hours without ventilator assistance.

William's older brother George died 2 years ago from complications of the same disease. His parents took care of him at home until his death. William's parents are preparing for a similar progression of the disease, which means that William will probably be maintained at home on a ventilator for many months until his death.

The case manager assigned to William is the same nurse who was assigned to his brother 2 years ago. This nurse, Ruth, was instrumental in helping the family cope with the technical issues of home ventilator management and total parenteral nutrition, as well as the stressors of caring for their dying child.

29. Ruth is concerned about crossing the boundary between collaborating with the Patterson family and becoming enmeshed in the family system as she did when George was dying. Ruth knows that the family is able to care technically for William, but she feels as if she also needs to be involved again in some way. Ruth has consulted her supervisor for advice. Based on the preceding information, the supervisor is *most* likely to suggest:
    a. reassignment.
    b. psychological counseling for Ruth.
    c. assessment of the therapeutic relationship.
    d. psychological counseling for the Pattersons.

30. If William suddenly becomes less active and demonstrates regressive behavior the nurse should implement a plan that addresses William's stage of development, and use strategies to better promote:
    a. oral-motor development.
    b. mobility and exploration.
    c. self-care.
    d. independence in home management.

31. The quality of William's home care would *best* be evaluated by asking:
    a. Ruth to review the goals.
    b. the Pattersons to review the goals.
    c. Ruth and the Pattersons to jointly review the goals.
    d. the Pattersons to complete an evaluation questionnaire.

CHAPTER 26

Family-Centered Care of the Child During Illness and Hospitalization

1. The following terms are related to children's reactions to hospitalization. Match each term with its description.

a. Stressors   e. Detachment   i. Depression
b. Anaclitic depression   f. Disbelief   j. Family-centered care
c. Protest   g. Anger, guilt   k. Self-care
d. Despair   h. Fear, anxiety, frustration

_____ The practice of activities that individuals initiate and perform on their own behalf to maintain life, health, and well-being

_____ The philosophy of care that recognizes the integral role of the family in a child's life and acknowledges the family as an essential part of the child's care and illness experience

_____ Usually occurs when the acute crisis is over; may be related to concerns for the child's future well-being, including negative effects produced by hospitalization and financial burden incurred

_____ Common feelings expressed by parents as they respond to their child's illness; often related to the type of trauma and pain inflicted on the child and lack of information provided to the parents

_____ Reactions that parents have following the realization of their child's illness; characterized by questioning their adequacy as caregivers

_____ The characteristic initial reaction parents have to their child's illness, especially if the illness is sudden and severe

_____ Also called "denial," the uncommon third phase of separation anxiety, in which superficially the child appears to have finally adjusted to the loss; behavior that is a result of resignation and not a sign of contentment

_____ The phase of separation anxiety in which the child stops crying, is much less active, and withdraws from others

_____ A phase of separation anxiety in which children cry loudly, scream for parents, refuse the attention of anyone else, and are inconsolable in their grief

_____ Separation anxiety; the major stress from middle infancy throughout the preschool years

_____ Events that produce stress

2. Match each pain management term with its description.

a. Pain
b. Narcotic addiction
c. Drug tolerance
d. Physical dependence
e. QUESTT
f. Pseudoaddiction
g. Pain assessment record
h. Titration
i. Ceiling effect
j. Nonopioids

k. Opioids
l. Coanalgesics
m. American Society of Pain Management Nurses
n. First pass effect
o. Equianalgesia
p. Patient-controlled analgesia
q. Epidural analgesia
r. Oral transmucosal/ trandermal routes

s. EMLA
t. Numby Stuff
u. Intradermal route
v. Buffered lidocaine
w. Around the clock (ATC)
x. Respiratory depression
y. Constipation
z. Pruritus
aa. Nausea/vomiting and sedation

_____ Physiologic, involuntary effect manifested by withdrawal symptoms when chronic use of opioid is abruptly discontinued or opioid antagonist such as naloxone is administered

_____ Equal analgesic effect; conversion factors developed for selected opioids when a change is made from intravenous to oral to account for the first pass effect

_____ Defined as "whatever the experiencing person says it is, existing whenever the person says it does"; implies to patients that they are believed

_____ The term used to indicate that doses higher than the recommended dose will not produce greater pain relief

_____ The phenomenon that occurs in individuals who have severe, unrelieved pain, in which they may become intensely focused on finding relief for their pain; includes behaviors that are suggestive of addiction, such as "clock watching"

_____ Behavioral, voluntary pattern characterized by compulsive drug-seeking behavior leading to overwhelming involvement with use and procurement of drug for purposes other than medical reasons, such as pain relief

_____ Suitable for mild to moderate pain; includes acetaminophen, nonsteroidal anti-inflammatory drugs

_____ Used to monitor the effectiveness of pain interventions and evaluate regimens to provide maximum pain relief with minimum side effects

_____ A specific approach to pain assessment

_____ Physiologic, involuntary need for larger dose of opioid to maintain original analgesic effect

_____ The gradual adjustment of drug dosage until optimum pain relief without excessive sedation is achieved

_____ Drugs that act primarily at site of the central nervous system; needed for moderate to severe pain

_____ Anesthetic cream; a eutectic mixture of local anesthetics (lidocaine 2.5% and prilocaine 2.5%); penetrates intact skin

_____ A procedure in which a catheter is usually placed into the space of the spinal column at the lumbar or caudal level in younger children; has recently increased in use for postoperative pain management in pediatric patients

_____ The professional organization that has issued a position statement against the use of placebos, because their use raises serious ethical and legal questions and can destroy the patient's trust in health care staff

_____ A common, sometimes serious, side effect of opioids that decreases peristaltic activity and increases anal sphincter tone, central nervous system

_____ Uses mild electrical current (iontophoresis) to actively push lidocaine with epinephrine into intact skin

_____ Provide nontraumatic preoperative and preprocedural analgesia and sedation

_____ Administration of parenteral analgesics in which the patient controls the amount and frequency of the analgesic

_____ Reduces the stinging sensation that initially occurs with injection

_____ Adjuvant analgesics; may be used alone or with opioids to control pain symptoms, although they may or may not have analgesic properties; e.g., Valium, Versed

_____ The rapid absorption from the gastrointestinal tract and partial metabolism in the liver before the drug reaches the central circulation, thus causing the loss of some of the drug's potency

_____ A preventive schedule of medication that is more effective than sporadic administration for continuous pain control

_____ Side effects of opioid administration that subside after about 2 days

_____ The most serious complication of pain medication administration; is most likely to occur in sedated patients

_____ A common side effect from epidural or IV infusions for pain; treated with low doses of naloxone infused slowly, with IV nalbuphine, or oral antihistamines

_____ Often used to inject a local anesthetic, typically lidocaine, into the skin to reduce pain from a procedure such as lumbar puncture, bone marrow aspiration, or venous arterial access

3. Match each hospitalization term with its description.

    a. Play therapy   d. Postvention

    b. Therapeutic play   e. Interdisciplinary team approach

    c. Child-life specialists

_____ An effective nondirective modality for helping children deal with their concerns and fears; often helps the nurse to gain insights into the child's needs and feelings

_____ A shift from the multidisciplinary team approach; team members typically share leadership, and decisions are made by consensus

_____ Technique used as an interpretive method with emotionally disturbed children by trained and qualified therapists

_____ Counseling subsequent to the event

_____ Health care professionals with intensive knowledge of child growth and development and the special psychosocial needs of children who are hospitalized and their families; help prepare children for hospitalization, surgery, and procedures

4. Separation anxiety would be _most_ expected in the hospitalized child at age:
    a. 3 to 6 months.
    b. 16 to 30 months.
    c. 30 months to 2 years.
    d. 2 to 4 years.

5. Match each phase of separation anxiety with the behaviors that are typical of that phase.

    a. Protest

    b. Despair

    c. Detachment

_____ Withdraws from others; is inactive, depressed, sad, uninterested in environment, uncommunicative, regressive

_____ Shows increased interest in surroundings; interacts with caregivers; appears happy; forms new but superficial relationships (rarely seen in hospitalized children)

_____ Cries continuously; screams; attacks stranger physically and verbally; attempts to escape

6. One difference between the toddler and the school-age child in their reactions to hospitalization is that the school-age child:
    a. does not experience separation anxiety.
    b. has coping mechanisms in place.
    c. relies on his or her family more than the toddler.
    d. experiences separation anxiety to a greater degree.

7. A toddler is most likely to react to short-term hospitalization with feelings of loss of control that are manifested by:
    a. regression.
    b. withdrawal.
    c. formation of new superficial relationships.
    d. self-assertion and anger.

8. The technique that is most appropriate to prepare a preschool-age child for a painful procedure is to:
    a. encourage the child to act grown up.
    b. demonstrate the procedure.
    c. verbally instruct the child.
    d. allow structured choices.

9. Which one of the following statements about getting a cold is *most* characteristic of the toddler?
    a. "I got this cold because I did not wear my hat."
    b. "I got this cold by breathing in bacteria."
    c. "I got this cold because I feel sick."
    d. "I got this cold from harmful germs."

10. The *most* consistent indicator of distress in infants is:
    a. initial cry.
    b. heart rate.
    c. facial expression.
    d. uncooperativeness.

11. School-age children with chronic illness are *most* likely to be concerned about which one of the following stressors?
    a. Pain
    b. Physical symptoms
    c. Strange surroundings
    d. Intrusive procedures

12. Which one of the following risk factors would make a child more vulnerable to the stresses of hospitalization?
    a. Urban dwelling
    b. Strong will
    c. Female gender
    d. Passive temperament

13. Complex care of the pediatric population in the hospital today differs from the pediatric population of 10 years ago in that the usual length of stay has:
    a. decreased and the acuity has increased.
    b. increased and the acuity has decreased.
    c. increased and the acuity has increased.
    d. decreased and the acuity has decreased.

14. Describe at least one of the possible psychological benefits a child might gain from hospitalization.

15. Which one of the following factors, according to Craft's 1993 framework, would be considered *most* likely to negatively influence the reactions of siblings to the hospitalized child?
    a. The sibling is an adolescent.
    b. Care providers are not relatives.
    c. The sibling has received information about the ill child.
    d. The ill child is cared for in the home.

16. Which one of the following statements is true in regard to parent participation in the hospitalized child's care?
    a. The parents need 24-hour responsibility to help maintain their feeling of importance to the child.
    b. Fathers and mothers need the same kind of support during the hospitalization of their child.
    c. Nurses may express support of parent participation but may not foster an environment that encourages parental involvement.
    d. Mothers feel comfortable assuming responsibility for their child's care.

17. List three strategies nurses can use to help minimize stresses for the parents of the hospitalized child.

18. To help the parent deal with issues related to separation while their child is hospitalized, the nurse should *not* suggest:
    a. using associations to help the child understand time frames.
    b. ways to explain departure and return.
    c. quietly leaving while the child is distracted or asleep.
    d. short frequent visits over an extended stay if rooming in is impossible.

19. Which one of the following strategies should the nurse use to help the hospitalized child adjust to the strange environment?
    a. Discontinue school lessons.
    b. Evaluate stimuli from the adult point of view.
    c. Send personal items home to prevent loss.
    d. Combine familiar sights with the unfamiliar.

20. Strategies used to minimize the hospitalized child's feelings of loss of control include attempts to:
    a. alter the child's schedule to match the hospital schedule.
    b. establish a daily schedule for the hospitalized child.
    c. eliminate rituals that have been used at home.
    d. perform all of the above.

21. The Joint Commission on Accreditation of Healthcare Organizations recommends that children's rights and responsibilities during hospitalization be:
    a. the same as those of adults.
    b. the same throughout the agency.
    c. different from those of adults.
    d. prominently displayed as a "Bill of Rights" for parents.

22. Whenever performing a painful procedure on a child, the nurse should attempt to:
    a. perform the procedure in the playroom.
    b. standardize techniques from one age to the next.
    c. perform the procedure quickly and safely.
    d. have the parents leave during the procedure.

23. After administering an intramuscular injection, the nurse would *best* reassure the young child with poorly defined body boundaries by:
    a. telling the child that the bleeding will stop after the needle is removed.
    b. using a large bandage to cover the injection site.
    c. using a small bandage to cover the injection site.
    d. using a bandage but removing it a few hours after the injection.

24. One way to evaluate whether a child fears mutilation of body parts is to:
    a. explain the procedure.
    b. ask the child to draw a picture of what will happen.
    c. stress the reason for the procedure.
    d. investigate the child's individual concerns.

25. Which of the following reactions to surgery is *most* typical of an adolescent's reaction of fear of bodily injury?
    a. Concern about the pain
    b. Concern about the procedure itself
    c. Concern about the scar
    d. Understanding explanations literally

26. List the six strategies used in the QUESTT approach to pain assessment.

    Q

    U

    E

    S

    T

    T

27. In regard to pain management, nurses tend to:
    a. overtreat children's pain more often than adults'.
    b. undertreat children's pain more often than adults'.
    c. overestimate the existence of pain in children but not in adults.
    d. overestimate the existence of pain in both children and adults.

28. Identify the following statements about pain in children as true or false.
    a. _____ Children may not realize how much they are hurting when they are in constant pain.
    b. _____ Children always tell the truth about pain.
    c. _____ Narcotics are no more dangerous for children than they are for adults.
    d. _____ Neonates have the mechanisms to transmit noxious stimuli by 20 weeks gestation.
    e. _____ Children cannot tell you where they hurt.
    f. _____ Younger children tend to rate procedure-related pain higher than older children.
    g. _____ A 3-year-old child can use a pain scale.

h. _____ Respirator depression is most likely to occur when the opioid is administered with another sedating drug.

i. _____ Children tolerate pain better than adults.

j. _____ Children may not admit having pain in order to avoid an injection.

k. _____ Infants do not feel pain if they are asleep.

l. _____ Children may believe that the nurse knows if they are hurting.

m. _____ Children become accustomed to pain or painful procedures.

n. _____ Children's signs of discomfort often increase with repeated painful procedures.

o. _____ The active resistant child may rate pain lower than the passive accepting child.

p. _____ Addiction from opioids used to treat pain is rare in children.

q. _____ Respiratory depression from opioids is uncommon in children.

r. _____ The child's behavior indicates the intensity of the pain.

s. _____ Infants 6 months of age or older metabolize opioids similarly to older children.

t. _____ An effective and safe combination of drugs for conscious sedation is Demerol, Phenergan, and Thorazine.

u. _____ A benefit of the sublingual route is direct absorption of the drug into the blood stream.

29. The Wong-Baker FACES pain rating scale:
    a. is easy to use but less reliable than other methods.
    b. is a rating of how children are feeling.
    c. has a coding system from .04 to .97.
    d. consists of six cartoon faces.

30. The Oucher rating scale:
    a. consists of six cartoon faces.
    b. consists of six photographs of faces.
    c. uses descriptive words.
    d. uses a straight line.

31. The Poker Chip Tool:
    a. is recommended for children who understand the value of numbers.
    b. does not offer an option for "no pain."
    c. uses a picture of four different colored poker chips.
    d. is recommended for children under 3 years of age.

32. In regard to behavioral and physiologic responses to pain, children:
    a. remain consistent from age to age.
    b. vary widely in their responses.
    c. exhibit typical behaviors at each developmental stage.
    d. are unaffected by temperament.

33. Which one of the following characteristics is *most* likely to be exhibited by an adolescent who is in pain?
    a. Decreased verbal expression and withdrawal
    b. Requests to terminate the procedure
    c. Verbal expression such as "You're hurting me!"
    d. Facial expression of pain and anger

34. The most reliable indicators of pain can be determined by verbal statements from the:
    a. Father
    b. Mother
    c. Nurse
    d. Child

35. Which one of the following pain assessment scales uses blood pressure as a variable?
    a. Behavior Pain Score (BPS)
    b. Children's Hospital of Eastern Ontario Pain Scale (CHEOPS)
    c. Nurses Assessment of Pain Inventory (NAPI)
    d. Objective Pain Score (OPS)

36. Which one of the following statements is true in regard to nonpharmacologic pain management?
    a. When used properly, nonpharmacologic measures are a good substitute for analgesics.
    b. Whenever possible, nonpharmacologic and pharmacologic measures should be combined to manage pain.
    c. Nurses and physicians are well educated about nonpharmacologic approaches to pain management.
    d. Nonpharmacologic approaches to pain management are not effective with children.

37. Identify three specific nonpharmacologic strategies that can be used to manage pain.

38. The Food and Drug Administration has recalled herbal pain management products that pose potential health risk and may cause kidney damage. The recalled products are those that contain:
    a. aristolochic acid.
    b. paracetamol.
    c. magnesium trisalicylate.
    d. acetylsalicylic acid.

39. Which one of the following opioids is considered the gold standard for severe pain management?
    a. Hydromorphone
    b. Fentanyl
    c. Oxycodone
    d. Morphine

40. If oral hydromorphone is *not* controlling the child's pain, which action should occur *first*?
    a. Change to morphine.
    b. Increase the dose.
    c. Change to fentanyl.
    d. Change to intravenous hydromorphone.

41. Describe the three typical methods of drug administration used with PCA devices.

42. When using patient-controlled analgesia (PCA) with children, the:
    a. drug of choice is meperidine.
    b. parent should control the dosing.
    c. nurse should control the dosing.
    d. drug of choice is morphine.

43. Which one of the following methods of analgesic drug administration is a liquid gel that provides anesthesia to nonintact skin in about 15 minutes?
    a. Midazolam
    b. EMLA
    c. LAT
    d. Numby Stuff

44. The anesthetic EMLA is used:
    a. before invasive procedures.
    b. as preoperative oral sedation.
    c. for chronic cancer pain.
    d. postoperatively.

45. Which one of the following guidelines should be followed when using EMLA?
    a. Explain that it is like "magic cream that takes hurt away."
    b. Apply a thin layer over intact skin.
    c. Leave the cream in place for about 20 to 30 minutes.
    d. Leave the cream in place for about 60 to 90 seconds.

46. For postoperative or cancer pain control, analgesics should be administered:
    a. whenever needed.
    b. around the clock.
    c. before the pain escalates.
    d. after the pain peaks.

47. The *most* common side effect from opioid therapy is:
    a. respiratory depression.
    b. pruritus.
    c. nausea and vomiting.
    d. constipation.

48. Treatment of tolerance to opioid therapy includes:
    a. discontinuing the drug.
    b. decreasing the dose.
    c. increasing the dose.
    d. increasing the duration between doses.

49. List three functions of play in the hospitalized child.

50. When helping parents to select activities for their hospitalized child, the nurse should recommend:
    a. simpler activities than would normally be chosen.
    b. new toys and games to help distract the child.
    c. challenging new games to keep the child engaged.
    d. games that can be played with adults.

51. List at least two ways that drawing or painting can be used by the nurse in caring for the hospitalized child.

52. The nurse can facilitate the hospitalized child's feelings of self-mastery by:
    a. acknowledging uncooperative behavior.
    b. acknowledging negative behavior.
    c. emphasizing aspects of the child's competence.
    d. providing emotional support to the family.

53. Preparation for hospitalization reduces stress in which of the following age groups?
    a. Infancy
    b. Toddlerhood
    c. Preschool
    d. All of the above

54. Define the role of a child-life specialist.

55. Questions related to activities of daily living at the time of admission are:
    a. inappropriate and should be saved for later.
    b. directed toward evaluation of the child's preparation for hospitalization.
    c. asked directly and in the order provided on the assessment form.
    d. designed to help the nurse develop appropriate routines for the hospitalized child.

56. Describe at least three strategies that can be used in the intensive care unit to support the child and family.

57. The question "How does your child act when annoyed or upset?" would be asked on admission to assess the child's:
    a. health perception-health management pattern.
    b. cognitive-perceptual pattern.
    c. activity-exercise pattern.
    d. self-perception/self-concept pattern.

58. The question "How does your child usually handle problems or disappointments?" would be asked on admission to assess the child's:
    a. role-relationship pattern.
    b. sexuality-reproductive pattern.
    c. coping-stress tolerance pattern.
    d. value-belief pattern.

59. The advantages of a hospital unit specifically for adolescents include:
    a. exclusive group membership.
    b. fewer preparation requirements.
    c. increased socialization with peers.
    d. all of the above.

60. The benefit of the ambulatory/outpatient setting is reduction of:
    a. stressors.
    b. infection risk.
    c. cost.
    d. all of the above.

61. Discharge instructions from the ambulatory setting should always include all of the following *except*:
    a. guidelines for when to call.
    b. dietary restrictions.
    c. activity restrictions.
    d. referral to a home health agency.

62. When caring for the child in isolation, the nurse should:
    a. spend as little time as possible in the room.
    b. teach the parents to care for the child to decrease the risk for spreading infection.
    c. let the child see the nurse's face before donning the mask.
    d. perform all of the above.

63. Define *postvention* and describe a situation in which it would be therapeutic.

64. The *most* ideal way to support parents when they first visit the child in the intensive care unit is:
    a. for the nurse to accompany them to the bedside.
    b. to use picture books of the unit in the waiting area.
    c. to limit the visiting hours so that parents are encouraged to rest.
    d. to expect parents to stay with their child continuously.

65. Transfer from the intensive care unit to the regular pediatric unit can be *best* facilitated by:
    a. discussing the details of the transfer at the bedside, where the child can listen.
    b. establishing a schedule that mimics the child's home schedule.
    c. assigning a primary nurse from the regular unit who visits the child before the transfer.
    d. explaining to the family that there are fewer nurses on the regular unit.

66. Transitional care, which is a trial period for the family to assume the child's care with minimum supervision, may take place:
    a. on the nursing unit.
    b. during a home pass.
    c. in a motel near the hospital.
    d. at or during any of the above.

Critical Thinking—Case Management

Peter Chen is an 8-year-old child who is admitted to the pediatric unit for an appendectomy. He is in the third grade and is very active in after-school activities. Recently he began to take karate lessons, and he also plays baseball. Peter loves school, particularly when he is able to read. He awakens every morning at 6 a.m. to read, and reading is the last thing he does before he falls asleep.

Peter's parents are with him during the admission interview. His mother works, but she has made arrangements to take some time off after surgery and during his hospital stay to be available to him.

67. Based on the preceding information, the nurse should expect:
    a. a normal response to hospitalization.
    b. more anxiety than would normally be seen.
    c. difficulty with the parents.
    d. cultural factors to take precedence.

68. The nurse identifies which of the following nursing diagnoses after surgery for Peter?
    a. Powerlessness related to the environment
    b. Activity intolerance related to pain or discomfort
    c. Anxiety/fear related to distressing procedures
    d. Any of the above

69. One reasonable expected outcome for Peter's diagnosis of powerlessness would be which of the following?
    a. Peter will tolerate increasingly more activity.
    b. Peter will remain injury-free.
    c. Peter will play and rest quietly.
    d. Peter will help plan his care and schedule.

70. Which one of the following interventions would be *best* for the nurse to incorporate into Peter's plan related to the diagnosis of activity intolerance?
    a. Organize activities for maximum sleep time.
    b. Keep side rails up.
    c. Choose an appropriate roommate.
    d. Assist with dressing and bathing.

Pediatric Variations of Nursing Interventions

1. The following terms are related to pediatric procedures. Match each term with its description.

a. Mature minors doctrine
b. Emancipated minor
c. Assent
d. Conscious sedation
e. Deep sedation

f. Nitrous oxide
g. Malignant hyperthermia (MH)
h. Compliance
i. Adherence

j. Organizational strategies
k. Educational strategies
l. Treatment strategies
m. Behavioral strategies
n. Contracting

_____ Interventions that are designed to modify behavior directly, with the goal of improving compliance; e.g., positive reinforcement and contracting

_____ Usually a verbal agreement; requires that the child be informed about the proposed treatment or research and that the child concurs with the decisions made by the person who gives consent

_____ One who is legally under the age of majority but is recognized as having the legal capacity of an adult under circumstances prescribed by state law

_____ Adherence; refers to the extent to which a patient follows medical advice in terms of taking medication, following diets, or executing other lifestyle changes

_____ Permits some patients who are not legally adults to give consent as long as they understand the consequences of their decisions

_____ Interventions that are related to the child's refusal or inability to take a prescribed medication or follow a prescribed treatment regimen; used to improve compliance

_____ Used to achieve conscious sedation; administered in concentrations of 50% or less, the balance of the mixture being oxygen

_____ A medically controlled state of depressed consciousness that allows protective reflexes to be maintained, retains the patient's ability to maintain a patent airway independently and continuously, and permits appropriate response by the patient to physical stimulation or verbal comment

_____ Interventions that are concerned with instructing the child and family about the treatment plan; used to improve compliance

_____ A potentially fatal genetic myopathy that occurs in the perioperative period and demands immediate attention; characterized by hypermetabolism, muscle rigidity, and an elevated temperature

_____ A process in which the exact elements of desired behavior are explicitly outlined in the form of a written agreement; a very effective method of shaping behavior, especially with older children who are involved in the process of defining the rules of the agreement; coincides with the prescribed regimen

_____ Interventions that are concerned with the care setting and the therapeutic plan; used to improve compliance

_____ A medically controlled state of depressed consciousness or unconsciousness from which the patient is not easily aroused

_____ Another term for compliance; refers to the extent to which the patient's behavior coincides with the prescribed regimen

222

2. The following terms are related to general hygiene and care. Match each term with its description.

a. Pressure ulcers
b. Pressure reduction device
c. Pressure relief device
d. Friction
e. Shear

f. Epidermal stripping
g. Set point
h. Fever
i. Hyperthermia
j. Chill phase

k. Plateau
l. Defervescence
m. Reactive hyperemia

_____ Flush; the earliest sign of tissue compromise and pressure-related ischemia

_____ Hyperpyrexia; an elevation in set point such that the body temperature is regulated at a higher level; may be arbitrarily defined as temperature above 38° C (100° F)

_____ The point in the febrile state in which shivering and vasoconstriction generate and conserve heat and raise the central temperatures to a level of the new set point

_____ The point during the febrile state in which the temperature stabilizes at the higher range

_____ Can develop when the pressure on the skin and underlying tissues is greater than the capillary closing pressure, causing capillary occlusion; results in tissue anoxia and cellular death; most commonly occurs over a bony prominence

_____ The result of the force of gravity pulling down on the body and friction of the body against a surface; occurs, for example, when a patient is in the semi-Fowler position and begins to slide to the foot of the bed

_____ A product used to decrease the pressure that occurs with a regular hospital bed or chair; usually consists of an overlay that is placed on top of the regular mattress

_____ Occurs when the surface of the skin rubs against another surface, such as the sheets on a bed

_____ A product that maintains pressure below the level that would cause capillary closing; usually consists of a high-technology bed used for patients who have multiple problems and cannot be turned effectively

_____ A situation in which body temperature exceeds the set point; usually occurs when the body or external conditions create more heat than the body can eliminate, such as in heat stroke, aspirin toxicity, or hyperthyroidism

_____ The point when the temperature is greater than the set point or when the pyrogen is no longer present

_____ Results when the epidermis is unintentionally torn away when tape is removed

_____ The temperature around which body temperature is regulated by a thermostat-like mechanism in the hypothalamus

3. The following terms are related to safety and collection of specimens. Match each term with its description.

a. Nosocomial
b. Standard precautions
c. Transmission-based precautions
d. Airborne precautions

e. Droplet precautions
f. Contact precautions
g. Direct contact transmission
h. Indirect contact transmission

i. Bladder catheterization
j. Suprapubic aspiration
k. Allen test
l. Gastric washings
m. Nasal washings

_____ Lavage; used to collect a sputum specimen from infants and small children who are unable to follow directions to cough effectively and who may swallow sputum produced when they do

_____ Designed to reduce the risk for transmission of infectious agents that are spread when large particles generated during coughing, sneezing, or talking come into contact with the conjunctiva or the mucous membrane of the nose or mouth of a susceptible person; suctioning or bronchoscopy generate these particles

_____ Designed to reduce the risk for transmission of microorganisms transmitted by direct or indirect contact

_____ Interventions that synthesize the major features of universal (blood and body fluid) precautions and body substance isolation (BSI); involve the use of barrier protection; designed for the care of all patients to reduce the risk for transmission of microorganism from both recognized and unrecognized sources of infection

_____ A sterile procedure in which a feeding tube or a Foley catheter is inserted into the urethra to obtain a sterile urine specimen when the child is unable to void or otherwise provide an adequate specimen

_____ Also referred to as *hospital-acquired*

_____ Involves skin-to-skin contact and physical transfer of microorganisms to a susceptible host from an infected or colonized person

_____ Designed for patients documented or suspected to be infected or colonized with highly transmissible or epidemiologically important pathogens for which interventions beyond standard precautions are needed to interrupt transmission in hospitals

_____ Involves contact of a susceptible host with a contaminated intermediate object, usually an inanimate object in the patient's environment

_____ A procedure that involves aspirating bladder contents by inserting a needle in the midline above the symphysis pubis and vertically downward into the bladder; used to obtain a urine specimen when the child is unable to void or otherwise provide an adequate specimen, when the bladder cannot be accessed through the urethra, and/or when use of a catheter poses too high a risk for contamination; useful in clarifying the diagnosis of suspected urinary tract infection in acutely ill infants

_____ A procedure in which 1 to 3 ml of sterile normal saline is instilled into one nostril and then aspirated; usually performed to diagnose an infection of respiratory syncytial virus (RSV)

_____ A procedure that assesses the circulation of the radial ulnar or brachial arteries

_____ Designed to reduce the transmission of infectious agents that remain suspended in air or by dust particles containing the infectious agent

4. The following terms are related to administration of medication and feeding techniques. Match each term with its description.

a. Body surface area (BSA)
b. West nomogram
c. Needleless injection system
d. Subcutaneous injections
e. Intradermal injection
f. Orogastric/nasogastric gavage
g. Enteral gavage
h. Gastrostomy
i. Jejunostomy
j. Skin-level device
k. Familial adenomatous polyposis (FAP)

_____ A long-term gastrostomy feeding device consisting of a small, flexible silicone tube that protrudes slightly from the abdomen; advantages—affords increased comfort and mobility to the child, is easy to care for, is fully water-immersible, has a one-way valve to minimize reflux, and eliminates the need for clamping; disadvantages—requires a well-established gastrostomy site and is expensive; examples—MIC-KEY, Bard Button, Gastroport

_____ Administered to the lateral side of the volar surface of the forearm

_____ The most reliable basis to use for calculating children's drug dosages from a standard adult dose

_____ Feeding by a tube inserted directly into the stomach

_____ Feeding by way of a tube inserted orally or nasally into the duodenum/jejunum

_____ Usually used to determine body surface area

_____ Condition that may require a colectomy with ileoanal reservoir to prevent or treat carcinoma of the colon

_____ Biojector; delivers intramuscular or subcutaneous injections without the use of a needle; eliminates the risk for accidental needle puncture

_____ Feeding by way of a tube inserted orally or nasally into the stomach

_____ Common injection sites include the center third of the lateral aspect of the upper arm, the abdomen, and the center third of the anterior thigh

_____ Feeding by a tube inserted directly into the jejunum

5. An informed consent is required for:
   a. an emergency appendectomy.
   b. a cutdown for intravenous medications.
   c. release of medical information.
   d. all of the above.

6. When parents are divorced, who is eligible to consent to medical treatment of their child?
   a. Only the custodial parent may consent.
   b. Only the noncustodial parent may consent.
   c. Both parents must consent.
   d. Either parent may consent.

7. The statutes for the mature minors doctrine vary from state to state. Based on the doctrine, a minor may be permitted to consent for:
   a. psychiatric care.
   b. treatment for any kind of health problem.
   c. treatment for sexually transmitted infections.
   d. routine physical exams only.

8. Although statutes vary from state to state, minors are usually recognized as having the legal capacity of an adult in all matters after they:
   a. have acquired a sexually transmitted infection.
   b. use contraceptives.
   c. use drugs or alcohol.
   d. become pregnant.

9. When preparing a child for a procedure, the nurse should:
   a. use abstract terms.
   b. teach based on the child's developmental level.
   c. use phrases with dual meanings.
   d. introduce anxiety-laden information first.

10. If a child needs support during an invasive procedure, the nurse should:
    a. insist that the parents participate in distraction techniques.
    b. instruct parents to stand quietly in back of the room and maintain eye contact with the child.
    c. respect parents' wishes and coach the parents about what to do.
    d. instruct parents to stay close by to console the child immediately following the procedure.

11. To prepare a toddler for an invasive procedure, the *best* strategy for the nurse to use would be to:
    a. give one direction at a time.
    b. prepare the child a day in advance.
    c. set up the equipment while the child watches.
    d. expect the child to sit still and cooperate.

12. Which of the following words or phrases is considered nonthreatening?
    a. "A little stick"
    b. "An owie"
    c. Die
    d. Deaden

13. According to Zain and colleagues (1996), who is *least* likely to believe that the parents' presence during a procedure is helpful?
    a. The child
    b. The mother
    c. The father
    d. The physician

14. List at least five strategies the nurse can use to support the child during and after a procedure.

15. Describe at least one play activity for each of the following procedures.

    a. Ambulation

    b. Range of motion

    c. Injections

    d. Deep breathing

    e. Extending the environment

    f. Soaks

    g. Fluid intake

16. The *most* effective method of preoperative preparation is:
    a. consistent supportive care.
    b. systematic preparation at specific stress points.
    c. offering parents the option of attending the induction of anesthesia.
    d. a single session of preparation.

17. The school-age child's perception of the surgical experience would include the concept that:
    a. fear is a major concern.
    b. most fearful events are remembered.
    c. children often remember waking up in pain.
    d. parental presence often increases the child's anxiety.

18. To prepare a breast-fed infant physically for surgery, the nurse would expect to:
    a. permit breast-feeding up to 4 hours before surgery.
    b. withhold breast-feeding from midnight the night before surgery.
    c. permit breast-feeding up to 6 hours before surgery.
    d. replace breast milk with formula and permit feeding up to 2 hours before surgery.

19. Preoperative sedation in children is *best* accomplished by:
    a. oral transmucosal fentanyl.
    b. intravenous midazolam.
    c. intravenous opioids.
    d. oral analgesics.

20. Early symptoms of malignant hperthermia include:
    a. anemia.
    b. enlarged lymph nodes.
    c. tachycardia.
    d. elevated temperature.

21. Fear of induction of anesthesia by mask can be minimized by applying:
    a. the mask quickly and with assurance.
    b. an opaque mask.
    c. the mask while the child is sitting.
    d. the mask while the child is supine.

22. A change in vital signs of the young child in the postanesthesia recovery room that demands immediate attention is:
    a. increased temperature.
    b. tachypnea.
    c. muscle rigidity.
    d. all of the above.

23. Noncompliant families:
    a. share typical characteristics.
    b. have less education than compliant families.
    c. often have complex medical regimens.
    d. often have an increased loss of control.

24. An example of an organizational strategy to improve compliance would be for the nurse to:
    a. incorporate teaching principles that are known to enhance understanding.
    b. encourage the family to adapt hospital medication schedules to their home routine.
    c. evaluate and reduce the time the family waits for their appointment.
    d. all of the above are organizational strategies.

25. In planning strategies to improve the child's compliance with the prescribed treatment, the nurse knows that:
    a. an every-8-hour schedule should be implemented.
    b. an every-6-hour schedule should be implemented.
    c. the child may not be able to swallow pills.
    d. the family usually does not remember or understand the instructions given.

26. General guidelines for care of a child's skin includes:
    a. covering the fingers of the extremity used for an intravenous line.
    b. lifting the child under the arms to transfer the child from the bed to a stretcher.
    c. placing a pectin-based skin barrier directly over excoriated skin.
    d. keeping the skin moist at all times.

27. A stage III pressure ulcer usually presents as:
    a. a deep crater.
    b. an abrasion.
    c. nonblanchable erythema.
    d. reactive hyperemia.

28. To prevent injuries from shearing, the nurse should avoid:
    a. using sheepskin over the elbows.
    b. pulling the patient up in bed without a lift sheet.
    c. pulling the patient up in bed with a lift sheet.
    d. using Montgomery straps.

29. The disadvantage that is associated with gel-filled or water-filled devices for pressure reduction is:
    a. the cost of electricity.
    b. that it is difficult to transfer the patient.
    c. that it is difficult to keep clean.
    d. that it is cold to touch.

30. When bathing an uncircumcised male child over the age of 3, the nurse should:
    a. gently remind the child to clean his genital area.
    b. not retract the foreskin.
    c. gently retract the foreskin.
    d. avoid cleansing between the skinfolds of the genital area.

31. Care for the hair of an African-American child includes braiding the hair:
    a. when it is wet.
    b. tightly.
    c. when it is dry.
    d. after petroleum jelly is applied.

32. To prevent a child from becoming dehydrated from diarrhea, the nurse should offer:
    a. gelatin.
    b. plain water.
    c. flavored fluids.
    d. carbonated beverages.

33. The *best* sample of adequate documentation of a child's food intake would be:
    a. "Child ate one bowl of cereal with milk."
    b. "Child ate an adequate breakfast."
    c. "Child ate 80% of the breakfast served."
    d. "Parent states that child ate an adequate breakfast."

34. During the chill phase of the febrile state:
    a. heat is generated and conserved.
    b. the temperature stabilizes at a higher range.
    c. a crisis of the temperature is occurring.
    d. the temperature is greater than the set point.

35. The *most* effective intervention for the treatment of fever in a 4-year-old child is to:
    a. administer a tepid sponge bath.
    b. administer ibuprofen.
    c. administer an alcohol sponge bath.
    d. administer acetaminophen.

36. Of the following strategies, the *best* intervention for the treatment of hyperthermia in a 4-year-old child is to administer:
    a. a tepid sponge bath.
    b. acetaminophen.
    c. an alcohol sponge bath.
    d. aspirin.

37. Ibuprofen oral drops are available in which one of the following strengths?
    a. 100 mg/1.25 ml
    b. 100 mg/ml
    c. 50 mg/1.25 ml
    d. 50 mg/ml

38. The revised CDC Guidelines for Isolation Precautions in Hospitals now contain:
    a. two levels.
    b. three levels.
    c. four levels.
    d. five levels.

39. To prevent spread of contamination from one patient to another after procedures, the *most* important strategy the nurse can use is to:
    a. follow disease-specific infection control guidelines.
    b. wear vinyl gloves.
    c. avoid wearing nail polish.
    d. wash the hands routinely after each patient contact.

40. List three acceptable methods to transport infants and children.

41. List five nursing interventions for the child who is restrained.

42. After mouth or lip surgery, the nurse would choose to restrain the child using:
    a. arm and leg restraints.
    b. elbow restraints.
    c. a jacket restraint.
    d. a mummy restraint.

43. Of the following techniques, the *best* strategy to use when performing venipuncture on a toddler is to:
    a. give simple instructions for the child to hold still.
    b. extend the neck and maintain head alignment to expose the jugular vein.
    c. place the child prone with legs in a frog position to expose groin the area.
    d. hold the child's upper body to prevent movement.

44. The *best* positioning technique for a lumbar puncture in a neonate is a:
    a. side-lying position with neck flexion.
    b. sitting position.
    c. side-lying position with modified neck extension.
    d. side-lying position with knees to chest.

45. The *most* frequently used site for bone marrow aspiration in children is the:
    a. femur.
    b. sternum.
    c. tibia.
    d. iliac crest.

46. To facilitate urination in a 12-month-old infant, the nurse could:
    a. wipe the abdomen with alcohol and fan it dry.
    b. elicit the Perez reflex.
    c. apply a urine collection device.
    d. wash and dry the genitalia thoroughly.

47. When applying a urine specimen bag to an infant boy, it is sometimes necessary to:
    a. oil the surface of the skin.
    b. place the scrotum inside the bag.
    c. remove and replace the bag often.
    d. restrain all four extremities tightly.

48. When necessary, suprapubic aspiration is used:
    a. to access the bladder through the urethra.
    b. to access the bladder in some congenital birth effects.
    c. even though it may increase the risk for contamination.
    d. for all of the above.

49. Suprapubic aspiration has a _____ success rate than catheterization of the bladder through the urethra.
    a. higher
    b. lower

50. To collect a blood culture specimen from an intermittent infusion device, the nurse should:
    a. use the first sample of blood.
    b. discard the first sample of blood.
    c. irrigate the device with D5W first.
    d. use a heparinized collection tube.

51. Of the following venipuncture techniques, the one that would be *most* important to use to avoid the complication of necrotizing osteochondritis would be to:
    a. warm the site with moist compresses.
    b. cleanse the site with alcohol.
    c. use an automatic lancet device.
    d. use the inner aspect of the heel.

52. After a venipuncture is performed in the young child, the nurse should:
    a. use a "spot" bandage for the day.
    b. extend the arm while pressure is applied.
    c. avoid the use of any bandage.
    d. flex the arm while pressure is applied.

53. To obtain a sputum specimen to test for tuberculosis or respiratory syncytial virus (RSV) in an infant, the nurse may need to:
    a. stimulate the infant's cough reflex.
    b. obtain mucus from the throat.
    c. insert a suction catheter into the back of the throat.
    d. perform gastric lavage.

54. The *most* accurate method for determining the safe dose of a medication for a child is to use:
    a. the body surface area formula.
    b. Clark's rule.
    c. Wright's rule.
    d. milligrams per kilogram.

55. The form of medication that is *best* to administer to a young child is the:
    a. intravenous preparation.
    b. intramuscular preparation.
    c. solid oral preparation.
    d. liquid oral preparation.

56. To administer one teaspoon of medication at home, the parent should use the:
    a. household soup spoon.
    b. household measuring spoon.
    c. hospital's molded plastic cup.
    d. household teaspoon.

57. All of the following techniques for medication administration in the infant are acceptable *except*:
    a. adding the medication to the infant's formula.
    b. allowing the infant to sit in the parent's lap during administration.
    c. allowing the infant to suck the medication from a nipple.
    d. inserting a needleless syringe into the side of the mouth while the infant nurses.

58. When determining the needle length for intramuscular injection into a child, the nurse should:
    a. grasp the muscle and use a length that is equal to the distance.
    b. use a needle length that is too short rather than one that is too long.
    c. choose a 1-inch needle for a 4-month-old infant.
    d. use a 25- to 30-gauge needle.

59. Which of the following intramuscular injection sites is generally reserved for children who have been walking for more than a year?
    a. Deltoid muscle
    b. Vastus lateralis
    c. Dorsogluteal
    d. Ventrogluteal

60. When administering intramuscular medications to infants and small children, the nurse should:
    a. depress the plunger at the same time the needle is inserted.
    b. use the dorsogluteal muscle in infants.
    c. instruct the small child to stand and lean against his or her parent for support.
    d. inject the medication slowly.

61. When administering intravenous medication to an infant, the nurse should:
    a. check site for patency before each dose.
    b. administer medications along with blood products.
    c. combine antibiotics to avoid fluid overload.
    d. use the maximum dilution of the drug permitted by the manufacturer.

62. When administering medications to a child through a gastric tube, the nurse should:
    a. use oily medications to ease passage through the tube.
    b. mix the medication with the enteral formula.
    c. use a syringe with the plunger in place to administer the drug.
    d. flush the tube well between each medication administration.

63. The rectal route of medication administration is used in children when the child:
    a. is not responding to oral antiemetic preparations.
    b. needs a reliable route of administration.
    c. is constipated.
    d. all of the above.

64. To instill eyedrops in an infant whose eyelids are clenched shut, the nurse should:
    a. apply finger pressure to the lacrimal punctum.
    b. place the drops in the nasal corner where the lids meet and wait until the infant opens the lid.
    c. administer the eye drops before nap time.
    d. use any of the above techniques.

65. During continuous enteral feedings, the nurse should:
    a. use the same pole as used for the intravenous line.
    b. use a burette to calibrate the feeding times.
    c. give the infant a pacifier for sucking.
    d. all of the above.

66. In the small infant, a feeding tube is usually inserted through the:
    a. nose.
    b. mouth.

67. One of the disadvantages of inserting a skin-level device for feeding a child is that the button device:
    a. clogs as easily as other devices.
    b. eliminates the need for frequent bubbling.
    c. is less expensive than the traditional devices.
    d. cannot be immersed in water.

68. When administering an enema to a small child, the nurse should use:
    a. a pediatric Fleet enema.
    b. a commercially prepared solution.
    c. an isotonic solution.
    d. plain water.

69. A young child with an ostomy pouch may need to:
    a. wear one-piece outfits.
    b. begin toilet training at a later than usual age.
    c. use an alcohol based skin sealant.
    d. use a rubber band to help the appliance fit.

Critical Thinking—Case Study

Janis Smith is a 6-year-old child admitted to the hospital for an emergency appendectomy. Her parents have been divorced for 4 years, and her mother accompanies her to the hospital. Janis has a sister who is 7 years old.

70. Based on Janis' developmental characteristics, the nurse's plan for preparing the girl for surgery should include:
    a. an emphasis on privacy.
    b. the correct scientific medical terminology.
    c. ways to help Janis accept new authority figures.
    d. teaching sessions that last no longer than 5 minutes.

71. One of the nursing diagnoses identified by the nurse for Janis is high risk for injury related to the surgical procedure and anesthesia. During the assessment interview, which of the following sets of facts would be *most* pertinent to this diagnosis?
    a. The nurse auscultated vesicular breath sounds.
    b. Janis' mother tells the nurse that the child's father is 27 years old and in good health but had some heart problems related to anesthesia after a minor surgical procedure last year.
    c. Janis' mother tells the nurse not to expect the child's father to participate in the preoperative preparation, because he lives in another state.
    d. The nurse assesses that the child has moist mucous membranes and no tenting of the skin.

72. The nursing diagnosis of anxiety related to the surgery and hospitalization is identified by the nurse. Which of the following strategies is the *best* one for the nurse to incorporate into the surgical care plan to address this diagnosis?
    a. Encourage Janis' mother to be present as much as possible.
    b. Administer analgesics around the clock.
    c. Teach Janis to use the incentive spirometer.
    d. Ambulate Janis as early as possible.

73. Which of the following findings represents the *most* appropriate measurable data to evaluate the care plan in regard to the nursing diagnosis of high risk for fluid volume deficit?
    a. The child has vesicular breath sounds.
    b. The child's father, who is 27 years old and in good health, had some heart problems with anesthesia after a minor surgical procedure last year.
    c. The child's father lives in another state.
    d. The child has moist mucous membranes and no tenting of the skin.

CHAPTER 28

Balance and Imbalance of Body Fluids

1. Match each term with its description or function.

   a. Total body water
   b. Intracellular fluid
   c. Extracellular fluid
   d. Osmotic pressure
   e. Diffusion
   f. Aldosterone

   g. Antidiuretic hormone
   h. Intravascular fluid
   i. Interstitial
   j. Transcellular fluid
   k. Insensible water loss
   l. Third-spacing

   m. Peripheral edema
   n. Ascites
   o. Pulmonary edema
   p. Oral rehydration solution

   _____ Constitutes about half of the total body water at birth
   _____ Fluid within the cells
   _____ Constitutes 45% to 75% of body weight
   _____ Enhances sodium reabsorption in renal tubules
   _____ Released from the posterior pituitary gland in response to increased osmolality and decreased volume of intravascular fluid
   _____ The physical pull created by a solution of higher concentration across a semipermeable membrane
   _____ Random movement of molecules from a region of greater concentration to regions of lesser concentration
   _____ Fluid loss through the skin and respiratory tract
   _____ Pooling of body fluids in a body space
   _____ Localized or generalized swelling of the interstitial space
   _____ Used to treat infants with dehydration
   _____ Surrounding the cell and the location of most extracellular fluid
   _____ Accumulation of fluid in the abdomen
   _____ Fluid contained within the body cavities; e.g., cerebrospinal fluid
   _____ Occurs when there is an increase in the interstitial volume
   _____ Fluid contained within the blood vessels

2. The nurse would expect which of the following conditions to produce an increased fluid requirement?
   a. Congestive heart failure
   b. High intracranial pressure
   c. Mechanical ventilation
   d. Tachypnea

3. The nurse recognizes which of the following individuals as having the *least* water content in relation to weight?
   a. Obese adolescent female
   b. Thin adolescent female
   c. Obese adolescent male
   d. Thin adolescent male

4. Infants and young children are at high risk for fluid and electrolyte imbalances. Which one of the following factors contributes to this vulnerability?
   a. Decreased body surface area
   b. Lower metabolic rate
   c. Mature kidney function
   d. Increased extracellular fluid volume

5. _____ dehydration occurs when electrolyte and water deficits are present in balanced proportion.

6. _____ dehydration occurs when the electrolyte deficit exceeds the water deficit. There is a greater proportional loss of extracellular fluid, and plasma sodium concentration is usually

   _____ than 130 mEq/L.

7. _____ dehydration results from water loss in excess of electrolyte loss. This is often

   caused by a large _____ of water and/or a large _____ of electrolytes. Plasma

   sodium concentration is _____ than 150 mEq/L.

8. In infants and young children, the *most* accurate means of describing dehydration or fluid loss is:
   a. as a percentage.
   b. by milliliters per kilogram of body weight.
   c. by the amount of edema present or absent.
   d. by the degree of skin elasticity.

9. An infant with moderate dehydration has what clinical signs?
   a. Mottled skin color, decreased pulse and respirations
   b. Decreased urine output, tachycardia, and fever
   c. Tachycardia, oliguria, capillary filling within 2 to 3 seconds
   d. Tachycardia, bulging fontanel, decreased blood pressure

10. Diagnostic evaluation of dehydration to initiate a therapeutic plan includes:
    i.   serum electrolytes.
    ii. acid-base imbalance determination.
    iii. physical assessment to determine degree of dehydration.
    iv. type of dehydration based on pathophysiology.

    a. i and ii
    b. i, ii, and iii
    c. i, ii, iii, and iv
    d. iii and iv

11. Johnny, age 13 months, is being admitted for parenteral fluid therapy because of excessive vomiting. The nurse would recognize which one of the following as *most* essential in implementing care for Johnny?
    a. Give Johnny oral fluids until the parenteral fluid therapy can be established.
    b. Question the physician's order for parenteral fluid therapy of glucose 5% in 0.22% sodium chloride.
    c. Withhold the ordered potassium additive until Johnny's renal function has been verified.
    d. Replace half of Johnny's estimated fluid deficit over the first 24 hours of parenteral fluid therapy.

12. Rapid fluid replacement is *contraindicated* in which one of following types of dehydration?
    a. Isotonic
    b. Hypotonic
    c. Hypertonic

13. Water intoxication can occur in children from:
    i.   excessive intake of electrolyte-free formula.
    ii.   administration of inappropriate hypotonic solutions.
    iii. dilution of formula with water.
    iv.   isotonic dehydration.
    v.   vigorous hydration with water following a febrile illness.
    vi.   fluid shifts from intracellular to extracellular spaces.

    a. i, ii, iii, and iv
    b. i, ii, iii, and v
    c. ii, iii, and iv
    d. ii, iii, v, and vi

14. Severe generalized edema in all body tissues is called _____.

15. Edema formation can be caused by which one of the following?
    a. Decreased venous pressure
    b. Alteration in capillary permeability
    c. Increased plasma proteins
    d. Increased tissue tension

16. How does the nurse assess for pitting edema?
    a. Measure abdominal girth.
    b. Observe for fluid retention in the lower extremities.
    c. Press fingertip against bony prominence for 5 seconds.
    d. Observe for loss of normal skin creases.

17. Match each term with its description.

    a. Respiratory acidosis   c. Metabolic acidosis
    b. Respiratory alkalosis   d. Metabolic alkalosis

    _____ Occurs when there is a reduction of hydrogen ion concentration or an excess of base bicarbonate

    _____ Caused by any process that reduces base bicarbonate concentration or increases metabolic acid formation

    _____ Results from factors that depress the respiratory center, factors that affect the lung, and factors that interfere with the bellows action of the chest wall

    _____ Results primarily from central nervous system stimulation

18. To obtain relevant information from the mother of a child with fluid and electrolyte disturbances, the nurse should question the parent about:
    a. the type and amount of intake and output.
    b. observations of general appearance.
    c. weight of the child.
    d. whether they have taken the child's temperature within the last 24 hours.

19. In measuring intake and output, the nurse often has to weigh the diaper. As a general rule, what is the wet diaper weight equivalent to in ml of urine?

20. Which symptoms would the nurse expect in a child with hypocalcemia?
    a. Abdominal cramps, oliguria
    b. Muscle cramps, hypertonic
    c. Thirst, low urine specific gravity
    d. Flushed, mottled extremities and weight gain

21. Joan, age 3, is admitted for fluid and electrolyte disturbances. The nurse's assessment should include:
    i.   general appearance observation.
    ii. vital signs.
    iii. intake and output measurements.
    iv. daily weights.
    v.   review of laboratory results.

    a. i, ii, iii, and iv
    b. ii, iii, and iv
    c. iii, iv, and v
    d. i, ii, iii, iv, and v

22. Johnny, age 2, presents with moderate dehydration from diarrhea. What would you expect to be the recommendation for replacement of fluid?

23. The American Academy of Pediatrics no longer advises withholding food and fluids for 24 hours after the onset of diarrhea or administering of the BRAT diet (bananas, rice, applesauce, and tea or toast).
    a. True
    b. False

24. Billy, age 3, has just been ordered NPO. To prevent intake of fluids, the nurse should do which of the following?
    a. Place an NPO sign over his bed and remove fluids from the bedside.
    b. Place him in a private room away from other children.
    c. Apply an elbow restraint jacket to keep Billy from being able to drink by himself.
    d. Provide administration of ice chips every 30 minutes.

25. In starting an IV infusion in most children, the nurse recognizes the plan of care should include which of the following?
    a. Interruptions during the procedure are kept to a minimum.
    b. Use of a 20-gauge over-the-needle catheter is preferred.
    c. Allow the child to handle the equipment before procedure.
    d. Before the procedure begins, prepare the IV fluid and tubing, set to deliver 20 drops/ml.

26. Identify the following statements as true or false.
    _____   Glucose 10% in water is a hypotonic solution.
    _____   One molecule of glucose has half the osmolality of one molecule of sodium chloride.
    _____   IV solutions given to infants and young children should contain at least 0.2% NaCl to prevent brain edema.

_____ IV infusion for children must be given with an apparatus that delivers a microdrop factor of 60 drops/ml and contains a calibrated volume control chamber.

_____ Pediatric patients receiving IV fluids via continuous infusion pumps need less monitoring.

_____ The IV infusion must be monitored every 4 hours for proper infusion rate and for site assessment.

_____ Chloraprep is approved for patients above the age of 2 months as a skin antisepsis before initiating a peripheral IV.

_____ Two recent improvements in IV therapy to help prevent needle sticks are over-the-needle safety catheters and the needle-less system.

_____ Peripherally placed catheters are associated with fewer complications than centrally placed catheters.

_____ When using safety catheters, the nurse reinserts the needle into the catheter after it is removed for inspection and before insertion.

_____ Safety catheters penetrate the skin easier because of their sharper needle.

_____ Phlebitis is the most important complication associated with the use of peripheral venous catheters.

_____ The peripheral lock should be flushed with saline before and after administration of medication.

27. What are intraosseous infusions and when are they used?

28. The nurse has orders to start an IV infusion in 4-year-old Martha. Which of the following does the nurse include in the plan?
    a. Gather supplies in Martha's room so that she will not have to be moved after the procedure.
    b. Gather supplies in the treatment room since this is not a "safe place" for Martha.
    c. Realize that Martha will need to be restrained before the procedure begins.
    d. Start at the proximal site of the vein and move to a more distal site if the first attempt fails.

29. What nursing action should be included in the plan of care for 10-year-old Debbie, who requires intravenous fluid therapy?
    a. Position the extremity in a natural anatomic position, with the fingers and thumb immobilized.
    b. Use an Ace bandage and completely encircle the extremity with tape to secure the IV line, insertion site, and extremity.
    c. Teach Debbie how to manipulate the IV safely when getting out of bed and ambulating.
    d. For the IV placement, use Debbie's dominant hand or the same extremity where her identification bracelet is located.

30. The nurse is removing the peripheral IV line from 10-year-old Debbie. Which of the following strategies is correct for this procedure?
    a. Exert firm pressure at the IV site while removing the catheter.
    b. Turn off the IV pump after removal of the catheter.
    c. Allow Debbie to help remove the tape from the site.
    d. All of the above are correct.

31. Which one of the following alerts the nurse to a potential problem in a child receiving IV fluids?
    a. Edema, blanching, and cool skin are evident at the IV insertion site.
    b. The IV tubing is not changed or replaced for 16 hours.
    c. Blood appears in the tubing when the IV bag is held below the IV site level.
    d. There is unrestricted flushing of the catheter.

32. An infiltration/extravasation is observed. The nurse should do all of the following *except*:
    a. stop the infusion immediately.
    b. remove the IV catheter immediately.
    c. elevate the extremity.
    d. notify the practitioner.

33. The nurse is starting an IV. Which of the following steps in insertion is *least* likely to prevent infection at the site?
    a. Wash hands before starting.
    b. Rigorously clean the skin with providone solution using a back-and-forth motion from the outside inward.
    c. Palpate the area for the vein before skin prep.
    d. Allow the antiseptic area to dry before site insertion.

34. Match each device with its description or safety guideline. (A device may be used more than once.)

    a.   Peripheral intermittent infusion device
    b.   Short-term or nontunneled catheters
    c.   Peripherally inserted central catheters (PICCs)
    d.   Long-term, tunneled catheters

    _____ Most contact sports are prohibited while using this device; examples include implanted infusion ports.
    _____ Placed by specially trained nurses in the antecubital area
    _____ A chest x-ray film should be taken to verify placement of the catheter tip before administration of medication.
    _____ These are used for infusion when extended access is necessary without the need for continuous fluid.
    _____ If catheter is threaded midline, TPN is not administered because it irritates the vessel.

35. Discuss ways to prevent catheter-related infections with the use of central line catheters.

36. A patient's central venous catheter is accidentally removed. Where is pressure applied?
    a. Exit site on the skin
    b. Entry site to the vein

37. Jamie, age 12 years, is receiving parenteral hyperalimentation. The nurse knows that which one of the following serum levels must be carefully monitored?
    a. White blood cell
    b. Calcium
    c. Bicarbonate
    d. Glucose

38. The practitioner has ordered cyclic total parenteral nutrition (TPN). The nurse understands that:
    a. the child will be off the machine at night.
    b. the child will have increased risk for TPN-induced liver damage.
    c. the child will be off the machine for a number of hours during the day.
    d. the child will have decreased blood glucose levels.

39. Before initiating home TPN, what factors should be assessed?

Critical Thinking—Case Study

Jennifer, age 4 months, is admitted to the hospital because of dehydration caused by diarrhea. Her mother has been giving her electrolyte-free solutions for volume replacement. Parenteral fluids have been ordered for Jennifer.

40. What type of dehydration does Jennifer *most* likely have?
    a. Isotonic
    b. Hypertonic
    c. Hypotonic
    d. Water intoxication

41. Diarrhea most commonly causes which one of the following?
    a. Respiratory acidosis
    b. Respiratory alkalosis
    c. Metabolic acidosis
    d. Metabolic alkalosis

42. Which of the following data about Jennifer should the nurse obtain during the admission history?
    a. Type and amount of food and fluid intake
    b. Urinary output amount or frequency
    c. Number and consistency of stools passed in the past 24 hours
    d. All of the above

43. Which of the following observations does the nurse recognize as the *best* indicator that Jennifer's dehydration is becoming more severe?
    a. Jennifer's cry is whining and low-pitched.
    b. Jennifer's activity level is decreased.
    c. Jennifer's appetite is diminished.
    d. Jennifer is becoming more irritable and lethargic.

44. A priority goal in the management of acute diarrhea is:
    a. determining the cause of the diarrhea.
    b. preventing the spread of the infection.
    c. rehydration of the child.
    d. managing the fever associated with the diarrhea.

45. The nurse's *most* critical responsibility when administering IV fluids to Jennifer is to:
    a. prevent IV infiltration.
    b. ensure sterility.
    c. prevent cardiac overload.
    d. maintain the fluid at body temperature.

46. Tim is a 1-month-old infant admitted for uncontrolled vomiting. The nurse will observe Tim for signs of which one of the following?
    a. Alkalosis
    b. Acidosis
    c. Hypocalcemia
    d. Hemodilution

47. An infant is to receive 500 ml of IV fluid per 24 hours. The drop factor of the microdropper is 60 gtts/ml. The nurse should regulate the IV to run at how many drops per minute?
    a. 15 gtts/min
    b. 60 gtts/min
    c. 21 gtts/min
    d. 27 gtts/min

CHAPTER 29

Conditions That Produce Fluid and Electrolyte Imbalance

1. Match each term with its description.

   a. Secretory diarrhea
   b. Cytotoxic diarrhea
   c. Osmotic diarrhea

   d. Dysenteric diarrhea
   e. Chronic diarrhea
   f. Acute diarrhea

   _____ Associated with inflammation of the mucosa and submucosa in the ileum and colon by infectious agents such as *Salmonella* or *Shigella*

   _____ Commonly seen in malabsorption syndromes such as lactose intolerance; occurs when the intestine cannot absorb nutrients

   _____ Leading cause of illness in children younger than 5 years of age

   _____ Usually due to bacterial enterotoxins, which stimulate fluid and electrolyte secretion from the small intestine

   _____ Viral destruction of the mucosal cells within the small intestine, resulting in a smaller intestinal surface area and decreased absorption of fluid and electrolytes

   _____ May be the result of inadequate management of acute diarrhea; increase in stool frequency and increased water content with a duration of more than 14 days

2. Which one of the following is *most* likely to develop acute diarrhea?
   a. The 2-month-old infant who attends daycare each day
   b. The 18-month-old infant who stays at home each day with his mother
   c. The 6-year-old child who attends public school
   d. The 24-month-old infant with two older brothers, ages 5 years and 8 years

3. Identify the following statements as true or false.

   _____ Rotavirus is the most common pathogen identified in young children hospitalized for diarrhea and dehydration in this country.

   _____ Acute diarrhea in children may be associated with respiratory infections, otitis media infections, and urinary tract infections.

   _____ Excessive ingestion of apple juice can cause osmotic dietary diarrhea.

   _____ Antibiotics are seldom associated with diarrhea in children because of their lower specific gravity.

   _____ *Clostridium difficile* produces a protective mechanism against diarrhea because it alters the intestinal flora increasing absorption surfaces.

   _____ Because the infant's metabolic rate is lower than the adult's, the infant is more rapidly depleted of nutritional reserves during periods of malabsorption and decreased intake and therefore more prone to the development of dehydration.

   _____ Continuing to feed breast milk to an infant during diarrhea illness results in reduced severity and duration of the illness.

4. Johnny, age 2 years, is diagnosed with uncomplicated diarrhea with no signs of dehydration. Diagnostic evaluation should include which one of the following?
   a. Cultures of the stool
   b. Presence of associated symptoms
   c. Complete blood count
   d. Urine specific gravity

5. Listed below are subjective and objective findings associated with diarrhea. For each finding, identify the suspected cause of diarrhea.

   a. _____ Administration of cefaclor for 1 month for recurrent ear infections

   b. _____ Neutrophils or red blood cells in the stool

   c. _____ Watery, explosive stools

   d. _____ Foul-smelling, greasy, bulky stools

   e. _____ High numbers of esinophils in the stools

6. What are the four major goals in the management of acute diarrhea?

7. What is the *most* appropriate therapeutic management for rehydration of Jenny, age 8 months, who has been diagnosed with acute diarrhea and has evidence of mild dehydration?
   a. Beginning oral rehydration therapy of 50 ml/kg within 4 hours
   b. Restarting lactose-free formula
   c. Encouraging oral intake of clear fluids, such as fruit juices and gelatin
   d. Feeding the BRAT diet, which consists of bananas, rice, apples, and toast or tea

8. Drug therapy for acute infectious diarrhea in young children should include:
   a. Kaopectate administered until the diarrhea has stopped.
   b. continuation of antibiotics for the presence of *C. difficile*.
   c. administration of sedatives to decrease bowel motility.
   d. antibiotic therapy based on culture results.

9. Which one of the following nursing interventions is *not* appropriate for 6-month-old Terry, admitted to the pediatric unit with acute diarrhea and vomiting?
   a. Ongoing assessment of Terry's intake and output and physical appearance
   b. Education of the parents about the necessity of administering oral rehydration solution
   c. Rectal temperatures at least every 4 hours to monitor fever elevations
   d. Gentle cleansing of perianal areas and application of protective topical ointments

10. What type of diarrhea occurs in the first few months of life, persists for longer than 2 weeks with no recognized pathogens, and is refractory to treatment?

11. The therapeutic management of chronic nonspecific diarrhea in children includes:
    a. increasing dietary intake of foods and liquids with sorbitol and fructose.
    b. increasing dietary fiber.
    c. decreasing dietary fat content.
    d. increasing total fluid intake.

12. The major emphasis of nursing care for the vomiting infant or child is:
    a. determining prior treatments used for the vomiting.
    b. preventing the spread of the infection.
    c. managing the fever associated with the vomiting.
    d. observation and reporting of vomiting behavior and associated symptoms.

13. Fill in the blanks to identify the type of shock described in each of the following statements.

    a. _____ shock follows a reduction in circulating blood volume, plasma volume, or extracellular fluid loss.

    b. _____ shock results from impaired cardiac muscle function resulting in reduced cardiac output.

    c. _____ shock results from a vascular abnormality that produces maldistribution of blood supply throughout the body.

    d. _____ shock is characterized by a hypersensitivity reaction, causing massive vasodilation and capillary leak.

    e. _____ shock is characterized by decreased cardiac output and derangements in the peripheral circulation in response to a severe, overwhelming infection.

14. Match each term with its description.

    a. Compensated shock   e. Acidosis   i. Enteritis
    b. Decompensated shock   f. Alkalosis   j. Hydrostatic edema
    c. Irreversible shock   g. Enteral   k. Permeable edema
    d. Colloids   h. Parenteral

    _____ By way of the alimentary tract
    _____ Serum pH equal to or less than 7.35
    _____ Serum pH equal to or greater than 7.45
    _____ Cardiovascular efficiency diminished; microcirculatory perfusion marginal despite compensatory adjustments; tissue hypoxia, metabolic acidosis, and impairment of organ systems function
    _____ Occurs from elevation of pulmonary microvascular pressure as a result of left ventricular dysfunction
    _____ Protein-containing fluids, often administered to children in shock; albumin
    _____ Not in or through the digestive tract
    _____ Condition in which vital organ function is maintained by intrinsic compensatory mechanism and blood flow is usually normal or increased but generally uneven or maldistributed in the microcirculation
    _____ Inflammation of the intestine
    _____ Condition in which actual damage to vital organs occurs and death ensues even if measurements return to normal with therapy
    _____ Occurs when damage to alveolar cells and pulmonary capillary epithelium causes fluid to leak into the interstitial space, resulting in ARDS

15. Clinical manifestations of pronounced tachycardia, narrowed pulse pressure, poor capillary filling, and increased confusion would suggest which of the following?
    a. Compensated shock
    b. Decompensated shock
    c. Irreversible shock

16. The position of choice for the child in shock is:
    a. Trendelenberg.
    b. head-down with feet straight.
    c. flat with the legs elevated.
    d. semi-Fowler's.

17. List the three major efforts in the treatment of shock.

18. Match each stage of septic shock with its characteristics.

    a. Hyperdynamic stage

    b. Normodynamic stage

    c. Hypodynamic stage

    _____ Progressive deterioration of cardiovascular function, hypothermia, cold extremities, weak pulses, hypotension
    _____ Warm, flushed skin with tachypnea, chills and fever, and normal urinary output
    _____ Duration of only a few hours; cool skin, normal pulses and BP, decreased urinary output, and depressed mental state

19. Which of the following describes the *most* common initial signs of anaphylaxis?
    a. Cutaneous signs and complaint of feeling warm
    b. Bronchiolar constriction with wheezing
    c. Vasodilation and hypotension
    d. Laryngeal edema and stridor

20. The sudden development of high fever, vomiting and diarrhea, profound hypotension, shock, olguria, and an erythematous macular rash with subsequent desquamation are clinical signs of which one of the following?
    a. Anaphylaxis
    b. Irreversible shock
    c. *C. difficile* infections
    d. Toxic shock syndrome

21. What should be included in the teaching plan for adolescent females to prevent toxic shock syndrome associated with tampon use?

22. Burns are caused by _____, _____, _____,

    and _____ agents.

23. Burn injury from child abuse is seen most often in children under 2 years of age and includes injury

    most often caused by _____.

24. Identify the following statements as either true or false.

    _____ The single most important factor in the decrease in fire-related deaths since 1978 is the use of smoke detectors.

    _____ Since electric current travels through the body on the path of least resistance, the area surrounding the long bones would be expected to experience the most damage.

    _____ An area of concern for electrical burns in the very young child is the possibility of the child chewing on electrical cords.

    _____ The physiologic responses, therapy, prognosis, and disposition of the injured child with burns is all directly related to the amount of tissue destroyed.

    _____ Children playing with matches accounts for 1 in 10 house fires.

    _____ The severity of injury in chemical burns is related to the chemical agent and the duration of contact.

    _____ Children who sustain a greater-than-40% TBSA burn show growth delays in height and weight and reduced bone mass.

    _____ Pulmonary complications remain the leading cause of death following thermal trauma associated with inhalation injury.

25. The standard adult rule of nines cannot be used to determine the total body surface area of a burn in a child because:
    a. the child has different body proportions than the adult.
    b. the child has different fluid body weight than the adult.
    c. the child's trunk and arm proportions are larger than the adult's.
    d. as the infant grows, the percentage alloted for the head increases while the percentages for the arms decrease.

26. Brock, 12 years old, has burns involving the epidermis and part of the dermis. Blister and edema formation are present, and the burns are extremely sensitive to temperature changes, exposure to air, and light touch. Brock has:
    a. superficial first-degree burns.
    b. partial-thickness second-degree burns.
    c. full-thickness third-degree burns.
    d. fourth-degree burns.

27. The severity of burn injury is determined by which of the following?
    i.   Pain associated with the burn, measured on a scale of 1 to 10
    ii. Percentage of body surface area burned
    iii. Level of consciousness of the victim
    iv. Depth of the burn
    v.   Vital sign measurements

    a. i, ii, and iii
    b. i, ii, iii, and v
    c. i, iii, iv, and v
    d. ii and iv

28. The expected predominant symptom of a superficial burn is:
    a. pain.
    b. significant tissue damage.
    c. absence of protective functions of the skin.
    d. blister formation.

29. The nurse recognizes that which one of the following pediatric patients is at higher risk for complications from burn injury?
    a. The 12-month-old infant who pulled a pan of hot water over on his chest
    b. The 12-month-old infant who is burned on his chest by gasoline
    c. The 9-month-old infant who is burned on the hands and feet with scalding water as a punishment
    d. The 12-year-old child who is burned on one side of the face as a result of playing with cigarettes

30. Jordan, age 12 years, has suffered severe burns, and now his chest appears constricted. What procedure should the nurse prepare for?
    a. Intubation
    b. Chest tube insertion
    c. Escharotomy
    d. Hydrotherapy

31. Systemic response to thermal injury would include:
    a. hypoglycemia.
    b. increased capillary permeability.
    c. myoglobinuria.
    d. decreased metabolic rate.

32. Decrease in cardiac output in the postburn period is caused by which of the following?
    a. Circulating myocardial depressant factor
    b. Fluid losses through denuded skin
    c. Vasodilation and increased capillary permeability
    d. All of the above

33. In the first few days after a major thermal burn injury, the nurse observes oliguria. What is the *most* likely cause for this finding?
    a. Acute renal failure
    b. Inadequate fluid replacement
    c. Blood urea nitrogen and creatinine elevations
    d. All of the above

34. Following a major burn injury, which of the following is the *most* common gastrointestinal systemic response?
    a. Gastric ileus
    b. Gastric ulcers
    c. Severe diarrhea
    d. Ulcerative colitis

35. The metabolic rate is affected in burn patients. Using knowledge about this system response, the nurse identifies which of the following as correct?
    a. Blood glucose levels may be elevated because of insulin resistance.
    b. Temperature may be elevated even in absence of infection.
    c. Medications may be used to help restore muscle mass, increase weight gain, and promote wound healing.
    d. All of the above are correct.

36. Thermally injured children have an immediate threat to life related to _____

_____ and _____. During healing, _____ is the primary complication.

37. What should be included in the plan for emergency care of the burned child?
    a. Apply large amounts of cold water over denuded areas.
    b. Apply ointments to the burned area.
    c. Remove jewelry and metal.
    d. Apply neutralizing agents to the skin of chemical burn areas.

38. Bobby, age 2 years, has suffered a minor burn injury. Expected management would include:
    a. redressing the wound with a gauze dressing every 5 days.
    b. soaking stuck dressings in hydrogen peroxide before removal.
    c. watching wound margins for redness, edema, or purulent drainage.
    d. administering narcotics for pain.

39. In major burn injuries of children weighing less than 30 kg, adequate fluid replacement during the emergent phase is *best* assessed by which one of the following?
    a. Urinary output of 30 ml an hour
    b. Urinary output of 1 to 2 ml/kg per hour
    c. Increasing hematocrit
    d. Normal blood pressure

40. To maintain adequate nutrition and promote healing in the child with a major burn injury, the nurse would recommend which one of the following nutrition plans?
    a. Diet high in proteins and calories
    b. Diet high in calories and low in proteins
    c. Diet high in fats and carbohydrates
    d. Diet high in vitamins A and D

41. Johnny, age 8 years, suffered partial-thickness second-degree burns of his chest, abdomen, and upper legs while on a recent camping trip. He is scheduled for hydrotherapy each morning for 20 minutes followed by further debridement. The *best* nursing action to assist Johnny at this time is to:
    a. ensure that pain medication is given before treatment.
    b. hold Johnny's breakfast until he returns from treatment.
    c. offer sedation after the procedure to promote rest.
    d. reassure Johnny that hydrotherapy and debridement are not painful.

42. Which of the following is a temporary graft obtained from human cadavers and used in burn treatment?
    a. Allograft
    b. Xenograft
    c. Autograft
    d. Isograft

43. A topical agent that is used in burn treatment and can cause transient neutropenia is:
    a. silver nitrate 0.5%.
    b. silver sulfadiazine 1%.
    c. mafenide acetate 10%.
    d. bacitracin.

44. In caring for the donor site following split-thickness skin graft, the nurse expects the dressing to be:
    a. changed daily.
    b. not changed for 10 to 14 days.

Critical Thinking—Case Study

Kenny, age 5 years, is brought to the emergency center after his clothes caught on fire while he was playing with matches in the family garage. He has partial-thickness second-degree burns and full-thickness third-degree burns on his anterior chest, anterior abdomen, upper right arm, both shoulders, and right hand. Singed nasal hair is evident on physical exam, and some minor burns apparent on his face. A Foley catheter is inserted, and a small amount of clear urine is obtained. Two IV routes are established for fluid replacement.

45. In conducting the physical examination of Kenny's burns, the nurse calculates the extent of body surface area involvement. How would the nurse best assess to see whether circulation to the area is intact?
    a. Touch the area to see whether Kenny feels pain.
    b. Test injured surfaces for blanching and capillary refill.
    c. Inspect the burns for eschar formation.
    d. Watch for edema of the affected part.

46. Based on the information given, the nurse should be careful to watch Kenny for immediate signs of which complication?
    a. Inhalation injury
    b. Facial deformities
    c. Sepsis
    d. Renal failure related to formation of myoglobin

47. During the acute phase of Kenny's burn management, the nursing plan indicates a need to administer pain medication by the intravenous route rather than by the intramuscular route. What is the rationale for this decision?
    a. Relieves pain more effectively
    b. Bypasses the impaired peripheral circulation
    c. Prevents further damage to sensitive tissue
    d. Reduces the risk for skin irritation and infection

48. Kenny has normal bowel sounds 24 hours following admission and is placed on a high-calorie, high-protein diet of which he eats very little. Kenny's hydrotherapy is scheduled right after breakfast and before supper. Which one of the following interventions by the nurse would *most* likely increase Kenny's dietary intake?
    a. Show Kenny a feeding tube and explain to him that if he does not eat more, the tube will need to be inserted.
    b. Maintain the current meal schedule and stay with Kenny until he eats all of his meal.
    c. Rearrange his meal and hydrotherapy schedule to prevent conflicts.
    d. Insist that Kenny stop snacking between meals.

49. Considering the extent and distribution of Kenny's burns, which one of the following nursing diagnoses would be recognized as having the highest priority for Kenny during the management phase of his illness?
    a. Impaired gas exchange related to inhalation injury
    b. High risk for altered nutrition: less than body requirements, related to loss of appetite
    c. Fluid volume deficit related to edema associated with burn injury
    d. High risk for infection related to denuded skin, presence of pathogenic organisms, and altered immune response

50. Kenny progressed well with skin grafts and healing and is now ready for discharge. The nurse will know that Kenny's parents understand discharge instructions by which one of the following statements?
    a. "Kenny will only need to wear this elastic support bandage for 1 month."
    b. "Kenny will not be able to participate in any sports until the grafts have taken hold firmly."
    c. "We will visit the teacher and Kenny's peers before Kenny returns to school to prepare them for his appearance."
    d. "We will need to protect Kenny from normal activities until he requires no further surgery."

CHAPTER 30

The Child with Renal Dysfunction

1. Identify the following statements as true or false.

_____ The primary responsibility of the kidney is to maintain the composition and volume of body fluids in excess of body needs.

_____ The kidney functions in the production of erythropoietin and thus in the formation of red blood cell production.

_____ Renin is secreted by the kidney in response to reduced blood volume, decreased blood pressure, or increased secretion of catecholamines.

_____ Approximately one-half of the total cardiac output makes up the blood flow to the kidneys.

_____ Protein is a normal finding in urine because it is too large a molecule to be reabsorbed in the proximal tubule.

_____ Glucose is reabsorbed in the proximal tubule and returned directly to the blood.

_____ Because there is a limit to the concentration gradient against which sodium can be transported out, when larger than normal amounts of sodium remain in the tubules, water is obliged to remain with the sodium.

_____ An end product of protein metabolism is urea.

_____ The newborn is unable to dispose of excess water and solute rapidly or efficiently because glomerular filtration and absorption do not reach adult values until the child is between 1 and 2 years of age.

_____ The loop of Henle, the site of urine-concentrating mechanism, is short in the newborn, thus reducing the ability to reabsorb sodium and water and produce a concentrated urine output.

_____ Newborn infants are unable to excrete a water load at rates similar to those of older persons.

_____ *Escherichia coli* is responsible for 80% of urinary tract infections.

_____ *Pseudomonas* is a nitrate-producing bacteria responsible for urinary tract infections.

2. Jordan is a 2-year-old who has had a clean-catch urinalysis done as part of a diagnostic work-up. The results of Jordan's urinalysis are listed below. Identify whether each result is normal (mark with an *N*) or abnormal (mark with an *A*).

_____ +1 Glucose

_____ Specific gravity 1.020

_____ RBC 3–4

_____ WBC greater than 10

_____ Occasional casts

_____ Trace protein

_____ + Nitrites

3. Match each term with its description.

a.	Bacteriuria	g.	Urethritis	m.	Uremia
b.	Efflux	h.	Pyelonephritis	n.	Hemodialysis
c.	Reflux	i.	Urosepsis	o.	Peritoneal dialysis
d.	Glomerular filtration rate	j.	Vesicoureteral reflux	p.	Hemofiltration
e.	Creatinine	k.	Azotemia		
f.	Cystitis	l.	Chronic glomerulonephritis		

_____ Backward flow of urine

_____ Inflammation of the bladder

_____ Inflammation of the upper urinary tract and kidneys

_____ Retrograde flow of bladder urine into the ureters

_____ Accumulation of nitrogenous waste within the blood resulting in elevated blood urea nitrogen and creatinine levels

_____ Forward movement of urine from kidney to bladder

_____ Measure of the amount of plasma from which a substance is cleared in 1 minute

_____ Febrile urinary tract infection coexisting with systemic signs of bacterial illness; blood culture reveals presence of urinary pathogen

_____ An end product of protein metabolism in muscle

_____ Inflammation of the urethra

_____ Presence of bacteria in the urine

_____ Toxic symptoms caused by retention of nitrogenous products in the blood

_____ A variety of different disease processes that may be distinguished from one another by renal biopsy

_____ Condition in which the abdominal cavity acts as a semipermeable membrane through which water and solutes of small molecular size move by osmosis and diffusion according to their respective concentrations

_____ Process by which blood is circulated outside the body through artificial cellophane membranes that permit a similar passage of water and solutes

_____ Process by which blood filtrate is circulated outside the body by hydrostatic pressure exerted across a semipermeable membrane and replaced simultaneously by electrolyte solution

4. The nurse, in preparing the child for a diagnostic test, explains that which one of the following tests provides direct visualization of the bladder through a small scope?
   a. Cystoscopy
   b. Voiding cystourethrogram
   c. IVP
   d. Renal biopsy

5. Preprocedural preparation of the child who is scheduled to have a cystourethrography includes:
   a. keeping the child NPO for 8 hours before the test.
   b. assessing for an allergy to iodine.
   c. administering a Fleet enema before the exam.
   d. preparing the child for catheterization.

6. Which one of the following does *not* predispose the patient to urinary tract infections?
   a. The short urethra in the young female
   b. The presence of urinary stasis
   c. Urinary reflux
   d. Lowering of urine pH

7. Symptoms of urinary tract infection often observed in children over age 2 years include:
   i.   incontinence in a child previously toilet trained.
   ii. abdominal pain.
   iii. strong or foul odor to the urine.
   iv. frequency of urination.
   v.   vomiting.

   a. i, ii, and iii
   b. iii and iv
   c. iii, iv, and v
   d. i, ii, iii, and iv

8. Three-year-old Ivy is brought to the clinic because of a suspected urinary tract infection. Which of the following is the correct method for collecting the urine specimen?
   a. Encourage large amounts of water because Ivy is unable to void at this time.
   b. Set Ivy on the toilet facing the tank to decrease likelihood of contamination.
   c. Wait until the first morning voided specimen can be collected.
   d. Bag Ivy with the bag covering the entire peritoneal area.

9. The treatment objectives for children with urinary tract infections include:

   a.

   b.

   c.

   d.

10. Which symptom suggests pyelonephritis in a 3-year-old child?
    a. Flank pain and tenderness
    b. Foul-smelling urine
    c. Dysuria or urgency
    d. Enuresis or daytime incontinence

11. The nurse is asked to obtain a urine specimen from 5-year-old Anne. Which of the following methods is the correct procedure?
    a. Place a urine bag on Anne to collect the next specimen.
    b. Obtain a catheterized specimen.
    c. Encourage Anne to drink large volumes of water in an attempt to obtain a specimen.
    d. Obtain a midstream specimen, preferably the first morning specimen.

12. Justin, age 8 years, has been diagnosed with pyelonephritis. The nurse would expect medical management to include:
    a. administration of oral nitrofurantoin.
    b. admission to the hospital with intravenous antibiotics administered for the first 24 hours.
    c. radiographic evaluation before antibiotic therapy.
    d. urine cultures repeated every month for 3 months.

13. The nurse is developing a preventive teaching plan for Tracy, a sexually active 16-year-old who has been diagnosed with a urinary tract infection. Which of the following should be included in the plan?
    a. Promote perineal hygiene by wiping back to front.
    b. Urinate as soon as possible after intercourse.
    c. Douche as soon as possible after intercourse to flush out bacteria.
    d. Eliminate all carbonated and caffeinated beverages because they irritate the bladder.

14. Vesicoureteral reflux is closely associated with which one of the following?
    a. Acute glomerulonephritis
    b. Nephrotic syndrome
    c. Renal scarring and kidney damage
    d. High alkaline content in the urine

15. Acute poststreptococcal glomerulonephritis (APSGN):
    i.   is the less common of the noninfectious renal diseases in children.
    ii. can occur at any age but primarily affects school-age children, the peak age of onset being 6 to 7 years.
    iii. is an immune complex disease related to a reaction that occurs as a byproduct from certain strains of group A b-hemolytic streptococcus.
    iv. follows a latent period of 10 to 14 days between the infection of the throat or skin and the onset of symptoms for APSGN.
    v.   most commonly occurs in fall and spring.

    a. i, ii, iii, iv, and v
    b. ii, iii, and iv
    c. i, iii, and iv
    d. ii, iii, and v

16. Which of the following clinical manifestations are associated with acute glomerulonephritis?
    a. Normal blood pressure, generalized edema, oliguria
    b. Periorbital edema, hypertension, dark-colored urine
    c. Fatigue, elevated serum lipid levels, elevated serum protein levels
    d. Temperature elevation, circulatory congestion, normal BUN and creatinine serum levels

17. The major complications that may develop during the acute phase of glomerulonephritis are:

18. Nursing interventions in caring for the child with acute glomerulonephritis include:
    a. enforced bed rest.
    b. daily weights.
    c. keeping the child NPO.
    d. high-sodium diet.

19. Which of the following diagnostic findings would suggest failing renal function?
    a. Decreased creatinine and elevated BUN
    b. Elevated BUN, creatinine, and uric acid levels
    c. Elevated potassium, phosphorus, and calcium
    d. Proteinuria and decreased creatinine and BUN

20. Clinical manifestations of nephrotic syndrome include:
    a. hypercholesterolemia, hypoalbuminemia, edema, and proteinuria.
    b. hematuria, hypertension, periorbital edema, flank pain.
    c. oliguria, hypocholesterolemia, and hyperalbuminemia.
    d. hematuria, generalized edema, hypertension, and proteinuria.

21. Which child is *most* at risk for minimal-change nephritic syndrome?
    a. A 4-year-old recovering from viral upper respiratory infection
    b. A 7-year-old who is post β-hemolytic group A strep throat infection
    c. A 6-year-old with AIDS
    d. A 2-year-old who recently received several bee stings

22. Therapeutic management in nephrotic syndrome includes the administration of prednisone. The nurse teaches which of the following as correct administration guidelines?
    a. Corticosteroid therapy is begun after BUN and serum creatinine elevation.
    b. Prednisone is administered orally in a dosage of 4 mg/kg of body weight.
    c. After the child is free of proteinuria and edema, the daily dose of prednisone is gradually tapered over several weeks to months.
    d. The drug is discontinued as soon as the urine is free from protein.

23. Drug side effects associated with cyclophosphamide are:
    i.   leukopenia.
    ii. azoospermia.
    iii. effects on gonadal function in females.
    iv. hypertenison.
    v.   mental retardation.

    a. i, ii, and iii
    b. i, iv, and v
    c. ii, iii, and v
    d. i, ii, iii, iv, and v

24. Identify the following statements as true or false

    _____   Proximal tubular acidosis is caused by the inability of the kidney to establish a normal pH gradient between tubular cells and tubular contents.

    _____   Primary functions of the distal renal tubules are acidification of urine, potassium secretion, and selective and differential reabsorption of sodium, chloride, and water.

    _____   Treatment of both proximal and distal disorders consists of administration of sufficient bicarbonate or citrate to balance metabolically produced hydrogen ions and maintain the plasma bicarbonate level within normal range.

    _____   In nephrogenic diabetes insipidus, the distal tubules and collecting ducts are insensitive to the action of antidiuretic hormone and vasopressin.

    _____   Nephrogenic diabetes insipidus occurs primarily in females and appears in the newborn period with vomiting, fever, failure to thrive, dehydration, and hypernatremia.

    _____   Hemolytic-uremic syndrome is characterized by acute renal failure, hemolytic anemia, and thrombocytopenia.

    _____   Alport syndrome is a condition of chronic hereditary nephritis, which consists of hematuria, high-frequency sensorineural deafness, ocular disorders, and chronic renal failure.

    _____   Transient proteinuria generally indicates renal disease.

25. Multiple cases of hemolytic uremic syndrome caused by enteric infection of the *E. coli* 0157:H7 serotype have been traced to:
    i.   undercooked meat, especially ground beef.
    ii. unpasteurized apple juice.
    iii. alfalfa sprouts.
    iv. public pools.

    a. i and iv
    b. i and ii
    c. i, ii, iii, and iv
    d. ii and iii

26. Diagnostic evaluation results for hemolytic uremic syndrome include which of the following?
    a. Proteinuria, hematuria, urinary cast, elevated BUN and serum creatinine, low hemoglobin and hematocrit, and a high reticulocyte count
    b. High potassium, low sodium, high hemoglobin and hematocrit, and proteinuria
    c. High number of urinary casts, low serum BUN and creatinine, and decreased sedimentary rates
    d. Urine negative for protein but positive for RBC, normal hemoglobin and hematocrit, and elevated serum BUN and creatinine

27. In evaluation of the child with possible renal trauma, which one of the following are usually indicative of kidney damage?
    a. Flank pain and hematuria
    b. Dysuria, proteinuria, and nausea
    c. Abdominal ascites, nausea, and hematuria
    d. Proteinuria and bladder spasms

28. What is the *most* frequent cause of prerenal failure in infants and children?
    a. Nephrotoxic agents
    b. Obstructive uropathy
    c. Dehydration related to diarrhea and vomiting
    d. Burn shock

29. The primary manifestation of acute renal failure is:
    a. edema.
    b. oliguria.
    c. metabolic acidosis.
    d. weight gain and proteinuria.

30. The *most* immediate threat to the life of the child with acute renal failure is:
    a. hyperkalemia.
    b. anemia.
    c. hypertension crisis.
    d. cardiac failure from hypovolemia.

31. Which drug therapy is used in the removal of potassium?
    a. Peritoneal dialysis
    b. Glucose 50% and insulin
    c. Kayexalate
    d. Calcium gluconate

32. The *major* nursing task in the care of the infant or child with acute renal failure is:

33. Which one of the following manifestations of chonic renal failure can have the *most* social consequences for the developing child?
    a. Anemia
    b. Growth retardation
    c. Bone demineralization
    d. Septicemia

34. Dietary regulation in the child with chronic renal failure includes:
    a. restriction of protein intake below the recommended daily allowance.
    b. protein in the diet of high biologic value.
    c. restriction of potassium when creatinine clearance falls below 50 ml/min.
    d. vitamin A, E, and K supplements.

35. Identify three goals for the child in ESRD.

36. Fill in the blanks in the following statements.

    a. Methods of dialysis for management of renal failure are _____,

    _____ _____, and _____.

    b. _____ is the preferred method for children with life-threatening hyperkalemia.

    c. In peritoneal dialysis, _____ _____ is greater than with hemodialysis.

    d. _____ is not recommended for small children because of the rapid changes in blood volume and systemic blood pressure and the difficulty of placing vascular access devices.

    e. The major complication associated with peritoneal dialysis is _____.

    f. The nurse can expect to see the child undergoing dialysis to have improved _____

    _____ and _____ _____ but not to recover to

    _____ _____.

    g. Continuous venovenous hemofiltration (CVVH) is an ideal form of dialysis for children with

    _____ _____ from _____ _____.

37. Johnny, age 12, had a renal transplant 5 months ago. He now presents to the hospital outpatient clinic with fever, tenderness over the graft area, decreased urinary output, and a slightly elevated blood pressure. The nurse's priority at this time is:
    a. to recognize that Johnny is probably undergoing acute rejection and to notify the physician immediately.
    b. to recognize that this is an episode of increased inflammation within the donor kidney because Johnny has probably been noncompliant with his immunosuppressant drugs. The nurse should educate Johnny regarding drug compliance and notify Johnny's physician when he makes rounds.
    c. to obtain a urine specimen for culture and sensitivity and a blood count to quickly identify Johnny's infection before alerting the physician.
    d. to recognize that Johnny is in chronic rejection and that no present therapy can halt the progressive process.

Critical Thinking—Case Study

Dean, age 3 years, is brought to the clinic by his mother. He has a history of a recent fever of 100.2° F, sore throat, and slight cough approximately 8 days ago that lasted about 3 days. Yesterday morning Dean's mother noticed "puffiness around his eyes" when he "got up" and then "swelling of his lower legs and scrotal area." Dean's appetite and activity level have decreased. This morning Dean's mother noticed that his urine was "darker in color" and "seemed to be less than usual." Physical examination of Dean reflects a child who does not appear acutely ill but who is irritable and seems fatigued, with pallor skin color. His blood pressure, pulse, and temperature are within normal limits. He has generalized edema. Laboratory findings of Dean's urine specimen include large amounts of protein and microscopic hematuria. Serum protein levels are very low with elevated lipid levels.

38. Based on the information given, the nurse would suspect that Dean has developed which one of the following conditions?
    a. Acute poststreptococcal glomerulonephritis
    b. Minimal-change nephrotic syndrome
    c. Acute renal failure
    d. Hemolytic-uremic syndrome

39. Dean is diagnosed by the health care provider as having nephrotic syndrome. Identify goals for restoring renal function in Dean.
    i.   Urine is protein-free.
    ii. Edema is resolved.
    iii. Fluid and electrolyte balance are restored.
    iv. Nutritional needs have returned to a state of positive nitrogen balance.

    a. i, ii, and iii
    b. i, ii, and iv
    c. ii and iii
    d. i, ii, iii, and iv

40. Which one of the following nursing diagnoses is of *least* benefit in planning for Dean's care?
    a. Impaired skin integrity related to edema, lowered body defenses
    b. Altered nutrition: less than body needs, related to decreased appetite
    c. Altered patterns of elimination related to obstruction
    d. Fluid volume excess related to fluid accumulation in tissues and third space

41. Which nursing intervention is appropriate for Dean's nursing diagnosis of impaired skin integrity?
    a. Administer corticosteroids on time with careful monitoring for infections.
    b. Monitor for complications, strict intake and output, daily checks of urine for protein, daily weight, and abdominal girth.
    c. Enforce bed rest during the edema phase of the disease.
    d. Support scrotum on small pillow.

42. Dean has progressed well and is being discharged. What teaching interventions will be necessary to prepare the family for discharge?

43. Darlene, age 15 years, has been diagnosed with chronic renal failure. She is being discharged and will need peritoneal dialysis at home. Describe the teaching interventions the nurse would include in the discharge plan for Darlene.

44. The nurse has developed the nursing diagnosis of altered nutrition related to restricted diet based on Darlene's diagnosis of chronic renal failure. Discuss expected nursing interventions to be used with this nursing diagnosis.

CHAPTER 31

The Child with Disturbance of Oxygen and Carbon Dioxide Exchange

1. The following terms are related to respiratory tract structure. Match each term with its description.

a. Respiratory tract	j. Empyema	s. Lower airway
b. Thoracic cavity	k. Barrel chest	t. Trachea
c. Mediastinum	l. Nasal structures	u. Carina
d. Parietal pleura	m. Upper airway	v. Bronchioles
e. Visceral pleural sac	n. Pharynx	w. Compliance
f. Pneumothorax	o. Larynx	x. Generations
g. Pleural effusion	p. Glottis	y. Alveoli
h. Hydrothorax	q. Epiglottis	z. Septa
i. Hemothorax	r. Cricoid cartilage	aa. Lung growth

_____ The diseases state in which there is fluid in the space between the visceral and the parietal pleura

_____ Encased in the bony framework provided by the ribs, vertebrae, and sternum; consists of three major partitions: the three-lobed lung on the right, the two-lobed lung on the left, and the space between them—the mediastinum

_____ The disease state in which there is blood in the space between the visceral and the parietal pleura

_____ Consists of many complex structures that function under neural and hormonal control, with the primary responsibility to distribute air and exchange gases so that cells are supplied with oxygen while carbon dioxide is removed

_____ Structure that encases each lung by only enough fluid to lubricate the surface for painless movement during filling and emptying of the lungs

_____ Pyothorax; the disease state in which there is pus in the space between the visceral and the parietal pleura

_____ Adheres to the ribs and superior surface of the diaphragm

_____ The condition in severe obstructive lung disease in which the anteroposterior measurement approaches the transverse (side to side) measurement

_____ Contains the esophagus, trachea, large blood vessels, and the heart; located in the thoracic cavity between the right and left lungs

_____ Affected by numerous pathologic conditions, such as kyphoscoliosis, coxsackievirus, hormone level changes, and biochemical substances

_____ Rigid passageways for air that warm and moisten the air, filter impurities, and destroy microorganisms

_____ Composed of smooth muscle supported by C-shaped rings of cartilage; ensures an open airway

_____ Oronasopharynx, pharynx, larynx, and upper part of the trachea; shared by both the respiratory and alimentary tracts; dilates during inspiration; constricts during exhalation

_____ The branch levels of the bronchioles that are divided into the two categories: the conducting airways and the terminal respiratory units

_____ The dividing point of the trachea into two primary bronchi

_____ A passageway for the entry and exit of air; plays a role in phonation; helps to produce vowel sounds

_____ The disease state in which there is serum in the space between the visceral and the parietal pleura

_____ The process of elasticity of the lungs which allows the lungs to expand and recoil; complimented by the concept of resistance, which affects the flow through the airways

_____ The part of the respiratory system one generation below the bronchi

_____ At the upper end of the trachea; constructed of a rigid circular framework of cartilage; contains the epiglottis and the glottis (vocal cords)

_____ The disease state in which there is air in the space between the visceral and the parietal pleura

_____ Airsacs; gas exchange occurs through these thin-walled sacs

_____ Vibrates to produce voice sounds; located closer to the head in infancy than in later childhood; very active reflexes in infancy

_____ Prevents solids or liquids from entering the airway during swallowing; is longer and projects further posteriorly in infants

_____ The term for the shared walls of the alveoli

_____ Location of the narrowest portion of the larynx

_____ Consists of the lower trachea, mainstem bronchi, segmental bronchi, subsegmental bronchioles, terminal bronchioles, and alveoli

2. The following terms are related to respiratory function. Match each term with its description.

a. Respiratory movements	j. Elastic recoil	r. Neural system
b. Ventilation	k. Resistance	s. Chemical system
c. Artificial ventilation	l. Partial pressures	t. Neural control
d. Positive pressure breathing devices	m. Torr	u. Proprioceptive vagal impulses
e. Negative pressure ventilator	n. Fraction of inspired air	v. Central chemoreceptors
f. Pneumotoxic center	o. Oxyhemoglobin	w. Peripheral chemoreceptors
g. Compliance	p. Oxyhemoglobin saturation	x. Acid-base balance
h. Alveolar surface tension	q. Oxyhemoglobin dissociation curve	
i. Surfactant		

_____ One of the major factors determining compliance; lowered by surfactant

_____ The passage of air in and out of the lungs; results from changes in pressure gradients created by changes in the size of the thoracic cavity

_____ A lipoprotein at the air-fluid interface that allows alveolar expansion and prevents alveolar collapse

_____ Based on the concept of air moving from higher pressure into the lungs, which have a lower pressure

_____ The tendency of the lungs to return to the resting state after inspiration; a major factor in determining compliance

_____ FIO$_2$; the term used for inspired oxygen; expressed as 1.0 for 100%, 0.21 for ambient air at 21%

_____ First evident at about 20 weeks gestation when amniotic fluid is exchanged in alveoli

_____ Determined primarily by airway size; caused during breathing by the chest wall, lungs, and flow in the airways; determined by flow rate velocity, gas viscosity, length of the airway, and airway diameter

_____ The neutral center that modulates respiratory depth and frequency

_____ The oxygen that is carried by hemoglobin; a large portion of oxygen is transported throughout the body this way

_____ Artificial respiratory devices that increase the pressure entering the air passages

_____ Tensions; expressed in torr

_____ Measure of chest wall and lung dispensability; represents the relative ease with which the chest and lungs expand with increasing volume and then collapse away from the pleural wall with decreasing volume (elastic recoil)

_____ Millimeters of mercury; partial pressures are expressed in this manner

_____ Arterial oxygen saturation (SaO_2); hemoglobin saturation

_____ Located in a pneumotaxic center, apneustic center, and the medullary respiratory centers

_____ Artificial respiratory device that lowers the atmospheric pressure around the body

_____ Nerve cells located in the medulla that mediate respiratory changes by responding to changes in pH, PCO_2, and PO_2

_____ The nonlinear relationship between PaO_2 and SaO_2

_____ Located in the great vessels; e.g., the carotid bodies; nerve cells that mediate respiratory changes by responding to changes in pH, PCO_2, and PO_2

_____ A process in which the lungs play an important role by acting as a chemical buffer; adjusts pH by eliminating or retaining PCO_2, acting within 1 to 3 minutes

_____ A signal that is generated by stretching of the lungs and is then transmitted to the respiratory center, which inhibits further inflation and prevents overdistention—e.g., the Hering-Breuer reflex (R1421), one of the categories that control respiration; maintains a coordinated, rhythmic respiratory cycle and regulates the depth of respiration

_____ Neurohumoral system that regulates alveolar ventilation and maintains normal blood gas pressure

_____ Maintains the coordinated rhythmic respiratory cycles and regulates the depth of respiration

3. The following terms are related to defenses of the respiratory tract. Match each term with its description.

a. Lymphoid tissues
b. Mucous blanket
c. Ciliary action
d. Cough
e. Tracheobronchial dynamics
f. Position change
g. Lymphatics
h. Humoral defenses

_____ Encourage drainage of tracheobronchial passages

_____ Tissues that localize and contain organisms to be destroyed by the humoral defense mechanisms

_____ The ability of the tracheobronchial tree to elongate and dilate on inspiration and shorten and narrow on expiration

_____ Remove invading organisms; drain the terminal bronchi

_____ Explosive force that propels foreign material out of the lower tract

_____ Epithelium that secretes a sticky mucus to which airborne organisms adhere

_____ Phagocytes, enzymes, and immunoglobulins secreted by the bronchial epithelium

_____ Keeps mucus flowing; carries microorganisms and other foreign agents away from the lungs to be coughed or swallowed

4. The following terms are related to physical assessment. Match each term with its description.

a. Auscultation

b. Palpation

c. Tachypnea

d. Hyperpnea

e. Hypopnea

f. Retractions

g. Nasal flaring

h. Head bobbing

i. Noisy breathing

j. Grunting

k. Skin color change

l. Chest pain

m. Parietal pleural pain

n. Diaphragmatic pleural irritation

o. Clubbing

p. Cough

q. Percussion

_____ An assessment technique that, along with palpation, provides information regarding areas of pain and tissue density

_____ Mottling, pallor, cyanosis; significant in the infant; suggests cardiopulmonary disease (except circulatory stasis or cyanosis from a cool environment)

_____ Respirations that are too deep

_____ Respirations that are too shallow

_____ May be a complaint of older children; may be caused by disease of any of the chest structures

_____ A sign of dyspnea in the infant who is sleeping or exhausted

_____ May be referred to the base of the neck posteriorly and anteriorly or to the abdomen

_____ An assessment technique that, along with percussion, provides information regarding areas of pain

_____ May be associated with disorders other than respiratory disease; serves as a protective mechanism; indicates irritation

_____ Sinking in of soft tissues relative to the cartilaginous and bony thorax; noted in some pulmonary disorders

_____ Physical assessment technique; helpful in identification of specific abnormalities and to assess response to treatment; used to determine airway patency

_____ Rapid ventilations; observed with anxiety, elevated temperature, severe anemia, and metabolic acidosis

_____ Significant finding in an infant; helps reduce resistance and maintain airway patency

_____ Proliferation of tissue at the terminal phalanges; associated with chronic hypoxia; does not reflect disease progression

_____ Frequently associated with hypertrophied adenoidal tissue, choanal obstruction, polyps, or foreign body in the nasal passages

_____ Usually localized over the affected area and aggravated by respiratory movement

_____ Frequently a sign of chest pain, suggests acute pneumonia, pleural involvement, pulmonary edema, or respiratory distress syndrome; increases end-respiratory pressure and prolongs gas exchange

5. The following terms are related to diagnostic procedures. Match each term with its description.

a. Pulse oximetry
b. Functional hemoglobin
c. Oxyhemoglobin
d. Deoxyhemoglobin

e. Transcutaneous monitoring
f. Arterial blood gas sampling
g. Allen test

_____ Performed to assess adequacy of collateral circulation
_____ Hemoglobin saturated with O_2
_____ A noninvasive method of determining SaO_2
_____ A noninvasive method of continually monitoring partial pressure of O_2 in arterial blood; may also be used to measure CO_2
_____ Performed on blood from an artery or capillary
_____ Hemoglobin capable of carrying O_2
_____ Hemoglobin that is not saturated with O_2

6. The following terms are related to respiratory therapy. Match each term with its description.

a. Hypoxemia
b. Plastic hood
c. Nasal cannula
d. Mask
e. Oxygen tent
f. Atelectasis
g. O_2-induced CO_2 narcosis
h. Hand-held nebulizer

i. Metered-dose inhaler (MDI)
j. Spacer device
k. Rotohaler/turbuhaler
l. Percussion
m. Vibration
n. Squeezing
o. Deep breathing

p. Breathing/postural exercises
q. Bag-valve mask
r. High-frequency ventilation
s. Extracorporeal membrane oxygenation (EMCO)
t. Endotracheal airway
u. Speaking valves

_____ The method of oxygen administration used for older infants and children; consists of two small tubes inserted into the nares; sometimes called *prongs*

_____ A method of oxygen administration that may be used for children beyond early infancy; advantage—does not require any device to come into direct contact with the face; disadvantage—difficult to control concentration of oxygen within the device

_____ Reduced blood oxygenation

_____ A hazard of oxygen therapy; may occur in persons with chronic pulmonary disease; seldom encountered in children except those with cystic fibrosis

_____ A self-contained, hand-held device that allows for intermittent delivery of a specified amount of medication

_____ Occurs as a result of the washing out of nitrogen from the alveoli by the high concentrations of oxygen; more likely to occur in persons with low tidal volume and retention of secretions

_____ A method of aerosolizing a medication; consists of a mask that the child holds over the nose and mouth

_____ Examples: Passy Muir, Kistner, and Tucker; not appropriate for use in seriously ill children, children using a tracheostomy cuff, or children with copious secretions

_____ Holding chamber to coordinate breathing and aerosol delivery

_____ A maneuver that is useful while the child is in the drainage position; increases the depth of the expiratory effort by brief, firm pressure from the practitioner's hands compressing the side of the chest

_____ Hand-operated self-inflating ventilation bag with a mask and a nonreturnable valve to prevent rebreathing

_____ Artificial airway that is most often used in association with artificial ventilation; e.g., nasal-tracheal, orotracheal, tracheostomy

_____ Used to help move secretions toward the head during exhalation

_____ A new type of metered-dose inhaler that does not require a space device

_____ Technique encouraged when the child is relaxed and in the desired position of drainage; uses diaphragmatic breathing; may stimulate a cough; may be facilitated by incentive spirometers, blow bottles, and games that involve blowing

_____ A form of cardiopulmonary bypass; provides both pulmonary and cardiac support

_____ Techniques that are useful with older motivated children with kyphoscoliosis, cystic fibrosis, asthma, or bronchiectasis

_____ Provides information regarding tissue density; the most common technique used in association with postural drainage; accomplished by the practitioner gently striking the chest wall with a cupped hand

_____ The method of oxygen administration that is best tolerated by infants

_____ A generic term for devices that use a rapid cycling rate and deliver small tidal volumes with each cycle

_____ A method of oxygen administration that is not usually well tolerated by children

7. The following terms are related to respiratory emergency. Match each term with its description.

a. Hypercapnea
b. Respiratory insufficiency
c. Respiratory failure
d. Respiratory arrest
e. Apnea
f. Central apnea
g. Obstructive apnea

h. Mixed apnea
i. Obstructive lung disease
j. Restrictive lung disease
k. Primary inefficient gas transfer
l. Respiratory center depression

m. Pulmonary diffusion defect
n. Head tilt
o. Chin lift
p. Jaw thrust
q. Back blows
r. Chest thrusts
s. Heimlich maneuver

_____ Absence of airflow (or absence of breathing that lasts for more than 15 seconds)

_____ Occurs in two conditions: (1) when there is increased work of breathing with near normal gas exchange function, and (2) when hypoxemia and acidosis develop secondary to CO_2 retention

_____ Absence of air flow that occurs when no respiratory efforts are present

_____ Components of central and obstructive apnea are present.

_____ The cessation of respiration

_____ Disease involving increased resistance to airflow

_____ Inadequate CO_2 removal

_____ Disease involving impaired lung expansion

_____ May be caused by cerebral trauma, intracranial tumors, central nervous system infection, tetanus

_____ The inability of the respiratory apparatus to maintain adequate oxygenation of the blood

_____ Includes pulmonary edema, fibrosis, embolism

_____ Used to relieve foreign body obstruction in infants; accomplished by placing hands on the sternum

_____ Absence of air flow that occurs when respiratory efforts are present

_____ Used to relieve foreign body obstruction in infants; involves hand placement over the spine between the shoulder blades

_____ Accomplished by placing one hand on the victim's forehead and applying firm, backward pressure with the palm

_____ Involves a series of nondiaphragmatic abdominal thrusts; recommended for children over 1 year of age

_____ Accomplished by placing fingers of the hand under the bony portion of the lower jaw to lift

_____ Insufficient alveolar ventilation due to dysfunction of the respiratory control mechanism or a diffusion defect

_____ Accomplished by grasping the angle of the victim's lower jaw and lifting with both hands

8. Of the following respiratory system structures, the one that does *not* distribute air is the:
   a. bronchiole.
   b. alveolus.
   c. bronchus.
   d. trachea.

9. The general shape of the chest at birth is:
   a. relatively round.
   b. flattened from side to side.
   c. flattened from front to back.
   d. the same shape as an adult's.

10. The infant relies primarily on:
    a. mouth breathing.
    b. intercostal muscles for breathing.
    c. diaphragmatic abdominal breathing.
    d. all of the above.

11. Because of the position of the diaphragm in the newborn:
    a. there is additional abdominal distention from gas and fluid in the stomach.
    b. the diaphragm does not contract as forcefully as that of an older infant or child.
    c. diaphragmatic fatigue is uncommon.
    d. lung volume is increased.

12. Which of the following statements is true in regard to the anatomy of an infant's nasopharyngeal area?
    a. The glottis is located deeper in infants than in older children.
    b. The laryngeal reflexes are weaker in infants than in older children.
    c. The epiglottis is longer and projects more posteriorly in infants than in adults.
    d. The infant and young child are both less susceptible than adults to edema formation in the nasopharyngeal regions.

13. List four anatomic factors that significantly affect the development of respiratory disorders in infants.

14. The condition that is *most* likely to reduce the number of alveoli in newborn is:
    a. maternal heroin use.
    b. increased prolactin.
    c. hyperthyroidism.
    d. kyphoscoliosis.

15. As the child grows, chest wall compliance:
    a. increases.
    b. decreases.

16. As the child grows, elastic recoil of the lungs:
    a. increases.
    b. decreases.

17. Relaxation of the bronchial smooth muscles occurs in response to:
    a. parasympathetic stimulation.
    b. inhalation of irritating substances.
    c. sympathetic stimulation.
    d. histamine release.

18. Room air consists of:
    a. 7% oxygen.
    b. 21% oxygen.
    c. 50% oxygen.
    d. 79% oxygen.

19. A child with anemia tends to be fatigued and breathes more rapidly, because the majority of oxygen is carried through the blood as:
    a. a solute dissolved in the plasma and the water of the red blood cell.
    b. bicarbonate and hydrogen ions.
    c. carbonic acid.
    d. oxyhemoglobin.

20. Retraction is defined as:
    a. the sinking in of soft tissues during the respiratory cycle.
    b. proliferation of the tissue near the terminal phalanges.
    c. an increase in the end expiratory pressure.
    d. contraction of the sternocleidomastoid muscles.

21. In a child, cough may be absent in the early stages of:
    a. cystic fibrosis.
    b. measles.
    c. pneumonia.
    d. croup.

22. Define the term *capacity* in relation to lung volume and pulmonary function.

23. Match each pulmonary function parameter with its description *and* its significance. Each parameter will be used twice.

    a.   Forced vital capacity (FVC), or peak flow

    b.   Tidal volume (TV or VT)

    c.   Functional residual volume (FRV); functional residual capacity (FRC)

Measurement:	**Significance:**
_____ Volume of air remaining in lungs after passive expiration	_____ Allows for aeration of alveoli; increased in hyperinflated lungs of obstructive lung disease
_____ Maximum amount of air that can be expired after maximum inspiration	_____ Information needed to determine rate and depth of artificial ventilation; multiplied by respiratory rate to provide minute volume
_____ Amount of air inhaled and exhaled during any respiratory cycle	_____ Reduced in obesity, obstructive airway disease

24. Match each diagnostic test with its description.

   a. Arterial blood gas
   b. Oximetry
   c. Transcutaneous CO_2 monitoring

   d. Radiography
   e. Magnetic resonance imaging
   f. Computerized tomography

   _____ Photometric measurement of O_2 saturation (SaO_2)
   _____ A sequence of pictures, each representing a cross-section or cut through lung tissue at a different depth
   _____ A sensitive indicator to monitor O_2, CO_2, and pH
   _____ Clearly identifies soft tissues with a two- or three-dimensional image
   _____ Produces images of internal structures of the chest, including air-filled lungs, vascular markings, heart, and great vessels
   _____ Provides a noninvasive, continuous, and reliable measurement of arterial carbon dioxide

25. When an infant's digits are connected to a pulse oximeter, the part of the sensor that is placed on the top of the nail is called the:
   a. photodetector.
   b. microprocessor.
   c. light-emitting diode (LED).
   d. electrode.

26. The nurse conducts a precautionary assessment of the collateral circulation when arterial puncture is performed on the child. This is called the:
   a. cover test.
   b. Allen test.
   c. Miller test.
   d. Weber test.

27. Of the following arterial blood gas results, the value that would indicate acidosis in an 8-year-old child is:
   a. pH of 7.32.
   b. pH of 7.47.
   c. PCO_2 of 44 mm Hg.
   d. O_2 of 75 mm Hg.

28. Oxygen delivered to infants is *best* tolerated when it is administered by:
   a. an oxygen mask.
   b. a plastic hood with humidified oxygen.
   c. delivery of oxygen directly into the incubator.
   d. nasal cannula or prongs.

29. The oxygen mist tent is a satisfactory means of O_2 administration for children past early infancy because it:
   a. comes into direct contact with the face.
   b. controls and maintains the oxygen above 50%.
   c. does not come into direct contact with the face.
   d. keeps the child warm and dry.

30. When caring for the child receiving oxygen via a mist tent, the nurse should:
   a. encourage the child to have a stuffed animal in the tent.
   b. open the tent as little as possible.
   c. open the tent at the bottom of the bed to allow as little oxygen to escape as possible.
   d. keep the child cool because the tent becomes very warm.

31. In children, oxygen-induced CO_2 narcosis is encountered *most* frequently with which one of the following disorders?
    a. Prematurity
    b. Asthma
    c. Cystic fibrosis
    d. Congenital heart disease

32. For a child under the age of 5 who needs intermittent delivery of an aerosolized medication, the nurse should consider using a:
    a. hand-held nebulizer.
    b. metered-dose inhaler with a spacer device.
    c. humidified mist tent with low-flow oxygen.
    d. metered-dose inhaler without a spacer device.

33. Postural drainage should be performed:
    a. before meals but following other respiratory therapy.
    b. after meals but before other respiratory therapy.
    c. before meals and before other respiratory therapy.
    d. after meals and after other respiratory therapy.

34. When performing postural drainage, special modifications of the usual techniques are necessary for:
    a. infants.
    b. children with head injuries.
    c. children in traction.
    d. all of the above.

35. The chest physiotherapy technique that has been shown through research to be an effective modality is
    a. postural drainage with forced expiration.
    b. postural drainage with percussion.
    c. percussion and vibration.
    d. all of the above.

36. Chest percussion is being performed correctly if:
    a. it makes a slapping sound.
    b. it is painful.
    c. a soft circular mask is used.
    d. it is performed over the rib cage and diaphragm.

37. The *best* method to stimulate deep breathing in a child is to:
    a. encourage the child to cover the mouth and suppress his or her cough.
    b. encourage the child to cough repeatedly.
    c. use games that extend expiratory time and pressure.
    d. leave some balloons at the bedside for the child to blow up.

38. To avoid barotrauma when using the bag-valve-mask device, the nurse should:
    a. use the type without a reservoir.
    b. use the type with a pop-off valve.
    c. use a low oxygen concentration.
    d. hyperextend the infant's neck.

39. In a younger child who weighs 30 kg, the urinary output value that *most* indicates a problem is:
    a. 100 ml from 2 a.m. to 3 a.m.
    b. 100 ml from 2 a.m. to 6 a.m.
    c. 200 ml from 2 a.m. to 4 a.m.
    d. 200 ml from 2 a.m. to 5 a.m.

40. The *most* severe complication that can occur during the intubation procedure is:
    a. infection.
    b. sore throat.
    c. laryngeal stenosis.
    d. hypoxia.

41. Of the following vacuum pressures, the *most* acceptable pressure to use to suction the tracheostomy of a child is:
    a. 30 mm Hg
    b. 50 mm Hg
    c. 70 mm Hg
    d. 120 mm Hg

42. When suctioning a child's airway, the nurse should always:
    a. use intermittent suction.
    b. inject saline into the tube.
    c. insert the catheter until it meets resistance.
    d. use continuous suction.

43. Suctioning obstructs the airway; therefore, the suction catheter should remain in the child's airway no longer than:
    a. 3 seconds.
    b. 5 seconds.
    c. 8 seconds.
    d. 10 seconds.

44. For a tracheostomy dressing, it would be *incorrect* to use:
    a. Duoderm CGF.
    b. Allevyn dressing.
    c. A 4 x 4 gauze pad cut into the needed shape.
    d. Hollister Restore.

45. After the initial postoperative change, the tracheostomy tube is usually changed:
    a. weekly by the surgeon.
    b. weekly by the nurse/family.
    c. monthly by the surgeon.
    d. monthly by the nurse/family.

46. Describe three factors in the home environment that need to be considered when discharging a child with a tracheostomy.

47. A tracheostomy with a speaking valve:
    a. decreases secretions.
    b. decreases the child's sense of taste and smell.
    c. limits gas exchange.
    d. has no effect on the ability to swallow.

48. List at least ten conditions that predispose a child to respiratory failure.

49. The pediatric nurse should know that the early subtle indication of hypoxia is:
    a. peripheral cyanosis.
    b. central cyanosis.
    c. hypotension.
    d. mood changes and restlessness.

50. Of the following strategies, the one that is *least* likely to decrease the oxygen demand of the child with respiratory distress is:
    a. maintain temperature within normal limits.
    b. place the child in the supine position.
    c. control pain.
    d. maintain an ambient room temperature.

51. Cardiac arrest in the pediatric population is *most* often a result of:
    a. atherosclerosis.
    b. congenital heart disease.
    c. prolonged hypoxia.
    d. undiagnosed cardiac conditions.

52. The *first* action the nurse should take when discovering a child in an emergency outside the hospital is to:
    a. transport the child to an acute care facility.
    b. determine whether the child is unconscious.
    c. administer rescue breathing.
    d. transport the child by car for help.

53. The nurse should place the bag-valve-mask device over both the mouth and the nose for individuals whose age is:
    a. birth to 1 year.
    b. 1 year to 3 years
    c. birth to 3 years
    d. birth to 2 years

54. The brachial pulse is the preferred site to use to assess circulation in the:
    a. infant.
    b. school-age child.
    c. adolescent.
    d. adult.

55. In a child who is conscious and choking, the nurse should attempt to relieve the obstruction if the victim:
    a. is making sounds.
    b. has an effective cough.
    c. has stridor.
    d. all of the above.

56. Match each drug with its use during pediatric emergency resuscitation.

    a. Sodium bicarbonate   d. Adenosine   g. Epinephrine

    b. Calcium chloride   e. Dopamine   h. Atropine

    c. Amiodarone   f. Lidocaine   i. Naloxone

    _____ Reverses respiratory arrest that is due to excessive opiate administration

    _____ Increases cardiac output and heart rate by blocking vagal stimulation in the heart

    _____ The first choice for ventricular tachycardia that is refractory to defibrillation

    _____ Used for hypermagnesemia; needed for normal cardiac contractility

    _____ Causes vasoconstriction and increases cardiac output

    _____ Used for ventricular dysrhythmias

    _____ Acts on alpha- and beta-adrenergic receptor sites, causing contraction, especially at the site of the heart, vascular, and other smooth muscle

    _____ Administered rapidly; causes a temporary block through the atrioventricular node

    _____ Used to buffer the pH

57. The Heimlich maneuver is recommended for children over the age of:
    a. 4 years.
    b. 3 years.
    c. 2 years.
    d. 1 year.

Critical Thinking

58. A 14-month-old male child is admitted to the pediatric unit with a respiratory infection. If he has a cough that is characteristic of croup syndromes, the nurse would expect to hear:
    a. paroxysmal cough with an inspiratory "whoop."
    b. a brassy cough.
    c. a very severe cough.
    d. a quiet cough.

59. If the child has no cough at all, the nurse would *most* likely suspect:
    a. cystic fibrosis.
    b. pertussis.
    c. pneumonia.
    d. measles.

60. The child is placed under a mist tent at 40% oxygen. Chest physiotherapy and intravenous antibiotics are started. The nurse is monitoring his oxygen saturation with pulse oximetry. The pulse oximeter alarm sounds, and the saturation registers at 76%. The nurse should begin the assessment with an evaluation for changes in:
    a. behavior.
    b. skin color.
    c. placement of the oximeter sensor.
    d. hemoglobin.

61. If the child were diagnosed as having pneumonia, which one of the following adjunctive techniques would be of *no* value?
    a. Intravenous antibiotics
    b. The mist tent at 40% oxygen
    c. Pulse oximetry
    d. Chest physiotherapy

CHAPTER 32

The Child with Respiratory Dysfunction

1. The following terms are related to respiratory infection. Match each term with its description.

a. Upper respiratory tract
b. Lower respiratory tract
c. Strep throat
d. Acute rheumatic fever (ARF)
e. Acute glomerulonephritis
f. Adenoids

g. Waldeyer tonsillar ring
h. Palatine tonsils
i. Pharyngeal tonsils
j. Lingual tonsils
k. Tubal tonsils
l. Tonsillectomy

m. Adenoidectomy
n. Epstein-Barr (EB)
o. Heterophil antibody test
p. Spot test (Monospot)
q. Antigenic shift
r. Antigenic drift

_____ One of the more serious sequelae of strep throat; an inflammatory disease of the heart, joints, and central nervous system

_____ Adenoids; located above the palatine tonsils on the posterior wall of the nasopharynx

_____ One of the more serious sequelae of strep throat; an acute kidney infection

_____ Removal of the adenoids; recommended for those children in whom hypertrophied adenoids obstruct nasal breathing

_____ The mass of lymphoid tissue that encircles the nasal and oral pharynx

_____ Consists of the alveoli, bronchi, and bronchioles (the reactive portion on the airway with smooth muscle and the ability to constrict)

_____ Faucial tonsils; located on either side of the oropharynx, behind and below the pillars of the fauces; usually visible during oral examination; removed during tonsillectomy

_____ A slide test of high specificity for the diagnosis of infectious mononucleosis

_____ Consists primarily of the nose and pharynx; upper airway

_____ Removal of the palatine tonsils; indicated for massive hypertrophy that results in difficulty breathing or eating

_____ Also known as the pharyngeal tonsils

_____ Major changes in viruses that occur at intervals of years (usually 5 to 10)

_____ A virus; the principal cause of infectious mononucleosis

_____ Group A β-hemolytic streptococcus (GABHS) infection of the upper airway

_____ Located at the base of the tongue

_____ Minor variations in viruses that occur almost annually

_____ Determines the extent to which the patient's serum will agglutinate sheep red blood cells; used to diagnose infectious mononucleosis (titer of 1:160 required for diagnosis); rapid, sensitive, inexpensive, and easy to perform

_____ Found near the posterior nasopharyngeal opening of the eustachian tubes; not a part of the Waldeyer tonsillar ring

2. The following terms are related to otitis media. Match each term with its description.

a. Otitis media
b. Acute otitis media (AOM)
c. Otitis media with effusion (OME)
d. Chronic otitis media with effusion
e. Hearing loss

f. Tympanic membrane retraction
g. Tympanosclerosis
h. Eardrum perforation
i. Adhesive otitis media
j. Chronic supportive otitis media

k. Labyrinthitis
l. Mastoiditis
m. Meningitis
n. Cholesteatoma
o. Pneumatic otoscopy
p. Tympanometry
q. Swimmer's ear

_____ An inflammation of the middle ear and mastoid otoscopy; characterized by perforation and discharge (otorrhea) lasting up to 6 weeks

_____ Assesses the mobility of the tympanic membrane, using air transmission

_____ Middle ear inflammation with rapid and short onset of signs and symptoms lasting approximately 3 weeks

_____ Infection of the inner ear

_____ One of the least common but potentially most dangerous sequelae of OME; the formation of a ketatinized epithelial cell lining that forms scales within the middle ear space; erodes all of the structures it encounters, especially bone

_____ An inflammation of the middle ear without reference to etiology or pathogenesis

_____ Eardrum scarring; the deposition of hyaline material into the fibrous layer of the tympanic membrane; associated with repeated inflammatory AOM or with repeated tympanoplasty tube placement

_____ Infection of the mastoid sinus

_____ One of the consequences of prolonged middle ear disorder, usually conductive and not severe

_____ A thickening of the mucous membrane by proliferation of fibrous tissue that can cause fixation of the ossicles with resultant hearing loss; sometimes called "glue ear"

_____ A suppurative intracranial complication from the extension of a middle ear or mastoid infection

_____ Middle ear effusion that persist beyond 3 months

_____ A common complication of AOM; often accompanies chronic disease; a complication of tympanoplasty tube placement

_____ Retraction pocket; occurs when continued negative middle ear pressure draws the tympanic membrane inward; may result in impaired sound transmission

_____ The test to asses mobility of the tympanic membrane using sound transmission

_____ Inflammation of the middle ear in which a collection of fluid is present in the middle ear space

_____ Otitis externa; inflammation that occurs when the external ear environment is altered during swimming, bathing, or conditions of increased humidity

3. The following terms are related to croup syndromes and other respiratory infections. Match each term with its description.

a. Croup
b. Racemic epinephrine
c. Tracheobronchitis
d. Respiratory syncytial virus (RSV)
e. Ribavirin
f. RespiGam
g. Meningism
h. Tubercle
i. Miliary TB

j. TB infection
k. TB disease
l. Purified protein derivative (PPD)
m. Tuberculin test
n. Positive reaction TB skin test
o. Negative reaction TB skin test

p. gastric washings
q. Reactive portion of the lungs
r. Pneumonitis
s. lobar pneumonia
t. bronchopneumonia
u. interstitial pneumonia
v. emphysemia

_____ Result that usually means the child has never been infected with the organism

_____ Responsible for at least 50% of children admitted for bronchiolitis

_____ Aspiration of lavaged contents from the fasting stomach; the best means for obtaining material for respiratory smears or culture

_____ The type of pneumonia in which the inflammatory process is confined within the alveolar walls and the peribronchial and interlobular tissues

_____ Nebulized epinephrine; used in children with stridor at rest, retractions, or difficulty breathing

_____ Meningeal symptoms

_____ A symptom complex characterized by hoarseness, a resonant cough described as "barking" or "brassy," inspiratory stridor, and respiratory distress from swelling in the region of the larynx

_____ Includes the bronchi and bronchioles in children because cartilaginous support of the large airways is not fully developed until adolescence

_____ Formed by epithelial cells surrounding and encapsulating multiplying bacilli in an attempt to wall off the invading organisms

_____ The type of pneumonia that begins in the terminal bronchioles, which become clogged with mucopurulent exudates to form consolidated patches in the nearby lobule;

_____ An antiviral agent; may be used to treat RSV

_____ Progressive overinflation of the lung caused by obstruction of the small airway passages, which prevents air from leaving the lungs

_____ Used widely; standard dose is 5 tuberculin units in 0.1 ml of solution, injected intradermally; Mantoux test

_____ Widespread dissemination of the tubercle bacillus to near and distant sites

_____ Result that indicates a person has been infected; does not confirm the presence of active disease

_____ The type of pneumonia in which all or a large segment of one or more pulmonary lobes is involved; known as "bilateral" or "double pneumonia" when both lungs are affected

_____ Respiratory syncytial virus immune globulin; has been used prophylactically to prevent RSV in high-risk infants

_____ The inflammation of the large airways, which is frequently associated with an upper respiratory infection; primarily caused by viral agents

_____ The localized acute inflammation of the lung without the toxemia associated with lobar pneumonia

_____ Manifested by a positive skin test; asymptomatic

_____ The single most important test to determine whether a child has been infected with the tubercle bacillus

_____ Diagnosed by positive chest radiograph, positive sputum culture, and presence of signs of the disease

4. The following terms are related to noninfectious irritants. Match each term with its description.

a. Aspiration pneumonia
b. Carbon monoxide (CO)
c. Carboxyhemoglobin (COHb)
d. Hyperbaric oxygen chamber
e. Cotinine

_____ Forms when carbon monoxide enters the bloodstream and binds with hemoglobin

_____ A colorless, odorless gas with an affinity for hemoglobin 200 to 250 times greater than that of oxygen

_____ A byproduct of nicotine that is considered a valid biochemical marker for environmental smoke exposure; urinary levels increased in children living with smokers

_____ Therapy for smoke toxicity that facilitates the breakdown of the carboxyhemoglobin bond and improves oxygen delivery to the tissues

_____ Occurs when food, secretions, inert material, volatile compounds, or liquids enter the lung and cause inflammation and a chemical pneumonitis

5. The following terms are related to long-term respiratory dysfunction. Match each term with its description.

a. Seasonal allergic rhinitis
b. House dust mites
c. Cockroach
d. Long-term control medications
e. Quick-relief medications
f. Nebulization
g. Exercise-induced bronchospasm
h. Written action plan
i. Peak expiratory flow meters
j. Spacers
k. Cystic fibrosis transmembrane regulator (CFTR)
l. Meconium ileus
m. Distal intestinal obstruction syndrome
n. Prolapse of the rectum
o. Chest physiotherapy
p. Flutter mucus clearance device
q. ThAIRapy vest
r. Dormase alfa
s. Lung transplantation
t. Specific tissue binding
u. Peak expiratory flow rate (PEFR)
v. Personal best value
w   Turbuhaler
x. Salmeterol
y. Status asthmaticus
z. Steatorrhea
aa. Azotorrhea
bb. Quantitative sweat chloride test

_____ Used daily to prevent infection and to maintain pulmonary hygiene in children with cystic fibrosis

_____ A method of medication administration in which the medication is mixed with saline and changed into an aerosol with a compressed air machine

_____ Used at home by the child with asthma to monitor personal best values

_____ Hay fever

_____ Holding chamber; devices that attach to a metered-dose inhaler and hold medication long enough for the patient to inhale slowly

_____ An important allergen in children with asthma; most common allergen in inner-city environments

_____ The protein product that is located on the long arm of chromosome 7; indicator of cystic fibrosis

_____ Rescue medications; used to treat acute symptoms and exacerbations of asthma

_____ Allergen identified most often in children allergic to inhalants

_____ Should be given to all children with asthma to use in the event of an exacerbation

_____ The earliest postnatal manifestation of cystic fibrosis; seen in 7% to 10% of newborns with the disease; occurs when thick, putty-like tenacious mucilaginous meconium blocks the lumen of the small intestine, usually at or near the ileocecal valve, giving rise to signs of intestinal obstruction

_____ Provides a high-frequency chest wall oscillation to help loosen secretions

_____ Small, hand-held plastic pipe with a stainless steel ball on the inside that facilitates removal of mucus

_____ Caused by a loss of heat and/or water from the lungs because of hyperventilation of air that is cooler and dryer than that of the respiratory tract

_____ The most common gastrointestinal complication associated with cystic fibrosis; occurs most often in infancy and early childhood and is related to large bulky stools and lack of supportive fat pads around the rectum

_____ Preventive medications; used to achieve and maintain control of inflammation in asthma

_____ A final therapeutic option for a few patients with end-stage cystic fibrosis

_____ Name given to a partial or complete intestinal obstruction that occurs in some children with cystic fibrosis

_____ Recombinant human deoxyribonuclease; an aerosolized medication that decreases the viscosity of mucus; available in brand name as Pulmozyme

_____ A chlorofluorocarbon (CFC)–propelled metered-dose inhaler that delivers powdered medication; eliminates the need to coordinate activation of the device with the breath

_____ Excessive protein in the stool

_____ The process whereby the antigen mediates a reaction; the antibody attaches to surfaces cells, where it reacts with the specific antigen to which they have developed a bonding capacity

_____ Serevent; a long-acting bronchodilator that is used twice a day; added to anti-inflammatory therapy for prevention of long-term symptoms

_____ A tool used to monitor pulmonary function; measures the maximum flow of air forcefully exhaled in 1 second; measured in liters per minute

_____ Excessive fat in the stool

_____ Established by measuring values during a 2- to 3-week period when asthma is stable; compared with current PEFR to make care management decisions

_____ A medical emergency in which the child continues to display respiratory distress despite vigorous therapeutic measures such as sympathomimetics

_____ Pilocarpine iontophoresis; a test that involves stimulating the production of sweat and measuring the seat electrolytes; used to determine presence of cystic fibrosis; should only be carried out by personnel skilled in performing the procedure

6. The largest percentage of respiratory infections in children are caused by:
   a. pneumococci.
   b. viruses.
   c. streptococci.
   d. *Haemophilus influenzae*.

7. The *most* likely reason that the respiratory infection rate increases drastically in the age range from 3 to 6 month is that the:
   a. infant's exposure to pathogens is greatly increased during this time.
   b. viral agents that are mild in older children are extremely severe in infants.
   c. maternal antibodies have disappeared and the infant's own antibody production is immature.
   d. diameter of the airways is smaller in the infant than in the older child.

8. A febrile seizure is *least* likely to be associated with:
   a. fever in a 2-year-old child.
   b. a family history of febrile seizures.
   c. fever in an 8-year-old child.
   d. all of the above.

9. When giving tips for how to increase humidity in the home of a child with a respiratory infection, the nurse should emphasize that the primary concern is to ensure that the child has:
   a. a steam vaporizer.
   b. a warm humidification source.
   c. a safe humidification source.
   d. a cool humidification source.

10. Bobby is a child with a respiratory disorder who needs bed rest but who is not cooperating. The nurse's *best* choice is to:
    a. be sure Bobby's mother takes the advice seriously.
    b. allow Bobby to play quietly on the floor.
    c. insist that Bobby play quietly in bed.
    d. allow Bobby to cry until he stays in bed.

11. For a child who is having difficulty breathing through his stuffy nose, the nurse should recommend:
    a. dextromethorphan nose drops.
    b. phenylephrine nose drops.
    c. dextromethorphan cough squares.
    d. steroid nose drops.

12. Children with nasopharyngitis may be treated with:
    a. decongestants.
    b. antihistamines.
    c. expectorants.
    d. all of the above.

13. The *best* technique to use to prevent spread of nasopharyngitis is:
    a. prompt immunization.
    b. to avoid contact with infected persons.
    c. mist vaporization.
    d. to ensure adequate fluid intake.

14. Group A β-hemolytic streptococci infection is usually a:
    a. serious infection of the upper airway.
    b. common cause of pharyngitis in children over the age of 15 years.
    c. brief illness that leaves the child at risk for serious sequelae.
    d. disease of the heart, lungs, joints, and central nervous system.

15. The American Academy of Pediatrics recommends that health care providers base their diagnosis of group A β-hemolytic streptococcus on:
    a. antibody responses.
    b. antistreptolysin O responses.
    c. complete blood count.
    d. throat culture.

16. A strategy for the prevention of streptococcal disease would be for the nurse to recommend that:
    a. a child with streptococcal infection should not return to school until after 48 hours of antibiotic therapy.
    b. children with streptococcal infection should discard their toothbrush and replace it with a new one after 24 hours of antibiotic therapy.
    c. children with streptococcal infection should not return to school until 36 hours of antibiotic therapy.
    d. children with streptococcal infection should discard their toothbrush and replace it with a new one as soon as the streptococcus is identified.

17. Offensive mouth odor, persistent dry cough, and a voice with a muffled nasal quality are commonly the result of:
    a. tonsillectomy.
    b. adenoidectomy.
    c. mouth breathing.
    d. otitis media.

18. An adenoidectomy would be *contraindicated* in a child:
    a. with recurrent otitis media.
    b. with malignancy.
    c. with thrombocytopenia.
    d. under the age of 3 years.

19. In the postoperative period following a tonsillectomy, the child should:
    a. be placed in Trendelenburg position.
    b. be encouraged to cough and deep breath.
    c. be suctioned vigorously to clear the airway.
    d. rest in bed the remainder of the day after the surgery.

20. Pain medication for the child in the postoperative period following a tonsillectomy should be administered:
    a. orally at regular intervals.
    b. orally as needed.
    c. rectally or intravenously at regular intervals.
    d. rectally or intravenously as needed.

21. Of the following foods the *most* appropriate to offer first to an alert child who is in the postoperative period following a tonsillectomy would be:
    a. ice cream.
    b. red gelatin.
    c. flavored ice pops.
    d. all of the above.

22. An early indication of hemorrhage in a child who has had a tonsillectomy is:
    a. frequent swallowing.
    b. decreasing blood pressure.
    c. restlessness.
    d. all of the above.

23. The finding that is almost always present in an adolescent with infectious mononucleosis is:
    a. skin rash.
    b. otitis media.
    c. hepatic involvement.
    d. failure to thrive.

24. Diagnosis of infectious mononucleosis is established when the:
    a. leukocyte count is elevated.
    b. leukocyte count is depressed.
    c. antibody testing is positive.
    d. antibody testing is negative.

25. Infectious mononucleosis is usually a:
    a. disease complicated with pneumonitis and anemia.
    b. self-limiting disease.
    c. disabling disease.
    d. difficult and prolonged disease.

26. Clinical manifestations of influenza usually include all of the following *except*:
    a. nausea and vomiting.
    b. fever and chills.
    c. sore throat and dry mucous membranes.
    d. photophobia and myalgia.

27. The infant is predisposed to developing otitis media because the eustachian tubes:
    a. lie in a relatively horizontal plane.
    b. have a limited amount of lymphoid tissue.
    c. are long and narrow.
    d. are underdeveloped.

28. List at least five complications of otitis media.

29. The clinical manifestations of otitis media include:
    a. purulent discharge in the external auditory canal.
    b. clear discharge in the external auditory canal.
    c. enlarged axillary lymph nodes.
    d. enlarged cervical lymph nodes.

30. An abnormal otoscopic exam would reveal:
    a. visible landmarks.
    b. a light reflex.
    c. dull gray tympanic membrane.
    d. mobile tympanic membrane.

31. Of the following antibiotics, the one that would most likely be prescribed for uncomplicated otitis media would be:
    a. tetracycline.
    b. amoxacillin.
    c. gentamicin.
    d. methicillin.

32. To help alleviate the discomfort and fever of otitis media, the nurse may administer:
    a. acetaminophen or ibuprofen.
    b. antihistamines and decongestants.
    c. analgesic ear drops.
    d. all of the above.

33. Recurrent otitis media in high-risk infants may be managed therapeutically by:
    a. tonsillectomy.
    b. steroids.
    c. polyvalent pneumococcal polysaccharide vaccine.
    d. immune globulin with antibodies.

34. Children with tympanostomy tubes should:
    a. never swim without earplugs.
    b. keep bath water out of the ear.
    c. notify the physician immediately if a grommet appears.
    d. never allow any water to enter their ears.

35. Which one of the following techniques would be *contraindicated* for the nurse to recommend to parents to prevent recurrent otitis externa?
    a. Administer a combination of vinegar and alcohol after swimming.
    b. Allow the child to swim every day.
    c. Dry the ear canal after swimming with a cotton swab.
    d. Use a hair dryer on low heat at 1-2 feet for 30 seconds several times a day.

36. Most children with croup syndromes:
    a. require hospitalization.
    b. will need to be intubated.
    c. can be cared for at home.
    d. are over 6 years old.

37. Of the following croup syndromes the one that is potentially life-threatening is:
    a. spasmodic croup.
    b. laryngotracheobronchitis.
    c. acute spasmodic laryngitis.
    d. epiglottitis.

38. The nurse should suspect epiglottitis if the child has:
    a. cough, sore throat, and agitation.
    b. cough, drooling, and retractions.
    c. absence of cough, drooling, and agitation.
    d. absence of cough, hoarseness, and retractions.

39. In the child who is suspected to have epiglottitis the nurse should:
    a. have intubation equipment available.
    b. prepare to immunize the child for *Haemophilus influenzae*.
    c. obtain a throat culture.
    d. all of the above.

40. Since the advent of immunization for *Haemophilus influenzae*, there has been a decrease in the incidence of:
    a. laryngotracheobronchitis.
    b. epiglottitis.
    c. Reye's syndrome.
    d. croup syndrome.

41. Of the following children, the one who is most likely to be hospitalized for treatment of croup is:
    a. a 2-year-old child whose croupy cough worsens at night.
    b. a 5-year-old child whose croupy cough worsens at night.
    c. a 2-year-old child using the accessory muscles to breath.
    d. a child with inspiratory stridor during the physical exam.

42. The primary therapeutic regimen for croup usually includes:
    a. vigilant assessment, racemic epinephrine, and corticosteroids.
    b. vigilant assessment, racemic epinephrine, and antibiotics.
    c. intubation, racemic epinephrine, and corticosteroids.
    d. intubation, racemic epinephrine, and corticosteroids.

43. The condition that is *most* likely to require intubation is:
    a. acute spasmodic laryngitis.
    b. bacterial tracheitis.
    c. acute laryngotracheobronchitis.
    d. acute laryngitis.

44. Respiratory syncytial virus is:
    a. an uncommon virus that usually causes severe bronchiolitis.
    b. an uncommon virus that usually does not require hospitalization.
    c. a common virus that usually causes severe bronchiolitis.
    d. a common virus that usually does not require hospitalization.

45. In the infant who is admitted with possible respiratory syncytial virus, the nurse would expect the lab to perform:
    a. the ELISA antibody test on nasal secretions.
    b. a viral culture of the stool.
    c. a bacterial culture of nasal secretions.
    d. an anaerobic culture of the blood.

46. Nurses caring for a child with respiratory syncitial virus should:
    a. have a skin test applied every 6 months.
    b. wear gloves and gowns when entering the room.
    c. turn off the aerosol machine before opening the tent.
    d. not take care of other children with respiratory syncitial virus at the same time.

47. Match the age of the child with the most common cause of pneumonia in that age group.

    a. *Haemophilus influenzae*

    b. *Streptococcus pneumoniae*

    c. *Mycoplasma pneumoniae*

    _____ Over 5 years of age
    _____ 3 months to 5 years old
    _____ Under 3 months

48. Closed chest drainage is most likely to be used with the type of pneumonia that is caused by:
    a. *Haemophilus influenzae.*
    b. *Mycoplasma pneumoniae.*
    c. *Streptococcus pneumoniae.*
    d. *Staphylococcal pneumoniae.*

49. Describe four nursing measures to use to care for the child with pneumonia.

50. In an 8-month-old infant admitted with pertussis, the nurse should particularly assess the:
    a. living conditions of the infant.
    b. labor and delivery history of the mother.
    c. immunization status of the infant.
    d. alcohol and drug intake of the mother.

51. The *best* test to screen for tuberculosis is the:
    a. chest x-ray.
    b. purified protein derivative (PPD) test.
    c. sputum culture.
    d. multipuncture tests (MPT), such as the tine test.

52. The recommended treatment for the child who has active tuberculosis includes:
    a. isoniazid.
    b. rifampin.
    c. pyrazinamide.
    d. all of the above.

53. Which one of the following Mantoux test results would be considered positive?
    a. Induration 5 mm in a 3-year-old child with HIV
    b. Induration 2 mm in a 5-year-old child without TB contacts
    c. Induration 7 mm in an 8-year-old child without any risk factors
    d. All of the above

54. The usual site of bronchial obstruction is the:
    a. left bronchus because it is shorter and straighter.
    b. left bronchus because it is longer and angled.
    c. right bronchus because it is shorter and straighter.
    d. right bronchus because it is longer and angled.

55. The *definitive diagnosis* of airway foreign bodies in the trachea and larynx requires:
    a. radiographic examination.
    b. fluoroscopic examination.
    c. bronchoscopic examination.
    d. ultrasonographic examination.

56. Parents may be taught to treat aspiration of a foreign body in an infant under 12 months old by using:
    a. back blows and chest thrusts.
    b. back blows only.
    c. the Heimlich maneuver only.
    d. a blind finger sweep.

57. The child who has ingested lighter fluid usually receives:
    a. the same treatment as a child who has hepatitis.
    b. medication to induce vomiting.
    c. the same treatment as a child who has pneumonia.
    d. activated charcoal.

58. List five strategies that may be used to manage acute respiratory distress syndrome in children.

59. Deaths from fires are most often a result of:
    a. full-thickness burns over 50% of the body.
    b. full-thickness burns to the chest and neck.
    c. noxious substances from incomplete combustion.
    d. injuries sustained in escape attempts.

60. Treatment of smoke toxicity with a COHb level of 10% would most likely consist of:
    a. humidified O_2 at 70%.
    b. humidified O_2 at 100%.
    c. intubation.
    d. use of a hyperbaric oxygen chamber.

61. The biochemical marker for environmental smoke exposure is called _____.

62. List at least five physical findings commonly seen in the child with allergic rhinitis.

63. Of the following children, the one who is *most* likely suffering from allergy rather than a cold would be the:
    a. two-year-old with fever and runny nose.
    b. adolescent with itchy eyes and constant sneezing without fever.
    c. two-year-old with sporadic sneezing and a runny nose.
    d. adolescent with sporadic sneezing and a runny nose.

64. The severity of asthma in a child with daily asthmatic symptoms would be classified as:
    a. mild intermittent.
    b. mild persistent.
    c. moderate persistent.
    d. severe persistent.

Critical Thinking—Case Study

Jason Wilson, 8 years old, is admitted to the pediatric unit with a diagnosis of reactive airway disease. This is his first hospitalization for this disorder. Both of Jason's parents smoke cigarettes, but they try to smoke outdoors. Jason usually does quite well, although his asthma tends to increase in severity during the winter months. Recently he has had several colds and his asthma has flared up each time. This time, however, he is quite uncomfortable. He has wheezes in all lung fields.

65. Of the following questions, the one that would be *most* important for the nurse to ask Jason's mother would be:
    a. "What brings you to the hospital?"
    b. "What is your ethnic background?"
    c. "Do you have any history of asthma in your family?"
    d. "Was your pregnancy and delivery uneventful?"

66. Mrs. Wilson wants the nurse to explain exactly what reactive airway disease is. She says she has been told many times, but it is always when Jason is in so much distress that she is not sure she hears it correctly. The nurse would respond, knowing that:
    a. asthma is caused by a certain inflammatory mediator.
    b. the one mechanism responsible for the obstructive symptoms of asthma is excess mucous secretion.
    c. the one mechanism responsible for the obstructive symptoms of asthma is spasm of the smooth muscle of the bronchi.
    d. most theories do not explain all types and causes of asthma.

67. In general Jason does not have difficulty with any food or emotional triggers for asthma. An asthmatic episode for Jason starts with itching all over the upper part of his back. He is usually quite irritable and very restless. He complains of headache, chest tightness, and feeling tired. He usually coughs, sweats, and sits in the tripod position with his shoulders in a hunched-over position. Today he has no fever, and he is sitting upright. His skin is not sweaty. Based on this information, the nurse would decide that Jason is:
    a. severely ill.
    b. moderately ill.
    c. mildly ill.
    d. not ill at all.

68. Jason's younger sister Tanya is an infant. Tanya's disease is much worse than Jason's. Mrs. Wilson states that Tanya often has movements of her chest muscles that make it appear that she is working very hard to breathe; however, her respiratory rate does not change. When this happens, Tanya is not exhaling a long breath like Jason. These differences between Jason and Tanya are confusing to Mrs. Wilson, and she asks the nurse for advice about what to do when this happens to Tanya. The nurse's response is based on the knowledge that:
    a. dyspnea is much more difficult to evaluate in an infant than in a young child.
    b. infants and young children's bodies respond to the asthmatic episode the same way.
    c. boys tend to have more severe symptoms of asthma than girls do.
    d. dyspnea is much more difficult to evaluate in a young child than in an infant.

69. The nurse examines Jason and finds that he has hyperresonance on percussion. His breath sounds are coarse and loud with sonorous crackles throughout the lung fields. Expiration is prolonged. There is generalized inspiratory and expiratory wheezing. Based on these findings, the nurse suspects that there is:
    a. minimal obstruction.
    b. significant obstruction.
    c. imminent ventilatory failure.
    d. an extrathoracic obstruction.

70. The nurse determines that Jason's peak expiratory flow rate is in the yellow zone. The nurse realizes this test result indicates that Jason's asthma control is about:
    a. 80% of his personal best and that his routine treatment plan can be followed.
    b. 50% of his personal best and that he needs an increase in his usual therapy.
    c. 50% of his personal best and that he needs immediate bronchodilators.
    d. less than 50% of his personal best and that he need immediate bronchodilators.

71. Jason's test results are back from the lab. The white blood cell count is 11,200/mm^3. The eosinophils are 728/mm^3. The chest x-ray shows hyperexpansion of the airways. The nurse knows that these findings:
    a. support the diagnosis of pneumonia without an episode of asthma.
    b. support the diagnosis of asthma complicated with pneumonia.
    c. do not support the diagnosis of an acute episode of asthma or pneumonia.
    d. support the diagnosis of an acute episode of asthma without pneumonia.

72. The physician orders albuterol via inhaler for Jason. Mrs. Wilson is very concerned, because she says that Jason usually receives theophylline intravenously. The nurse's response is based on the fact that:
    a. Jason's asthma episode is probably not as severe as usual.
    b. Jason's physician must be using information that is out of date.
    c. theophylline is a third-line drug that is a weak bronchodilator and not considered as effective as nebulized beta agonists.
    d. theophylline is a third-line drug because it has been shown to adversely affect school performance.

73. When preparing for discharge, the nurse would *most* likely plan to teach the Wilson family to:
    a. keep the humidity at home above 50%.
    b. vacuum the carpets at least twice weekly.
    c. treat carpets with a 3% tannic acid solution.
    d. launder sheets/blankets regularly in cold water.

74. Jason uses aerosolized steroids at home; therefore he should be taught to rinse his mouth thoroughly with water:
    a. before each treatment to increase absorption.
    b. after each treatment to minimize the risk for oral candidiasis.
    c. before each treatment to minimize the adverse effects of the drug.
    d. after each treatment to increase absorption.

75. Based on the nurse's assessment, a care plan is developed. Of the following nursing diagnoses, the one that would *least* likely appear on Jason's care plan is:
    a. activity intolerance related to imbalance between oxygen supply and demand.
    b. ineffective airway clearance related to allergenic response and inflammation in bronchial tree.
    c. high risk for infection related to the presence of infective organisms.
    d. altered family process related to a chronic illness.

76. One principle that should be a part of Jason's home self-management program is that:
    a. patients must learn not to abuse their medications so that they will not become addicted.
    b. it is easy to treat an asthmatic episode as long as the child knows the symptoms.
    c. although quite uncommon, asthma is very treatable.
    d. children with asthma are usually able to participate in the same activities as nonasthmatic children.

Andrea McCauley is an 8-year-old with cystic fibrosis. She is in the fifth percentile for both height and weight. This failure to thrive persists even though she has a voracious appetite. She has been managed at home most recently for about 6 months without the need for hospitalization. She is admitted today with blood-tinged sputum. The sputum culture obtained 2 days ago is positive for pseudomonas. The nurse hears crackles in both lungs, and Andrea has significant clubbing of her fingers with a capillary refill time of greater than 5 seconds.

77. Based on the information presented in Andrea McCauley's case, the nurse suspects that Andrea's:
    a. condition is improving and she will soon return to home care.
    b. condition is progressively worsening.
    c. condition is worse, but intravenous antibiotic therapy will correct the problem.
    d. family has been noncompliant, causing this set back.

78. The admission orders included an order for gentamicin at a dose that the nurse calculated to be higher than usual for a child of Andrea's size. Which of the following is an acceptable reason for the high dosage?
    a. The physician used Andrea's age rather than her size to determine the dose.
    b. The pharmacy has made an error.
    c. Children with cystic fibrosis metabolize antibiotics rapidly.
    d. Children with cystic fibrosis metabolize antibiotics slowly.

79. The use of which of the following strategies would most likely be *contraindicated* for Andrea?
    a. Forced expiration
    b. Aerobic exercise
    c. Chest physiotherapy
    d. High-flow oxygen therapy

80. The blood-tinged sputum progresses to an amount greater than 300 ml per day. The nurse recognizes that increased tendency to bleed may be a result of:
    a. iron deficiency anemia.
    b. vitamin K deficiency.
    c. thrombocytopenia.
    d. vitamin D deficiency.

81. At the present time, family support for Andrea will most likely include strategies to help her family cope with all of the following issues *except*:
    a. pregnancy and genetic counseling.
    b. relief from the continual routine with respite care.
    c. dealing with a chronic illness and anticipatory grieving.
    d. abnormal psychologic adjustment and dysfunctional family patterns.

82. Andrea takes seven pancreatic enzyme capsules about 30 minutes before each meal. She usually has two to three bowel movements per day. The nurse's action in regard to the pancreatic enzymes is based on the knowledge that the dosage:
    a. is adequate.
    b. should always be fewer than five capsules.
    c. should be seven to ten capsules.
    d. is adequate, but she should take it between meals.

CHAPTER 33

The Child with Gastrointestinal Dysfunction

1. Which one of the following is *not* a function of the GI system?
   a. Process and absorb nutrients necessary to support growth and development
   b. Maintain thermoregulatory functions
   c. Perform excretory functions
   d. Maintain fluid and electrolyte balance

2. Identify the following as true or false.
   _____ At birth the term infant has the ability to move food particles from the front of the mouth to the back of the mouth.
   _____ The infant has no voluntary control of swallowing for the first 3 months.
   _____ The chewing function is facilitated by eruption of the primary teeth.
   _____ The primary purpose of saliva in the newborn is to moisten the mouth and throat.
   _____ The infant's stomach is smaller in capacity but faster to empty than the child's stomach.
   _____ The infant's stomach at birth has an elongated shape.

3. Fill in the blanks in the following statements.

   a. Three processes, _____, _____, and _____, are necessary to convert nutrients into forms that can be used by the body.

   b. Chemical digestion involves five general types of GI secretions: _____,

   _____, _____ _____, _____,

   and _____ _____ _____.

   c. The _____ _____ is the principal absorption site in the GI system.

4. What are the five *most* important basic nursing assessments included in a thorough GI assessment?

5. The nurse is preparing Dottie, age 7, for an upper GI endoscopy. Which one of the following does the nurse recognize as *not* being an appropriate preparation for this test?
   a. Bowel cleansing with magnesium citrate or Golytely
   b. NPO for 8 hours before the procedure
   c. Dottie will need to be given sedation before the procedure is begun.
   d. The nurse will need to explain to Dottie in advance about the procedure by use of pictures or play with dolls and demonstration.

6. Match each term with its description.

a. Pica
b. Failure to thrive
c. Regurgitation
d. Projectile vomiting
e. Encopresis
f. Hematemesis

g. Hematochezia
h. Melena
i. Dysphagia
j. Occult blood guaiac test
k. Stool for O & P (ova and parasites)

l. Meconium
m. Peristalsis
n. Steatorrhea
o. Obstipation

_____ Appearance of ingested fat in the feces
_____ Detects presence of blood in the stool
_____ Vomiting of bright red blood as a result of bleeding in the upper GI tract or from swallowed blood from the upper respiratory tract
_____ Passage of bright red blood from the rectum
_____ Passage of dark-colored "tarry" stools
_____ Wavelike movements that squeeze food along the entire length of the alimentary tract
_____ Eating disorder in which there is compulsive eating of both food and nonfood substances
_____ Thick greenish-black secretions normally expelled from the intestine shortly after birth
_____ Having long intervals between bowel movements
_____ Accompanied by vigorous peristaltic waves
_____ Outflow of incontinent stool, causing soiling
_____ Deceleration from normal pattern of growth or growth below the 5th percentile
_____ Difficulty swallowing
_____ Aids in the diagnosis of parasitic infections
_____ A backward flowing as from the return of gastric contents into the mouth

7. Pica should be considered in which of the following children presenting to the health clinic?
   a. 7-year-old with nausea and vomiting for the past 3 days
   b. 4-year-old with history of celiac disease presenting with anemia and abdominal pain
   c. 2-year-old who is still drinking from a bottle and presents with anemia
   d. 4-month-old who presents with crying, irritability, and reddish-colored stools

8. Lance, a 2-year-old, has been brought to the clinic because his parents are afraid he has swallowed a small button battery from his father's watch, which he was playing with. The nurse recognizes which one of the following as the *most* appropriate nursing action at this time?
   a. Reassure the parents that Lance has probably not swallowed the battery because he has no symptoms, he is playing in the exam room, and his lung fields are clear.
   b. Explain to the parents that Lance will probably be allowed to normally pass the battery through the GI system because Lance has been able to eat and drink normally since the event.
   c. Start immediate teaching of Lance's parents on how to assess Lance's environment for hazardous objects, and how to assess Lance's toys and other items he might play with for safety.
   d. Explain to Lance's parents that x-ray examination will be conducted, and the battery will most probably need to be removed to prevent local damage.

9. John, age 16, asks the nurse why he has to have an endoscopy exam to determine whether he has helicobacter pylori. "Why can't they just do the blood test?" Formulate a correct response to this question.

10. After fecal impaction is removed, maintenance therapy for constipation may include laxative use. Why are milk of magnesia and polyethylene glycol considered the safest laxatives to use for pediatric patients?
    a. Decreases fluid in the colon
    b. Increases fluid in the colon
    c. Increases peristaltic stimulation
    d. Increases osmotic pressure and acidification of the colon contents

11. The nurse is counseling the mother of 12-month-old Brian on methods to prevent constipation. Which one of the following methods would be *contraindicated* for Brian?
    a. Add bran to Brian's cereal.
    b. Increase Brian's intake of water.
    c. Add prunes to Brian's diet.
    d. Add popcorn to Brian's diet.

12. Sally, age 5, is being started on bowel habit retraining program for chronic constipation. Instructions to the family should include which one of the following?
    a. Decrease the water and increase the milk in Sally's diet.
    b. Establish a regular toilet time twice a day after meals when Sally will sit on the toilet for 5 to 10 minutes.
    c. Withhold Sally's play time with her friend Julie if she does not have a daily bowel movement.
    d. Have Sally sit on the toilet each day until she has a bowel movement.

13. Which of the following is a congenital anomaly that results in mechanical obstruction from inadequate motility of part of the intestine?
    a. Intussusception
    b. Short bowel syndrome
    c. Crohn's disease
    d. Hirschsprung disease

14. To confirm the diagnosis of Hirschsprung disease, the nurse prepares the child for which one of the following tests?
    a. Barium enema
    b. Upper GI series
    c. Rectal biopsy
    d. Esophagoscopy

15. The nurse would expect to see what clinical manifestations in the older infant diagnosed with Hirschsprung disease?
    a. History of bloody diarrhea, fever, and vomiting
    b. Irritability, severe abdominal cramps, fecal soiling
    c. Decreased hemoglobin, increased serum lipids, and positive stool for O & P (ova and parasites)
    d. History of constipation, abdominal distention, and passage of ribbon-like, foul-smelling stools

16. Explain the defects present in Hirschsprung disease (congenital aganglionic megacolon).

17. The nurse would expect postoperative care for the child with Hirschsprung disease (megacolon) to include which of the following?
    i.   Nothing by mouth until return of bowel sounds
    ii. Measuring intake and output, including NG tube
    iii. Colostomy care
    iv. Monitoring intravenous fluids
    v.   Daily saline enemas
    vi. Explaining to the parents and child that the colostomy is permanent and encouraging them to assume care before discharge

    a. i, ii, iii, and iv
    b. ii, iii, and v
    c. i, ii, iii, iv, and vi
    d. i, ii, iv, and v

18. The passive transfer of gastric contents into the esophagus is termed:
    a. esophageal atresia.
    b. Meckel diverticulum.
    c. gastritis.
    d. gastroesophageal reflux.

19. To differentiate between gastroesophageal reflex (GER) and gastroesophageal reflex disease (GERD) the nurse knows that:
    a. GER includes symptoms of tissue damage.
    b. GERD includes development of complications such as failure to thrive, bleeding, and dysphagia.
    c. GER is associated with respiratory conditions such as bronchospasm and pneumonia.
    d. GERD may occur without GER.

20. The most common clinical manifestation of GER is _____.

21. The nurse instructs the parents of a 4-month-old with gastroesophageal reflux to include which one of the following in the infant's care?
    a. Stop breast-feeding since breast milk is too thin and easily leads to reflux.
    b. Place the infant in the prone position following feeding and at night.
    c. Increase the infant's intake of fruit and citrus juices.
    d. Try to increase feeding volume right before bedtime because this is the time when the stomach is more able to retain foods.

22. The child presenting with irritable bowel syndrome is *most* likely to represent which one of the following?
    a. History of alternating diarrhea and constipation, abdominal pain and bloating
    b. Alternating patterns of constipation and bloody diarrhea with little flatulence
    c. History of parasitic infections, poor nutrition, and low abdominal pain
    d. History of colic, laxative abuse, and growth retardation

23. Which one of the following would alert the nurse to possible peritonitis from a ruptured appendix in a child suspected of having appendicitis?
    a. Colicky abdominal pain with guarding of the abdomen
    b. Periumbilical pain that progresses to the lower right quadrant of the abdomen with an elevated WBC
    c. Low-grade fever of 100.6° F with the child demonstrating difficulty walking and assuming a side-lying position with the knees flexed toward the chest
    d. Temperature of 102° F, absent bowel sounds, and sudden relief from abdominal pain

24. a. What is the name given to the most intense site of pain in appendicitis?

    b. Where is this site located?

    c. What is the term used to describe pain elicited by light percussion around the perimeter of the abdomen, indicating the presence of peritoneal irritation?

25. The *most* common clinical manifestations expected with Meckel diverticulum include which of the following?
    a. Fever, vomiting, and constipation
    b. Weight loss, hypotension, and obstruction
    c. Painless rectal bleeding, abdominal pain, or intestinal obstruction
    d. Abdominal pain, bloody diarrhea, and foul-smelling stool

26. A common feature of inflammatory bowel diseases is:
    a. growth abnormalities.
    b. chronic constipation.
    c. obstruction.
    d. burning epigastric pain.

27. Describe the pathophysiologic differences between Crohn's disease (CD) and ulcerative colitis (UC).

28. Inflammatory bowel disease (IBD) can be treated with immunomodulators such as 6-mercaptopurine and azathioprine. When the patient is receiving these drugs, the nurse knows to watch for which of the following adverse effects?
    a. Anemia
    b. Splenomegaly
    c. Leukopenia
    d. Decreased serum calcium levels, leading to osteoporosis

29. Nursing considerations for the adolescent with inflammatory bowel disease include:
    a. assisting the adolescent to cope with negative self-esteem and feelings of being different from peers.
    b. encouraging three large meals a day of high-protein, high-caloric foods.
    c. stopping drug therapy with remission of symptoms.
    d. elimination of all high-fiber foods from the diet.

30. Billy, age 14, has an ulcer involving the mucosa of the stomach that has resulted from prolonged use of nonsteroidal antiinflammatory agents. The *best* term to describe the ulcer Billy has is:
    a. duodenal ulcer caused by secondary factors.
    b. duodenal ulcer caused by primary factors.
    c. gastric ulcer caused by secondary factors.
    d. gastric ulcer caused by primary factors.

31. Which one of the following is *not* thought to contribute to peptic ulcer disease?
    a. *Helicobacter pylori*
    b. Alcohol and smoking
    c. Caffeine-containing beverages and spicy foods
    d. Psychologic factors such as stressful life events

32. The current *most* effective treatment for *H. pylori* in children is a combination of what three drugs?

33. Common therapeutic management of peptic ulcer disease includes which of the following?
    a. Corticosteroids
    b. Cimetidine, ranitidine, or famotidine
    c. Acetaminophen
    d. Sulfasalazine and sucralfate

34. Which of the following is the term used to describe impaired motility of the GI tract?
    a. Pyloric stenosis
    b. Obstipation
    c. Abdominal distention
    d. Paralytic ileus

35. Justin, age 1 month, is brought to the clinic by his mother. The nurse suspects pyloric stenosis. Which of the following symptoms would support this theory?
    a. Diarrhea
    b. Projectile vomiting
    c. Fever and dehydration
    d. Abdominal distention

36. Preoperatively, the nursing plan for suspected pyloric obstruction should include which of the following?
    i.   Observation for dehydration
    ii. Keeping body temperature below 100° F
    iii. Parental support and reassurance
    iv. Observation for coughing and gagging after feeding
    v.   Observation of quality of stool

    a. i, ii, iii, iv, and v
    b. i, iii, and iv
    c. iii, iv, and v
    d. i, iii, and v

37. Postoperative feedings for the infant having undergone a pyloromyotomy include:
    a. keeping NPO for the first 24 hours, then introducing normal formula.
    b. glucose and electrolyte feedings beginning 4 to 6 hours after surgery and continuing for the first 72 hours.
    c. small, frequent feedings of glucose and electrolyte within 24 hours after surgery.
    d. thickened formula feeding within 24 hours after surgery.

38. An invagination of one portion of the intestine into another is called:
    a. intussusception.
    b. pyloric stenosis.
    c. tracheoesophageal fistula.
    d. Hirschsprung disease.

39. Al, age 5 months, is suspected of having intussusception. What clinical manifestations would he *most* likely have?
    a. Crying during abdominal exam; vomiting; currant jelly–appearing stools
    b. Fever, diarrhea, vomiting, and lowered WBC
    c. Weight gain, constipation, and refusal to eat
    d. Abdominal distention, periodic pain, hypotension

40. The use of barium as the contrast agent to reduce intussusceptions is being replaced in favor of water-soluble contrast and air pressure. Explain why.

41. Al's intussusception is reduced without surgery. The nurse should expect care for Al after the reduction to include:
    a. administration of antibiotics.
    b. enema administration to remove remaining stool.
    c. observation of stools.
    d. rectal temperatures every 4 hours.

42. Abnormal rotation of the intestine is called _____. When the intestine completely

    twists around itself, it is termed _____.

43. Symptoms in celiac disease include stools that are:
    a. fatty, frothy, bulky, and foul-smelling.
    b. currant jelly–appearing.
    c. small, frothy, and dark green.
    d. white with an ammonia-like smell.

44. The *most* important therapeutic management for the child with celiac disease is:
    a. eliminating corn, rice, and millet from the diet.
    b. adding iron, folic acid, and fat-soluble vitamins to the diet.
    c. eliminating wheat, rye, barley, and oats from the diet.
    d. educating the child's parents about the short-term effects of the disease and the necessity of reading all food labels for content until the disease is in remission.

45. The prognosis for children with short bowel syndrome has improved as a result of:
    a. dietary supplemental vitamin B_{12} additions.
    b. improvement in surgical procedures to correct the defect.
    c. improved home care availability.
    d. total parenteral nutrition and enteral feeding.

46. Jerry, a 4-year-old, is brought to the emergency department by his parents, who say he vomited a large amount of bright red blood. Jerry is pale, cool to the touch, and has increased respiratory rate and heart rate. The nurse expects priority care at this time to include:
    a. administration of intravenous fluids, usually normal saline or lactated Ringer's solution.
    b. stool testing for blood by hemocult.
    c. insertion of an NG tube for iced-water lavage.
    d. preparation for tracheostomy.

47. Match each type of viral hepatitis with its description. (Types may be used more than once.)

    a. Hepatitis A   d. Hepatitis D
    b. Hepatitis B   e. Hepatitis E
    c. Hepatitis C   f. Hepatitis G

    _____ Spread directly or indirectly by fecal-oral route and affects 25,000 people in the United States each year
    _____ Immunity by two inactivated vaccines given 6 to 12 months apart
    _____ Non-A, non-B with transmission through the fecal-oral route or with contaminated water
    _____ Spread directly and indirectly by the fecal-oral route
    _____ Occurs in children already infected with hepatitis B
    _____ Primary cause of posttransfusion hepatitis; often becomes a chronic condition and can cause cirrhosis
    _____ Incubation period 14 to 160 days; average 50 days
    _____ Universal vaccination recommended for all newborns
    _____ Blood-borne virus that affects high-risk groups, including individuals infected with HCV; transmitted also by organ transplantation; unknown incubation period

48. Sandy, age 2, is brought to the clinic by her mother because a toddler who attends Sandy's daycare center has been diagnosed with hepatitis A. Sandy's mother is concerned that Sandy might develop the disease. Which one of the following serum laboratory tests would indicate to the nurse that Sandy has immunity to hepatitis A?
    a. Anti-HAV IgG
    b. Anti-HAV IgM
    c. HAsAg
    d. HAcAg

49. Sandy's testing reflects that she has not had hepatitis A. Because her exposure to hepatitis A has occurred within the last 2 weeks, the nurse would expect the physician to order which one of the following for prophylactic administration?
    a. Hepatitis B immune globulin (HBIG)
    b. HBV vaccine
    c. Standard immune globulin (IG)
    d. HAV vaccine

50. What are the four major goals of management for viral hepatitis?

51. Which one of the following would *not* be expected in the child diagnosed with cirrhosis?
    a. Hepatospenomegaly
    b. Elevated liver function tests
    c. Decreased ammonia levels
    d. Ascites

Critical Thinking—Case Study

Danny, age 17, is a junior in high school. He comes to the clinic with complaints of right lower abdominal pain and slight fever.

52. What questions should be included in the history of present illness if appendicitis is suspected?

53. Danny should be advised to avoid which of the following until seen by the physician?
    a. All activity
    b. All laxatives
    c. Ice to the abdomen
    d. All of the above

54. Danny is admitted to the hospital with a diagnosis of acute appendicitis. The nurse should institute which one of the following independent nursing actions?
    a. Allow clear liquids only.
    b. Start intravenous fluids with antibiotics.
    c. Insert a nasogastric tube and connect to suction.
    d. Monitor closely for progression of symptoms.

55. What laboratory blood evaluation and results would the nurse expect to see in a patient with acute appendicitis?

56. Danny is now 2 hours postoperative. During surgery, his appendix was found to have ruptured before surgery. A priority nursing diagnosis at this time would be:
    a. high risk for spread of infection related to rupture.
    b. pain related to inflamed appendix.
    c. altered growth and development related to hospital care.
    d. anxiety related to knowledge deficit regarding disease.

57. Which of the following is the *most* critical outcome for Danny after surgery?
    a. Danny's peritonitis has resolved as evidenced by no fever, lack of elevated WBC, and a wound that is clean and healing.
    b. Danny's pain is relieved as evidenced by no verbalization of pain and the fact that Danny is resting quietly.
    c. Danny and his family demonstrate understanding of hospitalization.
    d. Danny is able to express feelings and concerns.

CHAPTER 34

The Child with Cardiovascular Dysfunction

1. The following terms are related to cardiac structure and function. Match each term with its description.

   a. Congenital heart defects
   b. Acquired cardiac disorders
   c. Mediastinum
   d. Myocardium
   e. Endocardium
   f. Pericardium

   g. Pericardial space
   h. Pericardial fluid
   i. Atria
   j. Ventricles
   k. Valves
   l. Tricuspid valve

   m. Mitral valve
   n. Atrioventricular (AV) valves
   o. Chordae tendineae
   p. Semilunar valves

   _____ Structures located in the pulmonary artery (pulmonic valve) and the aorta (aortic valve) that prevent backflow of blood

   _____ A few drops of serous fluid normally found between the two layers of membrane that cover the heart

   _____ Located between left atrium and the left ventricle; prevents flow from the right ventricle back into the left ventricle

   _____ The two bottom chambers of the interior of the heart

   _____ A double-walled membrane that forms a covering for the heart

   _____ The muscular tissue that forms the main mass of the heart

   _____ Disease processes or abnormalities that occur after birth; can be seen in the normal heart or in the presence of congenital heart defects

   _____ Prevent backflow in the heart

   _____ Anatomic abnormalities present at birth that result in abnormal cardiac function

   _____ Located between the right atrium and the right ventricle; prevents flow from the right ventricle back into the right ventricle

   _____ A thin layer of endothelial tissue that lines the inner surface of the myocardium

   _____ The two upper chambers of the interior of the heart

   _____ The space between the two pleural cavities

   _____ Term used to describe both the mitral valve and the tricuspid valve together

   _____ Cord-like structures that attach atrioventricular valves to the heart muscle

   _____ The slight space between the two layers of membrane that cover the heart

2. Match each of the following embryologic development terms with its description.

a. Endocardial cushions
b. Common atrium/ventricle
c. Bulbus cordis
d. Sinus venosus
e. Truncus arteriosus
f. Atrial septum
g. Foramen ovale
h. Ventricular septum
i. Muscular septum
j. Membranous septum
k. Ductus venosus
l. Ductus arteriosus
m. Coronary arteries
n. Coronary veins

_____ Develops into the inferior and superior vena cava

_____ The vessel that allows blood to travel directly to the inferior vena cava prior to birth

_____ Embryologic internal bulges that eventually merge to divide the heart chambers

_____ The structure that permits blood to be shunted to the descending aorta from the pulmonary artery prior to birth

_____ Eventually helps to form the outflow tracts of the ventricles

_____ Develops out of an intricate growth of the endocardial cushions, conal cushions, and conotruncal septum

_____ Collect blood and return it directly to the right atrium or through the coronary sinus that drains into the right atrium

_____ Divides into the pulmonary artery and aorta and gives rise to the aortic arch

_____ Structures that begin to be formed at about the 5th week of gestation; ultimately give rise to the heart chambers

_____ Develops from the joining of the muscular and membranous ventricular septa during the fourth to eighth week of embryologic growth

_____ A temporary flap opening that is formed from the overlapping of the septum primum and the septum secundum before they fuse

_____ Develops when the right and left ventricular chambers fuse

_____ Supply the heart muscle with its blood supply; arise above the aortic valve

_____ Formed by the growth of septum primum and septum secundum at about the fourth week of fetal growth

3. The following terms are related to the conduction system and physiology. Match each term with its description.

a. Cardiac cycle
b. Systole
c. Diastole
d. Cardiac output
e. Stroke volume
f. Preload
g. Afterload
h. Systemic vascular resistance
i. Pulmonary vascular resistance
j. Contractility
k. Starling's law
l. Tachycardia
m. Bradycardia
n. Tachypnea
o. Sinoatrial node
p. Atrioventricular node
q. Bundle of His
r. Purkinje fibers

_____ The efficiency of myocardial fiber shortening; the ability of the cardiac muscle to act as an efficient pump

_____ The amount of blood ejected by the heart in any one contraction

_____ Part of the cardiac conduction system; the heart's usual pacemaker; located within the right atrium near the opening of the superior vena cava

_____ Slow heart rate

_____ Composed of sequential contraction and relaxation of both the atria and the ventricles

_____ Fast heart rate

_____ The volume of blood ejected by the heart in 1 minute

_____ Part of the cardiac conduction system; extends from the atrioventricular node along each side of the interventricle septum and divides into right and left bundle branches

_____ Refers to the resistance against which the ventricles must pump when ejecting blood; blood pressure gives some indication of this resistance

_____ Contraction of both the atria and ventricles

_____ The resistance of the pulmonary circulation

_____ Relaxation of both the atria and the ventricles

_____ The volume of blood returning to the heart; the circulation blood volume

_____ Part of the cardiac conduction system; located within the right atrium at the low part of the septum

_____ The principle that demonstrates that an increase in ventricular end-diastolic volume somewhat increases stroke volume

_____ Part of the cardiac conduction system; these strands of conduction tissue extend from the AV bundle into the walls of the ventricles

_____ Resistance of the systemic circulation

_____ Fast respiratory rate

4. Match each wave form term with its description.

a. P wave
b. P-R interval
c. QRS complex
d. T wave
e. Q-T interval
f. S-T segment

_____ Represents ventricular repolarization

_____ Represents the spread of the impulse over the atria (atrial depolarization); sinus node's electrical activity not represented in the ECG

_____ Represents ventricular depolarization and repolarization; interval varies with heart rate—the faster the rate, the shorter the Q-T interval; in children interval normally shorter than in adults

_____ Represents the time that elapses from the beginning of atrial depolarization to the beginning of ventricular depolarization

_____ Represents the time that the ventricles are in absolute refractory period, the period between ventricular depolarization and repolarizaton

_____ Represents ventricular depolarization; actually composed of three separate waves that result from the currents generated when the ventricles depolarize before their contraction

5. Match each cardiac function term with its description.

a. Chest radiograph
b. Electrocardiography (ECG/EKG)
c. Holter monitor
d. Echocardiography
e. Transthoracic echocardiography
f. M-mode echocardiography
g. Two-dimensional echocardiography
h. Doppler echocardiography

i. Fetal echocardiography
j. Transesophageal echocardiography
k. Cardiac catheterization
l. Hemodynamics
m. Angiography
n. Biopsy
o. Electrophysiology (EPS)
p. Exercise stress test
q. Right-sided cardiac catheterization

r. Left-sided cardiac catheterization
s. Interventional cardiac catheterization
t. Diagnostic electrophysiologic catheterization
u. Interventional electrophysiologic catheterization
v. Cardiac magnetic resonance imaging

_____ Uses catheters with tiny electrodes that record the heart's electrical impulses directly from the conduction system to evaluate and treat dysrhythmias

_____ Newest noninvasive imaging technique; used in evaluation of vascular anatomy outside of heart (i.e., coarctation of the aorta, vascular rings) and in estimates of ventricular mass and volume; uses are expanding

_____ Venous; diagnostic catheterization of the venous side in which the catheter is introduced from a vein into the right atrium

_____ Type of echocardiography that uses real-time, cross-sectional views of heart; used to identify cardiac structures and cardiac anatomy

_____ An alternative to surgery in some congenital heart defects, such as isolated valvular pulmonic stenosis and patent ductus arteriosus

_____ Type of echocardiography that obtains a one-dimensional graphic view; used to estimate ventricular size and function

_____ Measures pressures and oxygen saturations in heart chambers

_____ Graphic measure of the electrical activity of the heart

_____ Type of echocardiography that images the fetal heart in utero

_____ Use of contrast material to illuminate heart structures and blood-flow patterns

_____ Use of high-frequency sound waves obtained by a transducer to produce an image of cardiac structures

_____ Type of echocardiography that uses a transducer placed in the esophagus behind the heart to obtain images of the posterior heart structures in patients with poor images from the chest approach

_____ Employs a special catheter with electrodes to record electrical activity from within heart; used to diagnose rhythm disturbances

_____ An alternative to surgery for some congenital heart defects

_____ Use of special catheter to remove tiny samples of heart muscle for microscopic evaluation; used for assessing infection, inflammation, or muscle dysfunction disorders; also used to evaluate for rejection following heart transplant

_____ Provides information about heart size and pulmonary blood flow

_____ Type of echocardiography done with transducer on chest

_____ Type of echocardiography that identifies blood-flow patterns and pressure gradients across structures

_____ Arterial; diagnostic catheterization of the arterial side in which the catheter is threaded retrograde into the aorta or from a right-sided approach to the left atrium by means of a septal puncture or through an existing septal opening

_____ 24-hour continuous ECG recording used to assess dysrhythmias

_____ Imaging study using radiopaque catheters placed in a peripheral blood vessel and advanced into the heart to measure pressures and oxygen levels in heart chambers and to visualize heart structures and blood-flow patterns

_____ Monitoring of heart rate, blood pressure, ECG, and oxygen consumption at rest and during progressive exercise on a treadmill or bicycle

6. Match each congenital heart disease term with its description.

a. Left-to-right shunt
b. Acyanotic-cyanotic defects
c. Hemodynamic characteristics
d. Cor pulmonale
e. Right-sided failure
f. Left-sided failure
g. Cardiac reserve

_____ Dysfunction that results in increased end diastolic pressure with lung congestion and pulmonary edema

_____ Term for congestive heart failure resulting from obstructive lung diseases such as cystic fibrosis or bronchopulmonary dysplasia

_____ Traditional categories of congenital heart defects that divide defects based on a physical characteristic; problematic because of the complexity of the many defects and the variability of their clinical manifestations

_____ Dysfunction that results in systemic venous hypertension that in turn causes hepatomegaly and edema

_____ The directional flow from an area of higher pressure to one of lower pressure in congenital heart disease

_____ The compensatory mechanisms that initially try to meet the body's demand for increased cardiac output, including hypertrophy and dilation of the cardiac muscle as well as stimulation of the sympathetic nervous system

_____ A useful classification system for congenital heart defects that uses movements involved in circulation of blood

7. The following terms are related to the clinical manifestations of congenital heart disease. Match each term with its description.

a. Gallop rhythm
b. Diaphoresis
c. Poor perfusion
d. Mild cyanosis
e. Dyspnea
f. Costal retractions
g. Pulmonary edema
h. Orthopnea
i. Wheezing
j. Cough
k. Hoarseness
l. Gasping/grunting respirations
m. Developmental delays
n. Hepatomegaly
o. Edema
p. Weight gain
q. Ascites/pleural effusions
r. Distended veins

_____ Dyspnea in the recumbent position

_____ Manifested by cold extremities, weak pulses, slow capillary refill, low BP, and mottled skin

_____ A late sign of heart failure

_____ Extra heart sounds S_3 and S_4 resulting from ventricular dilation and excess preload

_____ Occurs as the pliable chest wall in the infant is drawn inward during attempts to ventilate the noncompliant lungs

_____ Results from poor weight gain and activity intolerance

_____ Occurs when the pulmonary capillary pressure exceeds the plasma osmotic pressure and fluid is forced into the interstitial space

_____ Caused by mucosal swelling and irritation of the bronchial mucosa

_____ Result from a consistently elevated central venous pressure; venous return is slow; difficult to detect in the short, fat neck of infants; usually observed only in older children

_____ Occurs from pooling of blood in the portal circulation and transudation of fluid into the hepatic tissues

_____ Results from impaired gas exchange and is relieved with oxygen administration

_____ Caused by edema of the bronchial mucosa from obstruction to airflow

_____ Forms from sodium and water retention that causes systemic vascular pressure to rise

_____ Caused by pressure from edema on the laryngeal nerve

_____ Caused by decrease in the distensibility of the lungs; initially may be evident only on exertion; in infants may be accompanied by flaring nares

_____ The earliest sign of edema

_____ Often seen during exertion when myocardial function is impaired; in children especially noted on the head

_____ Later signs of gross fluid accumulation

8. The following terms are related to the therapeutic management of congestive heart failure. Match each term with its description.

a. Digoxin (Lanoxin)
b. Angiotensin-converting enzyme (ACE) inhibitors
c. Captopril/enalapril
d. Furosemide
e. Chlorothiazide
f. Spironolactone
g. Bumetanide
h. Metolazone

_____ Aldactone; blocks action of aldosterone to produce diuresis; allows retention of potassium

_____ Diuril; acts directly on distal tubules and possibly proximal tubules to decrease sodium, water potassium, chloride, and bicarbonate absorption; decreases urinary diluting capacity; may need to supplement potassium

_____ Causes vasodilation that decreases pulmonary and systemic vascular resistance, decreased blood pressure, a reduction in afterload, and decreased right and left atrial pressures

_____ Bumex; loop diuretic similar to, but more potent than, Lasix

_____ Lasix; blocks reabsorption of sodium and water to produce diuresis

_____ Zaroxolyn; unique thiazide diuretic; appears effective in patients with reduced renal function

_____ Used because of its rapid onset and decreased risk for toxicity; increases the force of contraction (positive inotropic effect), decreases the heart rate (negative chronotropic effect), slows the conduction of impulses through the AV note (negative dromotropic effect), and indirectly enhances diuresis

_____ ACE inhibitors that are frequently used in pediatrics

9. Match each term with its description.

a. Hypoxemia

b. Hypoxia

c. Cynaosis

d. Right-to-left shunting

e. Eisenmenger complex

f. Polycythemia

g. Clubbing

h. Squatting blue spells

i. Tet spells/hypercyanotic spells

j. Cerebrovascular accidents (CVAs)

k. Bacterial endocarditis

l. Shunt

m. Modified Blalock-Taussig shunt

_____ Uses a Gore-Tex or Impra tube graft to create a communication between the subclavian artery and the pulmonary artery to increase blood flow to the lungs; the preferred palliative treatment for severely hypoxemic newborns

_____ May occur in any child whose heart defect includes obstruction to pulmonary blood flow and communication between the ventricles; acute cyanotic episode with hyperpnea

_____ An increased number of red blood cells

_____ A reduction in tissue oxygenation that results from low SaO_2

_____ A palliative surgical procedure that serves the same purpose as the ductus arteriosus; increases blood flow to the lungs through a systemic artery-to-pulmonary artery connection

_____ Results from severe obstruction to pulmonary blood flow; desaturated venous blood enters the system circulation without passing through the lungs and cyanosis is present; tetralogy of Fallot is the most common cause of this type of obstruction

_____ Strokes; occurs in about 2% of the children with hypoxia

_____ An arterial oxygen tension (or pressure, PaO_2) that is less than normal and can be identified by decreased arterial oxygen saturation (SaO_2)or a decreased PaO_2

_____ A thickening and flattening of the tips of the fingers and toes; thought to occur because of chronic tissue hypoxemia and polycythemia

_____ Increased risk for this disorder in children who are cyanotic, especially those who have systemic-to-pulmonary shunts

_____ A syndrome in which a left-to-right shunt becomes a right-to-left shunt because of a progressive increase in pulmonary vascular resistance

_____ A blue discoloration in the mucous membranes, skin, and nail beds of the child with reduced oxygen saturation; results from the presence of deoxygenated hemoglobin

_____ Characteristically seen in children with unrepaired tetralogy of Fallot; an unconscious attempt to relieve chronic hypoxia; reduces the return of venous blood from the lower extremities and increases systemic vascular resistance

10. The following terms are related to acquired disorders. Match each term with its description.

a. Rheumatic heart disease
b. Aschoff bodies
c. Carditis
d. Polyarthritis
e. Erythema marginatum
f. Subcutaneous nodules
g. Chorea/Sydenham's chorea
h. Antistreptolysin-O (ASLO) titer
i. Ectasia
j. Hypertension
k. Primary hypertension

l. Secondary hypertension
m. Severe hypertension
n. Hyperlipidemia
o. Hypercholesterolemia
p. Atherosclerosis
q. Coronary artery disease
r. Cholesterol
s. Triglycerides
t. Chylomicrons
u. Very low-density lipoproteins

v. Low-density lipoprotein
w. High-density lipoproteins
x. Population approach
y. Individualized approach
z. Step one diet
aa. Step two diet
bb. Cholestyramine/colestipol
cc. Dilated cardiomyopathy
dd. Hypertrophic cardiomyopathy
ee. Restrictive cardiomyopathy

_____ Dietary restrictions that include a saturated fatty acid intake of 7% of calories and a cholesterol intake of less than 200 mg/day

_____ Fatty plaques on the arteries

_____ Measures the concentration of antibodies formed in the blood against a product that is present in streptococcal infection in children

_____ Primary cause of morbidity and mortality in the adult population

_____ Formed in rheumatic heart disease; inflammatory, hemorrhagic, bullous lesions; causes swelling, fragmentation, and alterations in the connective tissue

_____ Rare in children; describes a restriction to ventricular filling caused by endocardial or myocardial disease or both; characterized by diastolic dysfunction and absence of ventricular dilation or hypertrophy

_____ Dilation

_____ Major cardiac manifestation of rheumatic fever; involves the endocardium, pericardium, and myocardium

_____ A fat-like steroid alcohol; part of the lipoprotein complex in plasma that is essential for cellular metabolism

_____ Essential hypertension; no identifiable cause

_____ Caused by edema, inflammation, and effusions in joint tissue; reversible; migratory; favors large joints such as knees, elbows, hips, shoulders, and wrists; usually accompany the acute febrile period in rheumatic fever

_____ Characterized by an increase in heart muscle mass without an increase in cavity size, usually occurring in the left ventricle and associated with abnormal diastolic filling; idiopathic hypertrophic subaortic stenosis is a subgroup

_____ Contain low concentrations of triglycerides, high levels of cholesterol, and moderate levels of protein; high levels are a strong risk factor in cardiovascular disease

_____ Small, nontender swellings that persist indefinitely after the onset of rheumatic fever and gradually resolve with no resulting damage

_____ Characterized by ventricular dilation and greatly decreased contractility, resulting in symptoms of congestive heart failure

_____ A poorly understood autoimmune reaction to group A β-hemolytic streptococcal pharyngitis; self-limited disease that involves the joint, skin, brain, serous surface, and heart; cardiac valve damage is the most serious consequence

_____ St. Vitus dance; characterized by sudden, aimless, irregular movements of the extremities; involuntary facial grimaces, speech disturbances, emotional lability, and muscle weakness that can be profound in rheumatic fever; exaggerated by anxiety and attempts at deliberate fine motor activity and relieved by rest, especially sleep

_____ A general term for excessive lipids

_____ Contains very low concentrations of triglycerides, relatively little cholesterol, and high levels of protein; thought to protect against cardiovascular disease

_____ Natural fats synthesized from carbohydrates

_____ The consistent elevation of blood pressure beyond values considered the upper limits of normal

_____ A distinct erythematous macule with a clear center and wavy, well-demarcated border; transitory nonpruritic rash found most often on the trunk and proximal portion of the extremities in rheumatic fever

_____ Produced in the intestine in response to the intake of dietary fat; principal transporter of dietary fat

_____ Hypertension that has an identifiable cause; significant hypertension; a blood pressure that is consistently between the 95th and 99th percentile for age and sex

_____ A blood pressure persistently at or above the 99th percentile for age and sex

_____ Drugs recommended for the treatment of severe hypercholesterolemia

_____ An approach to controlling hypercholesterolemia, which is based on selective screening

_____ Refers to excessive cholesterol in the blood

_____ A diet that has the same nutrient intake as that of the general population (i.e., less than 10% of total calories from saturated fatty acids, no more than 30% of calories from total fat, less than 300 mg/day of cholesterol, and adequate calories to support growth and development and to reach or maintain desirable body weight)

_____ Contains high concentrations of triglycerides, moderate concentrations of cholesterol, and little protein

_____ Aims to lower the average levels of blood cholesterol among all American children through population-wide changes in nutrient intake and eating patterns

11. The following terms are related to the correction of defects. Match each term with its description.

a. Median sternotomy
b. Lateral thoracotomy
c. Intra-arterial monitoring
d. Intracardiac monitoring
e. Low cardiac output syndrome
f. Dysrhythmias
g. Cardiac tamponade
h. Paradoxical pulse pressure
i. Cerebral edema/brain damage
j. Seizure

_____ Decreased peripheral perfusion; symptoms are similar to the signs of shock

_____ Seen in approximately 10% of infants who require the use of cardiopulmonary bypass; may be focal or generalized

_____ Compression of the heart by blood and other effusion (clots) in the pericardial sac

_____ A type of incision that is made in heart surgery, where the sternum is split

_____ Characteristic sign of compression of the heart; systolic pressure drops during inspiration because of accumulated blood compressing the heart; results in drop in cardiac output

_____ Can result from electrolyte imbalance, especially hypokalemia, and surgical intervention to the septum or myocardium

_____ Almost always used following open heart surgery to measure blood pressure; more reliable than indirect blood pressure readings and provides continuous rather than intermittent monitoring

_____ May occur during open heart surgery; thought to be result of tissue ischemia or emboli; evidence is assessed by checking reflexes in both extremities, pupil size, equality and reaction to light and accommodation, and child's orientation to environment

_____   Provides data on cardiac function and output; allows assessment of pressures inside the cardiac chambers, giving information about blood volume, cardiac output, ventricular function, pulmonary artery pressures, and responses to drug therapy

_____   A type of incision that is made in heart surgery, which extends from the midaxillary line to the scapula

12. The following terms are related to cardiac dysrhythmias. Match each term with its description.

a. Sinus bradycardia
b. Sinus tachycardia
c. Supraventicular tachycardia
d. AV blocks
e. Electrophysiologic cardiac catheterization
f. Transesophageal recording

g. Vagal maneuvers
h. Transesophageal atrial overdrive pacing
i. Synchronized cardioversion
j. Pacemaker
k. Pulse generator

l. Lead
m. Epicardial leads
n. Orthotopic heart transplantation
o. Heterotopic heart transplantation

_____   Applying ice to the face, massaging the carotid artery on one side of the neck only, or having the child perform a Valsalva maneuver; used to treat supraventricular tachycardia

_____   Leaving the recipient's own heart in place and implanting a new heart to act as an additional pump or "piggyback" heart; rarely used in children

_____   One of the most common dysrhythmias found in children; a rapid, regular heart rate of 200 to 300 beats per minute

_____   Most often related to edema around the conduction system and resolved without treatment

_____   Implant made of a pulse generator and the lead

_____   Composed of a battery and the electronic circuitry

_____   Allow for identification of the conduction disturbance and immediate investigation of drugs that may control the dysrhythmia; selective induction of the dysrhythmia and treatment under observation

_____   Accomplished through placement of a protected lead into the esophagus behind the left atrium of the heart; lead then attached to a stimulator capable of pacing at a very rapid rate to interrupt the tachydysrhythmia

_____   An insulated, flexible wire that conducts electrical impulses

_____   An electrode catheter passed into the esophagus and, when in position at a point proximal to the heart, used to simulate and record dysrhythmias

_____   May result from the influence of the autonomic nervous system or in response to hypoxia and hypotension

_____   The timed delivery of a preset amount of energy through the chest wall in an attempt to reestablish an organized rhythm

_____   A wire that is directly attached to the heart and conducts impulses

_____   Removing the recipient's own heart and implanting a new heart from a donor

_____   Usually secondary to fever, anxiety, pain, anemia, dehydration, or any factor that requires an increased cardiac output

13. The embryologic development of the heart results in a heartbeat by the:
    a. fourth week.
    b. fifth week.
    c. sixth week.
    d. eighth week.

14. During the embryologic development of the lower heart, the muscular septum develops from:
    a. fusion of the chambers of the common ventricle.
    b. growth of endocardial cushions.
    c. growth of the conal cushions.
    d. fusion of the conotruncal septum.

15. The process of the formation of the heart's atrial septum results in a temporary flap called the:
    a. truncus arteriosus.
    b. foramen ovale.
    c. sinus venosus.
    d. ductus venosus.

16. In fetal circulation, the umbilical vein divides and sends blood directly to the inferior vena cava by way of the ductus venosus. This division occurs at the:
    a. heart.
    b. lungs.
    c. liver.
    d. placenta.

17. In fetal circulation the majority of the most oxygenated blood is pumped through the:
    a. foramen ovale.
    b. lungs.
    c. liver.
    d. coronary sinus.

18. When obtaining a history from the parents of an infant suspected to have altered cardiac function, the nurse would expect to hear:
    a. specific concerns related to palpitations the infant is having.
    b. vague, nonspecific complaints such as feeding difficulties.
    c. specific concerns about the infant's shortness of breath.
    d. all of the above.

19. A clue in the mother's history that is important to the diagnosis of congenital heart disease is:
    a. rheumatoid arthritis.
    b. rheumatic fever.
    c. streptococcal infection.
    d. rubella.

20. Coarctation of the aorta should be suspected when:
    a. the blood pressure in the arms is different from the blood pressure in the legs.
    b. the blood pressure in the right arm is different from the blood pressure in the left arm.
    c. apical pulse is greater than the radial pulse.
    d. point of maximum impulse is shifted to the left.

21. Of the following descriptions, the heart sound that would be considered normal in a young child is:
    a. splitting of S_1.
    b. splitting of S_2.
    c. splitting of S_3.
    d. splitting of S_4.

22. The standard pediatric electrocardiogram has:
    a. 6 leads.
    b. 12 leads.
    c. 15 leads.
    d. 18 leads.

23. The test that requires intravenous sedation and has been used increasingly in recent years to confirm the diagnosis of a congenital heart defect without a cardiac catheterization is the:
    a. electrocardiogram.
    b. echocardiogram.
    c. transesophageal echocardiogram.
    d. two-dimensional echocardiogram.

24. In children, the usual approach to the left ventricle of the heart in a cardiac catheterization is through the:
    a. left side of the heart.
    b. right side of the heart.

25. List at least five of the most significant complications following a cardiac catheterization in an infant or young child.

26. If bleeding occurs at the insertion site after a cardiac catheterization, the nurse should apply:
    a. warmth to the unaffected extremity.
    b. pressure one inch below the insertion site.
    c. warmth to the affected extremity.
    d. pressure one inch above the insertion site.

27. When children develop congestive heart failure from a congenital heart defect, the failure is usually:
    a. right-sided only.
    b. left-sided only.
    c. cor pulmonale.
    d. both right- and left-sided.

28. Which one of the following heart rates would be considered tachycardia in an infant?
    a. A resting heart rate of 120 beats per minute
    b. A crying heart rate of 200 beats per minute
    c. A resting heart rate of 170 beats per minute
    d. A crying heart rate of 180 beats per minute

29. Labored breathing in an infant may be identified by:
    a. inability to feed.
    b. circumoral cyanosis.
    c. costal retractions.
    d. all of the above.

30. Developmental delays in the infant with congestive heart failure are *most* pronounced in the:
    a. fine motor areas.
    b. gross motor areas.
    c. social skill areas.
    d. cognitive areas.

31. Evaluation of the infant for edema is different from the older child in that:
    a. weight is not reliable as an early sign.
    b. pedal edema will be most pronounced in the newborn.
    c. edema is usually generalized and difficult to detect.
    d. distended neck veins are the most reliable sign.

32. In the child taking digoxin, electrocardiographic signs that the drug is having the intended effect are:
    a. prolonged P-R interval and slowed ventricular rate.
    b. shortened P-R interval and slowed ventricular rate.
    c. prolonged P-R interval and faster ventricular rate.
    d. shortened P-R interval and faster ventricular rate.

33. The two main angiotensin-converting enzyme (ACE) inhibitors *most* commonly used for children with congestive heart failure are:
    a. digoxin and captopril.
    b. enalapril and captopril.
    c. enalapril and furosemide.
    d. spironolactone and captopril.

34. The electrolyte that is usually depleted with most diuretic therapy is:
    a. sodium.
    b. chloride.
    c. potassium.
    d. magnesium.

35. The nutritional needs of the infant with congestive heart failure are usually:
    a. the same as an adult's.
    b. less than a healthy infant's.
    c. the same as a healthy infant's.
    d. greater than a healthy infant's.

36. The calories are usually increased for an infant with congestive heart failure by:
    a. increasing the number of feedings.
    b. introducing solids into the diet.
    c. increasing the density of the formula.
    d. gastrostomy feeding.

37. Chronic hypoxemia is manifested clinically by which of the following signs?
    a. Squatting
    b. Polycythemia
    c. Clubbing
    d. All of the above

38. Prostaglandin is administered to the newborn with a congenital heart defect to:
    a. close the patent ductus arteriosus.
    b. keep the ductus arteriosus open.
    c. keep the foramen ovale open.
    d. close the foramen ovale.

39. Dehydration must be prevented in children who are hypoxemic because the dehydration places the child at risk for:
    a. infection.
    b. cerebrovascular accident.
    c. fever.
    d. air embolism.

40. Air embolism may form in the venous system, traveling directly to the brain by way of the arterial, of the child with:
    a. a right-to-left shunt.
    b. a left-to-right shunt.
    c. dehydration and hypoxemia.
    d. hypernatremia and hypopotassemia.

41. Match the type of defect with the specific disorder. (Defects may be used more than once.)

    a. Defects with decreased pulmonary blood flow
    b. Mixed defects
    c. Defects with increased pulmonary blood flow
    d. Obstructive defects

    _____ Patent ductus arteriosus
    _____ Coarctation of the aorta
    _____ Ventricular septal defect
    _____ Subvalvular aortic stenosis
    _____ Hypoplastic left heart syndrome
    _____ Atrioventricular canal defect
    _____ Pulmonic stenosis
    _____ Tetralogy of Fallot
    _____ Aortic stenosis
    _____ Tricuspid atresia
    _____ Valvular aortic stenosis
    _____ Truncus arteriosus
    _____ Atrial septal defect
    _____ Transposition of the great vessels
    _____ Total anomalous pulmonary venous connection

42. Which one of the following defects has the *best* prognosis?
    a. Tetralogy of Fallot
    b. Ventricular septal defect
    c. Atrial septal defect
    d. Hypoplastic left heart syndrome

43. Which of the following defects has the *worst* prognosis?
    a. Tetralogy of Fallot
    b. Atrial ventricular canal defect
    c. Transposition of the great vessels
    d. Hypoplastic left heart syndrome

44. Which one of the following sets of assessment findings are the *most* frequent clinical manifestations of congenital heart disorders in an infant or child?
    a. Decreased cardiac output and low blood pressure
    b. Congestive heart failure and murmurs
    c. Increased blood pressure and pulse
    d. All of the above

45. Surgical intervention is always necessary in the first year of life when an infant is born with:
    a. atrial septal defect.
    b. ventricular septal defect.
    c. transposition of the great vessels.
    d. patent ductus arteriosus.

46. The *best* approach for the nurse to use in regard to advising parents about how to discipline the child with a congenital defect is to:
    a. provide the parents with anticipatory guidance.
    b. teach the parents to overcompensate.
    c. help the parents focus on the child's defect.
    d. teach the parents to use benevolent overreaction.

47. Parents of the child with a congenital heart disorder are usually interested primarily in information about:
    a. the anatomy and physiology of the heart.
    b. the pathophysiology and morbidity of the disorder.
    c. the prognosis and surgical correction of the disorder.
    d. all of the above.

48. Parents of the child with a congenital heart defect should know the signs of congestive heart failure, which include:
    a. poor feeding.
    b. sudden weight gain.
    c. increased efforts to breathe.
    d. all of the above.

49. List at least three major categories that should be included in a teaching plan for parents of a child with a congenital heart disorder.

50. A visit to the intensive care unit prior to open heart surgery should take place:
    a. several days before the surgery.
    b. at a busy time with a lot to see and hear.
    c. the day before surgery.
    d. several weeks before the surgery.

51. Children who will undergo cardiac surgery should be informed about:
    a. the location of the intravenous lines.
    b. the pain at the intravenous insertion sites.
    c. the need to lie still at all times after surgery.
    d. all of the above.

52. Which one of the following patterns is indicative of infection in the postoperative period following cardiac surgery?
    a. Temperature of 38.6° C (101.5° F) 72 hours after surgery
    b. Temperature of 37.7° C (100° F) 36 hours after surgery
    c. Hypothermia in the early postoperative period
    d. All of the above

53. Following cardiac surgery in a child, congestive heart failure would be suspected if the central venous pressure catheter (CVP) readings begin to:
    a. fall with a rise in blood pressure.
    b. rise with a rise in blood pressure.
    c. fall with a fall in blood pressure.
    d. rise with a fall in blood pressure.

54. While suctioning an infant after cardiac surgery, the nurse should:
    a. hyperoxygenate before suctioning.
    b. suction for no more than 5 seconds.
    c. provide supplemental O_2.
    d. perform all of the above.

55. List five observations the nurse should be making while suctioning an infant after cardiac surgery.

56. Which one of the following reasons is *not* a common reason for chest tube drainage in the child following cardiac surgery?
    a. Removal of secretions
    b. Removal of air
    c. Prevention of pneumothorax
    d. Removal of an empyema

57. Which one of the following strategies is *not* acceptable to include in the care of the child prior to removing chest tube(s) after cardiac surgery?
    a. Explain that the removal is uncomfortable but not painful.
    b. Administer intravenous fentanyl.
    c. Administer intravenous morphine sulfate.
    d. Use a topical anesthetic on the site.

58. The *most* painful part of cardiac surgery for the child is usually the:
    a. thoracotomy incision site.
    b. graft site on the leg.
    c. sternotomy incision site.
    d. intravenous insertion sites.

59. An infant who weighs 7 kg has just returned to the intensive care unit following cardiac surgery. The chest tube has drained 30 ml in the past hour. In this situation, what is the *first* action for the nurse to take?
    a. Notify the surgeon.
    b. Identify any other signs of hemorrhage.
    c. Suction the patient.
    d. Identify any other signs of renal failure.

60. An infant who weighs 7 kg has just returned to the intensive care unit following cardiac surgery. The urine output has been 20 ml in the past hour. In this situation, what is the *first* action for the nurse to take?
    a. Notify the surgeon.
    b. Identify any other signs of hypervolemia.
    c. Suction the patient.
    d. Identify any other signs of renal failure.

61. Following cardiac surgery, fluid intake calculations for a child would include:
    a. intravenous fluids.
    b. arterial and CVP line flushes.
    c. fluid used to dilute medications.
    d. all of the above.

62. Following cardiac surgery, fluid output calculations in a child would include:
    a. nasogastric secretions.
    b. blood drawn for analysis.
    c. chest tube drainage.
    d. all of the above.

63. One of the factors that increases blood volume in open heart surgery in children is the postoperative:
    a. reabsorption of potassium.
    b. secretion of antidiuretic hormone.
    c. inhibition of aldosterone.
    d. diffusion of fluid into the interstitial spaces.

64. One of the strategies the nurse can use to progressively increase a child's activity in the postoperative period after cardiac surgery is to plan:
    a. to expect some degree of dyspnea.
    b. to ambulate on the first day.
    c. to ambulate after analgesic medication.
    d. all of the above.

65. List at least five complications of cardiac surgery in children.

66. Techniques to provide emotional support to the child and family following cardiac surgery include:
    a. realizing that some procedures are too difficult for the child to perform.
    b. encouraging the child to keep being brave.
    c. reassuring the parents that a child's anger or rejection of them is normal.
    d. all of the above.

67. Which one of the following patients with bacterial endocarditis (BE) is at highest risk for mortality?
    a. A 15-year-old with BE caused by a bacterium that is susceptible to ampicillin
    b. A 2-month-old infant with no cardiac problems
    c. A 5-year-old child with BE following a mitral valve replacement
    d. A 9-year-old with BE and aortic stenosis

68. One of the *most* important factors in preventing bacterial endocarditis is:
    a. administration of prophylactic antibiotic therapy.
    b. surgical repair of the defect.
    c. administration of prostaglandin to correct patent ductus arteriosus.
    d. administration of antibiotics after dental work.

69. One of the *most* common findings on physical examination of the child with acute rheumatic heart disease is:
    a. a systolic murmur.
    b. pleural friction rub.
    c. an ejection click.
    d. a split S_2.

70. The test that provides the *most* reliable evidence of recent streptococcal infection is the:
    a. throat culture.
    b. Mantoux test.
    c. elevation of liver enzymes.
    d. antistreptolysin-O test.

71. Children who have been treated for rheumatic fever:
    a. do not need additional prophylaxis against bacterial endocarditis.
    b. are immune to rheumatic fever for the rest of their lives.
    c. will have transitory manifestations of chorea for the rest of their lives.
    d. may need antibiotic therapy for years.

72. The peak age for the incidence of Kawasaki disease is in the:
    a. infant age group.
    b. toddler age group.
    c. school-age group.
    d. adolescent age group.

73. Which one of the following doses of aspirin would be considered adequate for the initial treatment of Kawasaki disease for a child who weighs 20 kg?
    a. 80 mg every 6 hours
    b. 100 mg every 6 hours
    c. 500 mg every 6 hours
    d. 2000 mg every 6 hours

74. Kawasaki disease is treated with:
    a. aspirin and gamma globulin.
    b. aspirin and cryoprecipitate.
    c. meperidine hydrochloride and gamma globulin.
    d. meperidine hydrochloride and cryoprecipitate.

75. Because of the drug used for long-term therapy, children with Kawasaki disease are at risk for:
    a. chicken pox.
    b. influenza.
    c. Reye syndrome.
    d. myocardial infarction.

76. Most cases of hypertension in children are a result of:
    a. essential hypertension.
    b. secondary hypertension.
    c. primary hypertension.
    d. congenital heart defects.

77. Most children with essential hypertension that is resistant to nonpharmacologic intervention are managed with:
    a. diuretics.
    b. calcium channel blockers.
    c. ACE inhibitors.
    d. any of the above.

78. The nurse's role in relation to hypertension may include:
    a. routine accurate assessment of blood pressure in infants and children.
    b. providing information.
    c. follow-up of the child with hypertension.
    d. all of the above.

79. Elevated cholesterol in childhood:
    a. can predict the long-term risk for heart disease for the individual.
    b. can predict the risk for hypertension in adulthood.
    c. is a major predictor of the adult cholesterol level.
    d. is usually symptomatic.

80. The National Cholesterol Education Program recommends screening for cholesterol in:
    a. children over 5 years of age.
    b. children with a family history of premature cardiovascular disease.
    c. children with congenital heart disease.
    d. all children.

81. The *most* common kind of cardiomyopathy found in children is:
    a. dilated cardiomyopathy.
    b. hypertrophic cardiomyopathy.
    c. restrictive cardiomyopathy.
    d. secondary cardiomyopathy.

82. The heart transplant procedure that is used *most* often in children is the:
    a. heterotopic heart transplantation.
    b. orthotopic heart transplantation.

83. Which one of the following dysrhythmias would be included on a list of dysrhythmias commonly seen in children?
    a. Ventricular tachycardia
    b. Asystole
    c. Supraventricular tachycardia
    d. All of the above

Critical Thinking—Case Study

Pauline Smith is a 3-year-old child admitted for repair of an atrial septal defect. Her parents have known about the defect since her birth. She has had numerous respiratory infections with occasional episodes of congestive heart failure in the past year. Pauline has taken digoxin and furosemide in the past but currently takes only vitamins with iron. Her parents state that they are anxious to have the surgery over with, so that they can treat Pauline like the other children. They have three other children who are all older than Pauline.

84. On admission Pauline is afebrile and playful and has no signs of congestive heart failure. As part of the admission process, the nurse would want to be sure to have a baseline assessment of:
    a. Pauline's sucking and swallowing abilities.
    b. Pauline's reading ability.
    c. Pauline's exercise tolerance level.
    d. all of the above.

85. When developing a nursing care plan for Pauline's admission for the surgical repair of the atrial septal defect, the nurse would *most* likely have identified a nursing diagnosis of:
    a. interrupted family process.
    b. impaired skin integrity.

86. One of the *best* ways for the nurse to provide emotional support for Pauline and her family in the stressful postoperative period is to:
    a. facilitate a swift transfer out of ICU.
    b. expect courage and bravery from Pauline.
    c. limit Pauline's expression of anger toward her parents.
    d. praise Pauline for her efforts to cooperate.

CHAPTER 35

The Child with Hematologic or Immunologic Dysfunction

1. Identify the following statements as true or false.

   _____ The major physiologic component of red cells is erythropoietin.

   _____ A complete blood count with differential describes the components of blood known as platelets.

   _____ A child with a suspected bacterial infection would have a differential count that shows a shift to the left with more mature cells present.

   _____ Erythrocytes supply oxygen and remove CO_2 from cells.

   _____ The mature RBC has no nucleus.

   _____ Reticulocytes indicate active RBC production.

   _____ The regulator of erythrocyte production is tissue oxygenation and renal production of erythropoietin.

   _____ The regulatory mechanism for the production of erythrocytes is their circulating numbers.

   _____ The absolute neutrophil count reflects the body's ability to handle bacterial infection.

   _____ Monocytes and lymphocytes are granulocytes.

   _____ In the child with increased numbers of eosinophils, the nurse should suspect allergies or parasite infection.

   _____ Monocytosis is more evident in acute inflammation.

   _____ The hematocrit is approximately three times the hemoglobin content.

   _____ The mean corpuscular hemoglobin is the average volume of a single RBC.

   _____ Mean corpuscular hemoglobin concentration is the average concentration of hemoglobin in a single cell.

   _____ Bands are immature neutrophils, and they increase in number during bacterial infections.

2. The nurse would expect laboratory results for the patient with chronic blood loss to include:
   a. high iron levels.
   b. macrocytic and hyperchromic erythrocytes.
   c. microcytic and hypochromic erythrocytes.
   d. normocytic and normochromic erthrocytes.

3. What are the main causes of anemia?

4. What is the basic physiologic defect caused by anemia?

5. Match the term with its description.

a. Normocytes   g. Normochromic   m. Polycythemia
b. Macrocytes   h. Hypochromic   n. Fetal Hgb
c. Microcytes   i. Hemolysis   o. MCH
d. Spherocytes   j. MCHC   p. Granulocytes
e. Poikilocytes   k. MCV   q. Agranulocytes
f. Drepanocytes   l. Hemostasis

_____ Indicates the average volume or size of a single RBC
_____ Reduced amount of hemoglobin concentration
_____ Sickle-shaped cells
_____ Indicates the average concentration of Hgb in the RBC
_____ Process that stops bleeding when a blood vessel is injured
_____ Excessive destruction of red blood cells
_____ Indicates the average weight of Hgb in each RBC
_____ Neutrophils, basophils, eosinophils
_____ Monocytes, lymphocytes
_____ Larger than normal cell size
_____ Smaller than normal cell size
_____ Normal cell size
_____ Sufficient or normal hemoglobin concentration
_____ Two alpha and two gamma chains; has a greater affinity for oxygen
_____ Increase in the number of erythrocytes
_____ Globular-shaped cells
_____ Irregular-shaped cells

6. When the hemoglobin level falls sufficiently to produce clinical manifestations of anemia, the patient experiences:
   a. cyanosis.
   b. tissue hypoxia.
   c. nausea and vomiting.
   d. feelings of anxiety.

7. Which of the following does the nurse expect to include in the care plan of a patient with anemia?
   i.   Prepare the child for laboratory tests.
   ii. Observe for complications of therapy.
   iii. Decrease tissue oxygen needs.
   iv. Implement safety precautions.

   a. i and iv
   b. i, ii, iii, and iv
   c. ii and iii
   d. i and ii

8. The nurse is scheduled to administer 100 ml of packed red blood cells to 3-year-old Amy. Which one of the following is *not* a correct guideline when administering the blood?
   a. Take vital signs before administration.
   b. Infuse the blood through an appropriate filter.
   c. Administer 50 ml of the blood within the first few minutes to detect for possible reactions before proceeding with the remainder of the infusion.
   d. Start the blood within 30 minutes of its arrival from the blood bank or return it to the blood bank.

9. Lucas, age 7 years, is receiving a transfusion of packed red blood cells. After 45 minutes, he begins to have chills, fever, a sensation of tightness in his chest, and headache. The priority action of the nurse is to:
   a. stop the transfusion and administer acetaminophen.
   b. stop the transfusion and notify the practitioner.
   c. slow the transfusion rate until the symptoms subside.
   d. slow the transfusion and send a sample of the patient's blood and urine to the laboratory.

10. At birth the normal full-term newborn has maternal stores of iron sufficient to last how long?
   a. The first 5 to 6 months of life
   b. The first 2 to 3 months of life
   c. The first 8 months of life
   d. Less than 1 month of life

11. Which one of the following laboratory values is diagnostic of anemia caused by inadequate intake or absorption of iron?
   a. Elevated TIBC and reduced SIC
   b. Reduced TIBC and SIC
   c. Elevated TIBC and SIC
   d. Reduced TIBC and elevated SIC

12. Angie, age 11 months, is brought into the clinic by her mother for a routine checkup. On physical exam, the nurse observes that Angie appears chubby; that her skin looks pale, almost porcelain-like; and that Angie has poor muscle development. Based on these observations, which one of the following questions is *most* important for the nurse to include when completing Angie's history?
   a. "Did you have any complications during pregnancy or delivery of Angie?"
   b. "Tell me about what you are currently feeding Angie."
   c. "Has Angie had any recent infections or high fevers?"
   d. "Have you noticed if Angie is having difficulty with her movements or advancing in her growth and development abilities?"

13. The nurse is instructing a new mother in how to prevent iron deficiency anemia in her new premature infant when she takes her home. The mother intends to breast-feed. Which one of the following statements reflects a need for further education of the new mother?
   a. "I will use only breast milk or formula as a source of milk for my baby until she is at least 12 months old."
   b. "My baby will need to have iron supplements introduced when she is 2 months old."
   c. "As my baby is able to tolerate other foods, such as cereal, I should limit her formula intake to about 1 L/day to encourage intake of iron-rich cereals."
   d. "I will need to add iron supplements to my baby's diet when she is 6 months old."

14. When teaching the parents of 4-year-old Tony how to administer the iron supplement ordered for his iron deficiency, the nurse should include which one of the following in the teaching plan?
   a. Give the iron twice daily in divided doses with orange juice.
   b. Give the iron twice daily with milk.
   c. Administer the oral liquid iron preparation with the use of a syringe or medicine dropper directly into each side of the mouth in the cheek areas.
   d. Make sure parents have at least 3 months' supply of the iron preparation on hand so that they will not run out.

15. On a return clinical visit after Tony has been taking the iron supplement, his mother tells the nurse that Tony's stools are now greenish-black in color and she is concerned. What would your response be?

16. Hereditary spherocytosis (HS) is:
   a. transmitted as an autosomal recessive disease.
   b. a hemolytic disorder caused by a defect in the proteins that form the RBC membrane.
   c. rarely evident until the infant is 4–6 months of age.
   d. usually resolved when additional folic acid supplements are administered.

17. Sally and David Brown are returning with Jason, their 6-week-old infant, for a routine newborn exam. Sally is a carrier for sickle cell anemia; David is not. What is the chance that Jason was born with sickle cell anemia?
   a. 25% chance
   b. 50% chance
   c. 75% chance
   d. 0% chance

18. Infants are often not diagnosed with sickle cell anemia until they are 1 year of age. Why?
   a. Usually there are no symptoms until after age 1 year.
   b. High intake of fluids from formulas prevents sickle cell crises during this age.
   c. Fetal hemoglobin is present during the first year of life.
   d. Increased hemoglobin and hematocrit amounts compensate during this period.

19. Under conditions of _____, _____, _____, and

    _____ _____, the relatively insoluble HbS changes its molecular structure to filamentous crystals that cause distortion of the cell membrane to a sickle-shaped RBC.

20. Bruce, age 12 years, is admitted to your unit with a diagnosis of sickle cell crisis. Which one of the following activities is *most* likely to have precipitated this episode?
   a. Attending the football game with his friends
   b. Going camping and hiking in the mountains with his friends
   c. Going to the beach and surfing with his friends
   d. Staying indoors and reading for several hours

21. Pat is a 5-year-old being admitted because of diminished RBC production triggered by a viral infection. What type of sickle cell crisis is she *most* likely experiencing?
   a. Vasoocclusive crisis
   b. Splenic sequestration crisis
   c. Aplastic crisis
   d. Hyperhemolytic crisis

22. Therapeutic management of sickle cell crisis generally includes which one of the following?
   a. Long-term oxygen use to enable the oxygen to reach the sickled RBCs
   b. Decrease in fluids to increase hemoconcentration
   c. Diet high in iron to decrease anemia
   d. Bed rest to minimize energy expenditure

23. In controlling pain related to vasoocclusive sickle cell crisis, which one of the following can the nurse expect to be included in the plan of care?
    a. Administration of long-term oxygen
    b. Application of cold compresses to the area
    c. Meperidine (Demerol) to be titrated and administered to a therapeutic level
    d. Adding codeine to acetaminophen or ibuprofen if neither one of these is effective in relieving the pain alone

24. In planning for a child's discharge after a sickle cell crisis, the nurse recognizes which one of the following as a critical factor to include in the teaching plan?
    a. Ingestion of large quantities of liquids to promote adequate hydration
    b. Rigorous exercise schedule to promote muscle strength
    c. A high-caloric diet to improve nutrition
    d. At least 12 hours of sleep per night

25. Norma, age 2 years, is to begin therapy for beta-thalassemia. Which one of the following would be appropriate for the nurse to include in the educational session held with the parents?
    a. Norma will need frequent blood transfusions to keep her Hgb level above 12 g/dl.
    b. Large doses of vitamin C will be needed throughout the disease.
    c. Chelation therapy is delayed until after 6 years of age to promote normal physical development.
    d. To minimize the effect of iron overload, deferoxamine (Desferal), an iron-chelating agent, will be given intravenously or subcutaneously.

26. A diagnostic evaluation used to distinguish the type and severity of the various thalassemias is:
    a. hemoglobin electrophoresis.
    b. Sickledex.
    c. stained blood smear.
    d. microscopic exam of RBC.

27. What are the two etiologies of aplastic anemia?

28. a. How is a definite diagnosis of aplastic anemia determined?

    b. Acquired aplastic anemia presents with clinical manifestations of _____,

    _____, and _____ _____

    _____.

    c. Identify two main approaches aimed at restoring function to the marrow in aplastic anemia.

29. Danny is scheduled to receive antithymocyte globulin (ATG) for treatment of his aplastic anemia. Based on knowledge about this therapy, which one of the following does the nurse recognize as true?
    a. ATG is administered intramuscularly every 3–4 weeks.
    b. ATG is administered intravenously in a peripheral vein over a 3-hour period.
    c. All reactions to ATG will occur within the first hour of administration and include skin rash and fever.
    d. ATG suppresses T-cell-dependent autoimmune responses but does not cause bone marrow suppression.

30. Match the term with its description.

    a. Bleeding time
    b. Prothrombin time (PT)
    c. Partial thromboplastin time (PTT)
    d. Thromboplastin generation test (TGT)

    e. Fibrinogen level
    f. Hemophilia A
    g. Hemophilia B

    _____ Allows for determination of specific factor deficiencies, especially factors VIII and IX
    _____ Directly measures fibrinogen level in blood
    _____ Function depends on platelet aggregation and vasoconstriction
    _____ Measures factors necessary for prothrombin conversion to thrombin and fibrinogen
    _____ Measures the activity of thromboplastin and specific for factor deficiencies except factor VII
    _____ Factor IX deficiency
    _____ Factor VIII deficiency

31. When discussing hemophilia with the parents of a child recently diagnosed with this disease, the nurse tells the parents that:
    i. hemophilia is an x-linked disorder in which the mother is the carrier of the illness but is not affected by it.
    ii. hemophilia is a recessive disorder carried by either the mother or the father.
    iii. all of the daughters of the parents will be carriers.
    iv. each of their sons has a 50% chance of being affected and each of their daughters has a 50% chance of being a carrier.

    a. i and iv
    b. ii and iii
    c. i and iii
    d. ii and iv

32. Which one of the following is the *most* frequent form of internal bleeding in the child with hemophilia?
    a. Hemarthrosis
    b. Epistaxis
    c. Intracranial hemorrhage
    d. Gastrointestinal tract hemorrhage

33. Which one of the following is no longer recommended for use in treating factor VIII deficiency because the risk for hepatitis or HIV cannot be safely eliminated?
    a. Factor VIII concentrate
    b. Cryoprecipitate
    c. DDAVP (1-deamino-8-D-arginine vasopressin)
    d. Epsilon aminocaproic acid (Amicar, EACA)

34. Donald, age 5 and previously diagnosed with hemophilia A, is being admitted with bleeding into the joints. The nurse knows that which of the following is *contraindicated* in the plan of care for Donald?
    i.   Ice packs to the affected area
    ii. Application of a splint or sling to the area
    iii. Administration of corticosteroids
    iv. Administration of aspirin, indocin, or butazolidin
    v.   Passive range-of-motion exercises
    vi. Active range-of-motion exercises
    vii. Teaching Donald how to administer AHF to himself

    a. i, iii, and vi
    b. ii, iii, iv, and vi
    c. i, v, and vii
    d. iv, v, and vii

35. Which one of the following statements about von Willebrand disease is true?
    a. The characteristic clinical feature is an increased tendency toward bleeding from mucous membranes.
    b. It affects females but not males.
    c. It will be unsafe for the female affected with the disease to have children because of hemorrhage.
    d. It is an inherited autosomal recessive disease.

36. An acquired hemorrhagic disorder characterized by excessive destruction of platelets and a discoloration caused by petechiae beneath the skin is called _____

    _____ _____.

37. Which one of the following does the nurse recognize as true when administering anti-D antibody for idiopathic thrombocytopenic purpura?
    a. The platelet count will increase immediately after administration.
    b. Eligible patients include those with lupus.
    c. Bone marrow examination to first rule out leukemia is necessary before administration.
    d. Premedicate the patient with acetaminophen before medication is infused.

38. In severe cases of disseminated intravascular coagulation, treatment may include the administration of heparin. What is the rationale for this therapy?
    a. Inhibit thrombin formation
    b. Decrease platelet count
    c. Increase bleeding time
    d. All of the above

39. The *most* common manifestations of chronic benign neutropenia are _____

    _____ and _____ _____ .

40. What are the four characterizations of Henoch-Schonlein purpura?

41. In children, HIV is likely to be transmitted by which of the following methods?
    a. Exposure in utero by an infected mother or through breast milk of an infected mother
    b. Receiving infected blood products by transfusion before 1985
    c. Adolescent engagement in high-risk behaviors (sexual or IV drugs)
    d. All of the above

42. What are the seven *most* common clinical manifestations of HIV infection in children?

43. Goals of therapy for HIV infection in children are:

44. Identify the following as true or false.

    _____ Combinations of antiretroviral drugs are more likely to delay the emergence of drug resistance in the treatment of HIV than is single-drug therapy.

    _____ *Pneumocystis carinii* pneumonia is the most common opportunistic infection of children infected with HIV.

    _____ Prophylaxis antibiotic therapy is rarely recommended for children with HIV until after the age of 1 year.

    _____ The ELISA and Western blot immunoassay tests are not accurate in infants since these tests may be positive up to the age of 18 months because of maternal antibodies.

    _____ Developmental delay in children with AIDS includes receptive language delays rather than expressive language delays.

45. Immunization needs of the child with HIV infection include which one of the following?
    a. Delay of all immunizations until the child has the HIV infection under control
    b. Withholding of pneumococcal and influenza vaccines
    c. Administration of varicella vaccine at the age of 12 months
    d. Provision of MMR vaccine to children receiving IV gamma globulin prophylaxis

46. Nursing strategies to improve the growth and development of the child with HIV infection include which one of the following?
    a. Provide high-fat and high-calorie meals and snacks to meet body requirements for growth.
    b. Provide only those foods that the child feels like eating.
    c. Fortify foods with nutritional supplements to maximize quality of intake.
    d. Weigh the child and measure height and muscle mass on a daily basis.

47. Nursing strategies to improve school and peer interactions of the child with HIV infection would *best* include which one of the following?
    a. Encouraging the child to have one best friend to whom he or she relates
    b. Assisting the child in identifying personal strengths to facilitate coping
    c. Telling the child that the hospitalization will not contribute to isolation from peers and allowing the child's friends to send letters
    d. Discouraging the child's parents from allowing school friends to visit the child at home recuperating because rest is especially important to the HIV-infected child

48. Why are the ELISA and Western blot immunoassay tests not used to determine HIV infection in infants born to HIV-infected mothers?

49. Two-year-old Jennifer is HIV-infected. Her mother is concerned about placing Jennifer in daycare and is discussing this with the nurse at a routine pediatric follow-up visit. Which of the following is the *best* information to provide Jennifer's mother?
    a. The risk for HIV transmission is significant in daycare centers. Jennifer should not go to daycare until she is older.
    b. It will be all right for Jennifer to attend the daycare, but Jennifer's mother must tell the daycare that Jennifer is infected.
    c. Jennifer can go to daycare but will not be allowed to participate in sports or physical activity that could lead to injury.
    d. Jennifer should be admitted to the daycare without restrictions and allowed to participate in all activities as her health permits.

50. In Wiskott-Aldrich syndrome, the *most* notable effect of the disease at birth is which one of the following?
    a. Bleeding
    b. Infection
    c. Eczema
    d. Malignancy

51. What are the clinical manifestations associated with Wiskott-Aldrich syndrome?

Critical Thinking—Case Study

Mary, age 9, has sickle cell anemia. She is admitted to the hospital with knee and back pain and is diagnosed as being in vasoocclusive crisis.

52. The nurse, in developing a plan of care for Mary, formulated a diagnosis of pain. The nurse understands that Mary's pain is related to which one of the following?
    a. Pooling of large amounts of blood in the liver and spleen
    b. Shorter life span of the RBCs and the fact that the bone marrow cannot produce enough RBCs
    c. Tissue anoxia brought on by sickle cells occluding blood vessels
    d. RBC destruction related to a viral infection or transfusion reaction

53. Describe interventions that the nurse can include in the plan of care to control pain during this vaso-occlusive crisis in order to prevent undermedicating.

54. The nurse is developing an educational plan about sickle cell anemia for Mary and her parents. In order to prevent recurrence of this type of crisis, which one of the following is *most* important to include in the educational session?
    a. Explaining the signs of dehydration
    b. Explaining that frequent rest periods are required when the child is in a low-oxygen atmosphere
    c. Explaining that the child should avoid injury to joints to decrease sickling of blood cells
    d. Explaining the importance of avoiding infection by routine immunization and protection from known sources of infection

55. Evaluation of Mary's progress is best based on which one of the following observations?
    a. Mary's verbalization that she no longer has pain or need for pain medication
    b. Mary's ability to perform active range-of-motion exercises
    c. Mary's desire to drink the required level of fluids for hydration
    d. Mary's verbalization of how to prevent future sickle cell crisis

56. Cindy is a 12-month-old being treated for HIV infection. Describe nursing interventions to prevent the spread of the disease to others.

57. In preparing a nursing care plan for Cindy, expected goals would be:

CHAPTER 36

The Child with Cancer

1. The following terms are related to the etiology and diagnosis of cancer. Match each term with its description.

   a. Biologic cure
   b. Oncogenes
   c. Retroviruses
   d. Carcinogenic
   e. Cancer classification
   f. Tumor staging
   g. Bone marrow test
   h. Aspiration
   i. Biopsy

   _____ Refers to the biologic characteristics of the tumor
   _____ Obtaining a piece of tissue through a special type of needle
   _____ Used to determine the extent of bone marrow involvement by malignant cells
   _____ Not an absolute term; the complete eradication of all cancer cells
   _____ Obtaining a sample through a large- or fine-bore needle
   _____ Genes having the potential to transform normal cells into malignant ones
   _____ RNA tumor viruses; have the ability to translate RNA back to DNA
   _____ Refers to the extent of the disease at the time of diagnosis
   _____ Capable of producing cancer

2. The following terms are related to modes of therapy and complications of therapy. Match each term with its description.

   a. Clinical trials
   b. Protocol
   c. Alkylating agents
   d. Antimetabolites
   e. Plant alkaloids
   f. Antitumor antibiotics
   g. Hormones
   h. Lethal damage
   i. Sublethal damage
   j. Total body irradiation (TBI)
   k. Monoclonal antibody
   l. Mono
   m. Clone
   n. Human leukocyte antigen (HLA) system complex
   o. Haplotype
   p. Graft-versus-host disease (GVHD)
   q. Allogenic BMT
   r. Umbilical cord blood stem cell transplantation
   s. Autologous BMTs
   t. Peripheral stem cell transplants (PSCTs)
   u. Acute tumor lysis syndrome
   v. Hyperleukocytosis
   w. Obstruction
   x. Superior vena cava syndrome
   y. Overwhelming infections

   _____ Genes inherited as a single unit
   _____ Natural products that interfere with cell division by reacting with DNA in such a way as to prevent further replication of DNA and transcription of RNA
   _____ Autologous transplant; stem cells first stimulated to grow, then collected and filtered from whole blood; whole blood then returned to the patient; performed without problems on very small children
   _____ The system used to select a suitable donor
   _____ The name given to the formalized treatment plan that is derived from clinical trials
   _____ Adrenal and gonadal are used; have antineoplastic properties; precise mechanism of action unclear; may bind with DNA to alter the transcription process

_____ Resemble essential metabolic elements needed for cell growth but are sufficiently altered in molecular structure to inhibit further synthesis of DNA and/or RNA

_____ Refers to the death of the cell

_____ Comparative evaluations of different types of treatment; may involve any aspect of cancer care; frequently concerned with evaluating investigational drugs

_____ Damage to injured cells that may subsequently be repaired

_____ Replace a hydrogen atom of a molecule by an alkyl group; irreversible; cause unbalanced growth of unaffected cell constituents so that the cell eventually dies; similar action as irradiation

_____ Associated with the most severe reactions and employed to prepare the immune system for bone marrow transplantation

_____ Arrests cells in metaphase by binding to microtubular protein needed for spindle formation

_____ Antibodies that recognize a single specific antigen

_____ Condition wherein donor's bone marrow may contain antigens that are not matched to the recipient's antigens and that begin attacking body cells

_____ A new source of hematopoietic stem cells for use in children with cancer; allows for partially matched unrelated transplants to be successful; lowers risk for GVHD-related problems

_____ Life-threatening condition; peripheral white blood cell count greater than $100,000/mm^3$; can lead to capillary obstruction, microinfarction, and organ dysfunction

_____ Also means one

_____ Compression of the mediastinal structures, leading to airway compromise and potentially to respiratory failure

_____ Exact duplicate

_____ Caused by space-occupying lesions such as Hodgkin's disease and non-Hodgkin's lymphoma structures

_____ Involves the matching of a histocompatible donor with the recipient

_____ May constitute an emergency situation; can result in complications such as disseminated intravascular coagulation (DIC), hemorrhage, thrombocytopenia, and leukocytosis

_____ Uses the patient's own marrow that was collected from disease-free tissue, frozen, and sometimes treated to remove malignant cells; has been used to treat neuroblastoma, Hodgkin's disease, non-Hodgkin's lymphoma, rhabdomyosarcoma, Ewing sarcoma, and Wilms tumor

_____ Life-threatening condition caused by the rapid release of intracellular metabolites during the initial treatment of malignancies such as Burkitt's and T-cell lymphomas and acute leukemia; leads to hyperuricemia, hypocalcemia, hyperphosphatemia, and hyperkalemia

3. The following terms are related to the signs and symptoms of cancer. Match each term with its description.

a. Pain

b. Fever

c. Skin assessment

d. Anemia

e. Abdominal mass

f. Swollen lymph glands

g. White reflection

_____ Classic sign of retinoblastoma; cat's eye reflex or leukokoria

_____ Common finding in children; if enlarged and firm for more than a week, may indicate a serious disease

_____ Typical finding in children with Wilms tumor and neuroblastoma

_____ Caused by the replacement of normal cells with malignant cells in the bone marrow

_____ May show signs of low platelet count; ecchymosis; petechiae

_____ A frequent occurrence caused by numerous illnesses other than cancer; with cancer usually caused by infection secondary to the malignant process

_____ May be an early or late initial sign of cancer

4. The following terms are related to the nursing care of children with cancer. Match each term with its description.

a. Absolute neutrophil count
b. Colony-stimulating factors
c. Granulocyte colony-stimulating factor
d. Postirradiation somnolence
e. Mood changes
f. Moon face

_____ Neupogen; directs granulocyte development and can decrease the duration of neutropenia following immunosuppressive therapy

_____ One of the effects of long-term steroid treatment that can be extremely distressing to older children; child's face becomes rounded and puffy

_____ May be experienced shortly after beginning steroid therapy; range from feelings of well-being and euphoria to depression and irritability

_____ If lower than 500/mm^3, risk for infection and major complications

_____ A neurologic syndrome that may develop 5 to 8 weeks after central nervous system irradiation; characterized by somnolence with or without fever, anorexia, and nausea and vomiting; may be an early indicator of long-term neurologic sequelae after cranial irradiation

_____ A family of glycoprotein hormones that regulate the reproduction, maturation, and function of blood cells; used as a supportive measure to prevent the side effects caused by low blood counts

5. Match each term with its description.

a. Leukemia
b. Induction
c. Intensification
d. Central nervous system prophylactic therapy
e. Maintenance phase
f. Ann Arbor staging classification
g. Leukokoria
h. Sternberg-Reed cell
i. Involved field radiation
j. Extended field radiation
k. Total nodal irradiation
l. Burkitt lymphoma
m. Brain tumors
n. Neuroblastoma
o. Infratentorial
p. Supratentorial
q. Astrocytes
r. Astrocytomas
s. Stereotactic surgery
t. Lasers
u. Brain mapping
v. Phantom limb pain
w. Somatic mutations
x. Germinal mutations
y. Plaque brachytherapy
z. Photocoagulation
aa. Cryotherapy

_____ Vaporize tumor tissue

_____ Consolidation therapy; the phase of leukemia treatment that decreases the tumor burden

_____ The phase of leukemia therapy that serves to maintain the remission of the disease

_____ Determines the precise location of critical brain areas that are avoided during surgery

_____ Cat's eye reflex; a whitish glow in the pupil that is a sign of retinoblastoma and is often visualized first by the parent

_____ A broad term given to a group of malignant diseases of the bone marrow and lymphatic system; in children acute lymphoid leukemia (ALL) and acute mylogenous leukemia (AML) generally recognized

_____ The phase of leukemia therapy that prevents leukemic cells from invading the central nervous system

_____ The phase of leukemia treatment that achieves a complete remission or disappearance of leukemic cells

_____ Children with stage I Hodgkin's disease candidates for this treatment

_____ A staging system to classify Hodgkin's disease

_____ Entire axial lymph node system irradiated; usually combined with chemotherapy

_____ A type of cancer that is rare in the United States; endemic in parts of Africa; a rapidly growing neoplasm that is most commonly seen as a mass in the jaw, abdomen, or orbit

_____ A giant cell with a dark-staining nucleolus; considered diagnostic of Hodgkin's but may occur in mononucleosis

_____ The most common solid tumors that occur in children; second only to leukemia as a form of cancer

_____ Indicated for stage II or stage III Hodgkin's disease; involved areas and adjacent nodes irradiated

_____ The most common malignant tumors of infancy and are second only to brain tumors as the type of solid malignancy seen during the first 10 years

_____ May develop following amputation; characterized by sensations such as tingling, itching, and more frequently, pain felt in the amputated limb; amitriptyline may decrease the pain

_____ Below the tentorium cerebelli

_____ Those retinoblastomas occurring in the general body cells as opposed to the germ cells or gametes; sporadic, nonhereditary events; result in unilateral retinoblastoma tumors

_____ Within the anterior two-thirds of the brain, mainly the cerebrum

_____ Passed to future generations; bilateral retinoblastomas considered hereditary; 15% of unilateral disease possibly hereditary; transmitted as an autosomal dominant trait

_____ Cells that form most of the supportive tissue for the neurons

_____ Surgical implantation of an iodine-125 applicator on the sclera until the maximum radiation dose has been delivered to the tumor

_____ The most common glial tumor

_____ Freezing the tumor; destroys the microcirculation to the tumor and the cells themselves through microcrystal formation

_____ Involves the use of CT and MRI in conjunction with other special computer techniques to reconstruct the tumor in three dimensions

_____ Use of a laser beam to destroy retinal blood vessels that supply nutrition to the tumor

6. The cancer that occurs with the most frequency in children is:
   a. lymphoma.
   b. neuroblastoma.
   c. leukemia.
   d. melanoma.

7. Which one of the following carcinogenic agents has been definitely implicated in the development of childhood cancer?
   a. Low doses of radiation
   b. Excessive sun exposure
   c. Exposure to cigarette smoke
   d. Intramuscular vitamin K at birth

8. Of the following assessment findings, the one that would *most* likely be seen in a child with leukemia is:
   a. weakness of the eye muscle.
   b. bruising, nosebleeds, paleness, and fatigue.
   c. wheezing and shortness of breath.
   d. abdominal swelling.

9. When a clinical trial is used to evaluate an aspect of childhood cancer care, the parents can expect that treatment the child receives will always be:
   a. better than the current treatment usually used.
   b. an evaluation of an investigational drug.
   c. intermittent intravenous infusion of drugs.
   d. at least as good as the best possible treatment presently known.

10. The use of clinical trials and protocols for cancer treatment has resulted in an increased use of:
    a. intermittent intravenous therapy.
    b. continuous intravenous therapy.
    c. lower doses of single-drug therapy.
    d. prolonged duration of maintenance therapy.

11. The severe cellular damage that is caused by chemotherapy drugs infiltrating into surrounding tissue occurs when the chemotherapeutic agent is a(n):
    a. hormone.
    b. steroid.
    c. vesicant.
    d. antimetabolite.

12. Match each type of chemotherapeutic agent with the side effect or nursing consideration that *most* pertains to that type of drug.

    a. Alkylating agents   d. Hormones
    b. Antimetabolites   e. Enzymes
    c. Plant alkaloids

    _____ Neurotoxicity
    _____ Renal toxicity or hemorrhagic cystitis
    _____ Usually no short-term acute toxicity
    _____ Mucosal ulceration/stomatitis
    _____ Allergic reactions

13. A candidate for bone marrow transplant is the child who:
    a. is unlikely to be cured by other means.
    b. has acute leukemia.
    c. has chronic leukemia.
    d. has a compatible donor in his or her family.

14. Name four types of early side effects of radiation therapy, and describe one nursing intervention for each type.

15. A major benefit of using umbilical cord blood for stem cell transplantation is:
    a. stem cells are found in low frequency in newborns.
    b. umbilical cord blood is relatively immunodeficient.
    c. there is a lower risk for acute tumor lysis syndrome.
    d. all of the above.

16. List five cardinal symptoms of cancer in children.

17. The family of glycoprotein hormones that regulate the function of blood cells is called

_____.

18. A child who is anemic from myelosuppression should:
    a. strictly limit activities.
    b. regulate his or her own activity with adult supervision.
    c. receive transfusions until the hemoglobin level reaches 12.
    d. receive chemotherapy until the hemoglobin level reaches 10.

19. The nursing intervention that would be *most* helpful to use for the child who has stomatitis from cancer chemotherapy would be:
    a. an anesthetic preparation without alcohol.
    b. viscous xylocaine.
    c. lemon glycerin swabs.
    d. a mild sedative.

20. Describe three strategies the nurse can use to prevent sterile hemorrhagic cystitis.

21. Parents sometimes view the child's moon face from steroids as an appearance of:
    a. an anorexic, undernourished child.
    b. a malnourished child with a swollen abdomen.
    c. an overweight but undernourished child.
    d. a well-nourished, healthy child.

22. The child who receives a bone marrow transplant will require:
    a. meticulous skin care.
    b. multiple peripheral sites for intravenous therapy.
    c. less chemotherapy prior to the transplant.
    d. a room with laminar air flow.

23. After a bone marrow aspiration is performed on a child, the nurse should:
    a. apply an adhesive bandage.
    b. place the child in Trendelenburg position.
    c. ask the child to remain in the supine position.
    d. apply a pressure bandage.

24. Dental care for a child whose platelet count is 32,000/mm^3 and granulocyte count is 450/mm^3 should include daily:
    a. toothbrushing with flossing.
    b. toothbrushing without flossing.
    c. flossing without toothbrushing.
    d. wiping with moistened sponges.

25. Although the immune response is likely to be suboptimal in the immunosuppressed child, it is considered safe to administer:
    a. any vaccines.
    b. any live attenuated vaccines.
    c. any inactivated vaccines.
    d. the varicella vaccine.

26. Leukemia is characterized by:
    a. a high leukocyte count.
    b. destruction of normal cells by abnormal cells.
    c. low numbers of blast cells.
    d. overproduction of white blood cells.

27. Name the three main consequences of bone marrow dysfunction, and list their causes.

28. Staging the child with leukemia by using initial white blood cell count, the patient's age, sex, and the histologic type of the disease is used to:
    a. determine potential chemotherapy side effects.
    b. estimate long-term survival.
    c. make a definitive diagnosis.
    d. determine whether metastases have occurred.

29. Children who receive reinduction therapy for a relapse in their acute lymphocytic leukemia are likely to:
    a. recover rapidly.
    b. receive vincristine and prednisone.
    c. receive a bone marrow transplant.
    d. relapse 5 years after a complete remission.

30. Which one of the following children with acute lymphoid leukemia has the *best* prognosis?
    a. A 1-year-old girl with a leukocyte count of 30,000/mm^3
    b. A 6-year-old boy with a leukocyte count of 120,000/mm^3
    c. A 6-year-old boy with a leukocyte count of 30,000/mm^3
    d. A 1-year-old girl with a leukocyte count of 120,000/mm^3

31. To attempt to prevent central nervous system invasion of malignant cells, children with leukemia usually receive prophylactic:
    a. cranial/spinal irradiation.
    b. intravenous steroid therapy.
    c. intrathecal chemotherapy.
    d. intravenous methotrexate and cytarabine.

32. The fact that 95% of children with acute lymphoid leukemia will achieve an initial remission should be interpreted as:
    a. the percentage of children who will live 5 years or longer.
    b. an estimate that applies to children treated with the most successful protocols since diagnosis.
    c. the number to use only for the low-risk group of children.
    d. the estimate that may be used to determine the probability of a cure.

33. Hodgkin's disease increases in incidence in children between the ages of:
    a. 1 and 5 years.
    b. 5 and 10 years.
    c. 11 and 14 years.
    d. 15 and 19 years.

34. Using present treatment protocols, prognosis for Hodgkin's disease may be estimated with:
    a. the Ann Arbor Staging Classification.
    b. histologic staging.
    c. degree of tumor burden.
    d. initial leukocyte count.

35. A child with Hodgkin's disease who has lesions in both the left and the right supraclavicular area, the mediastinum, and the lungs would be classified as:
    a. stage I.
    b. stage II.
    c. stage III.
    d. stage IV.

36. The Sternberg-Reed cell is a significant finding, because it:
    a. is absent in all diseases other than Hodgkin's disease.
    b. is absent in all diseases other than the lymphomas.
    c. eliminates the need for laparotomy to determine the stage of the disease.
    d. is absent in all lymphomas other than Hodgkin's disease.

37. A particular area of concern for the adolescent receiving radiation therapy is:
    a. frequent vomiting.
    b. altered sexual function.
    c. the high-risk for sterility.
    d. precocious puberty.

38. Burkitt lymphoma is a type of:
    a. Hodgkin's disease.
    b. non-Hodgkin's lymphoma.
    c. acute myleocytic leukemia.
    d. neuroblastoma.

39. The early signs and symptoms of brain tumor in the infant:
    a. are similar to those of a young child's.
    b. may be undetectable while the sutures are open.
    c. will be demonstrated as vomiting after feedings.
    d. will be demonstrated as headache and vomiting.

40. Match each major brain tumor of childhood with its corresponding characteristics.

    a. Medulloblastoma   d. Ependymoma

    b. Cerebral astrocytoma   e. Brainstem glioma

    c. Low-grade astrocytoma

    _____ Poor prognosis, because tumor is located in vital brain centers

    _____ The most common pediatric brain tumor; infiltrates brain parenchyma without distinct boundaries

    _____ Usually invades the ventricles and obstructs the cerebrospinal fluid flow

    _____ Slow-growing tumor (if low-grade); has a 70%–90% likelihood of cure (without residual tumor postoperatively)

    _____ Fast-growing, highly malignant tumor with a high risk for recurrence

41. The surgical technique that uses computerized tomography and magnetic resonance imaging is called:
    a. sclerotherapy.
    b. microsurgery.
    c. laser surgery.
    d. stereotactic surgery.

42. An assessment finding that is consistent with the presence of a brain tumor is increased:
    a. temporal headaches.
    b. appetite.
    c. pulse rate.
    d. blood pressure.

43. Describe three strategies the nurse can use to help prepare the child for shaving the hair prior to surgery to remove a brain tumor.

44. If a child vomits in the postoperative period following surgery for a brain tumor, it may predispose the child to:
    a. incisional rupture.
    b. increased intracranial pressure.
    c. aspiration.
    d. all of the above.

45. Of the following assessment findings in the postoperative care of the a child who had surgery to remove a brain tumor, the one with the most serious implications is:
    a. a comatose child.
    b. serous sanguinous drainage on the dressing.
    c. colorless drainage on the dressing.
    d. decreased muscle strength.

46. Neuroblastoma is often classified as a silent tumor because:
    a. diagnosis is not usually made until after metastasis.
    b. the primary site is intracranial.
    c. the primary site is the bone marrow.
    d. diagnosis is made based on the location of the primary site.

47. The peak age for the appearance of bone tumors is:
    a. 5 to 9 years of age.
    b. 10 to 14 years of age.
    c. 15 to 19 years of age.
    d. 20 to 24 years of age.

48. The most common bone cancer in children has a peak incidence at the age of:
    a. birth to 4 years.
    b. 4 years to 8 years.
    c. 8 years to 10 years.
    d. over 11 years.

49. Treatment for Ewing sarcoma usually involves:
    a. radiation alone.
    b. radiation and chemotherapy.
    c. amputation and chemotherapy.
    d. chemotherapy alone.

50. Wilms tumor in children is based on clinical stage and histologic pattern and treated with:
    a. chemotherapy and radiation.
    b. radiation alone.
    c. surgery, chemotherapy, and radiation.
    d. surgery alone.

51. Rhabdomyosarcoma is a:
    a. malignant bone neoplasm.
    b. nonmalignant soft tissue tumor.
    c. nonmalignant solid tumor.
    d. malignant solid tumor of the soft tissue.

52. With a multimodal approach to treatment, 5-year survival rates for rhabdomyosarcoma have improved to:
    a. 15%.
    b. 35%.
    c. 50%.
    d. 65%.

53. Bilateral malignant retinoblastoma is almost always considered to be transmitted by:
    a. an autosomal dominant trait.
    b. a somatic mutation.
    c. a chromosomal aberration.
    d. an autosomal recessive trait.

54. Instructions for the parents of a child who has an eye enucleation performed should be based on the fact that:
    a. there will be a cavity in the skull where the eye was.
    b. the child's face may be edematous and ecchymotic.
    c. the eyelids will be open and the surgical site will be sunken.
    d. all of the above.

55. A nodule discovered on an adolescent male's testicle should be evaluated because a tumor in this location:
    a. usually causes infertility.
    b. is usually malignant in this age group.
    c. has usually metastasized by the time of discovery.
    d. could not be felt using testicular self-exam.

56. Which one of the following children would be most likely to develop malignancies as a result of their cancer treatment?
    a. An 18-year-old who receives radiation for treatment of Hodgkin's disease
    b. A 2-year-old who receives interthecal chemotherapy
    c. A 4-year-old who receives radiation for treatment of leukemia
    d. A 15-year-old who receives interthecal chemotherapy

Critical Thinking—Case Study

Cory is a 6-year-old child who is diagnosed with acute lymphoid leukemia. She receives chemotherapy regularly. Her parents are divorced, and she is an only child. She lives with her mother and rarely sees her father.

Cory attends first grade when she can. She had little difficulty with school before her diagnosis, but lately she has had trouble keeping up with the activities, because she is so tired.

57. Today Cory arrives at the chemotherapy clinic for her regular medication regimen. A complete blood count shows that her white blood count is lower than expected. The *best* nursing diagnosis for the nurse to use for Cory today based on the above information would be:
    a. altered family process related to the therapy.
    b. high risk for hemorrhagic cystitis related to white cell proliferation.
    c. high risk for infection related to depressed body defenses.
    d. altered mucous membranes related to administration of chemotherapy.

58. Cory's mother tells the nurse that she has noticed that after the chemotherapy, Cory's appetite is usually quite poor. She knows that nutrition is essential, so she is trying everything to get Cory to eat even during those times when she is nauseated after the chemotherapy. Strategies the nurse might suggest include:
    a. gargling with viscous xylocaine to relieve pain.
    b. permitting only nutritious snacks.
    c. establishing regular meal times.
    d. offering small snacks frequently.

59. To plan for the body image disturbance related to loss of hair, moon face, and debilitation, which of the following actions by Cory's mother would be considered *most* beneficial?
    a. Emphasize the benefits of the therapy.
    b. Encourage Cory to select a wig to wear.
    c. Suggest that Cory keep her hair long for as long as possible.
    d. All of the above

60. Which one of the following expected outcomes would be appropriate for the nurse to use to measure Cory's mother's progress toward coping with the possibility of her child's death?
    a. Cory's mother frequently talks to the staff about her fear of living without her daughter.
    b. Cory's mother is able to verbalize an understanding of the procedures and tests that have been performed.
    c. Cory's mother is able to provide the care at home that is needed.
    d. Cory's mother complies with the suggestions the nurses make.

CHAPTER 37

The Child with Cerebral Dysfunction

1. Match each term with its description.

   a. Central nervous system
   b. Peripheral nervous system
   c. Autonomic nervous system
   d. Meninges
   e. Dura mater
   f. Epidural space
   g. Falx cerebri

   h. Falx cerebelli
   i. Tentorium
   j. Tentorial hiatus
   k. Arachnoid membrane
   l. Subdural area
   m. Pia mater
   n. Subarachnoid space

   o. Arachnoid trabeculae
   p. Longitudinal fissure
   q. Corpus callosum
   r. Basal ganglia
   s. Brainstem
   t. Autoregulation

   _____ Cerebral nuclei; situated deeply within each hemisphere and on each side of the midline; serve as vital sorting areas for messages passing to and from the hemispheres

   _____ The large gap through which the brainstem passes; the site of herniation in untreated intracranial pressure

   _____ The part of the nervous system that is composed of the sympathetic and parasympathetic systems, which provide automatic control of vital functions

   _____ A potential space that normally contains only enough fluid to prevent adhesion between the arachnoid and the dura mater

   _____ A double-layered membrane that serves as the outer meningeal layer and the inner periosteum of the cranial bones

   _____ Located between the pia mater and the arachnoid membrane; filled with cerebrospinal fluid, which acts as a protective cushion for the brain tissue

   _____ A segment of the sheet of dura that separates the cerebral hemispheres

   _____ Connected to the hemispheres by thick bunches of nerve fibers; all nerve fibers traverse through this structure as they pass from the hemispheres to the cerebellum and the spinal cord; extends from the base of the hemispheres through the foramen magnum, where it is continuous with the spinal cord

   _____ A segment of the sheet of dura that separates the cerebellar hemispheres

   _____ The part of the nervous system that is composed of the cranial nerves that arise from or travel to the brainstem and the spinal nerves that travel to or from the spinal cord and which may be motor (efferent) or sensory (afferent)

   _____ A segment of dura that separates the cerebellum from the occipital lobe of the cerebrum; a tent-like structure

   _____ Separates the outer meningeal layer and the inner periosteum of the cranial bones

   _____ The middle meningeal layer; a delicate, avascular, weblike structure that loosely surrounds the brain

   _____ The innermost covering layer of the brain; a delicate, transparent membrane that, unlike other coverings, adheres closely to the outer surface of the brain, conforming to the folds (gyri) and furrows (sulci)

   _____ The unique ability of the cerebral arterial vessels to change their diameter in response to fluctuating cerebral perfusion pressure

   _____ Fibrous filaments that provide protection by helping to anchor the brain

_____ The membranes that cover and protect the brain; the dura mater, arachnoid membranes, and pia mater

_____ Separates the upper part of the two large cerebral hemispheres that occupy the anterior and medial fossae of the skull

_____ The part of the nervous system that is composed of two cerebral hemispheres, the brainstem, the cerebellum, and the spinal cord

_____ The largest fiber bundle in the brain; joins the central part of the cerebral hemispheres; interconnects cortical areas of the right and left hemispheres

2. The following terms are related to the evaluation of neurologic status. Match each term with its description.

a. Neurologic physical examination
b. Cranial nerve involvement
c. Level of development
d. Alertness
e. Cognitive power
f. Unconsciousness
g. Coma

h. Comatose state
i. Glasgow Coma Scale
j. Brain death
k. Reproducible
l. Pulse/respiration/blood pressure
m. Autonomic activity

n. Body temperature
o. Corneal reflex
p. Doll's head maneuver
q. Caloric test
r. Papilledema
s. Decorticate posturing
t. Decerebrate posturing

_____ Indicated by abnormal eye movements, an inability to suck or swallow, lip smacking, asymmetric contraction of facial muscles, and yawning

_____ An arousal-waking state that includes the ability to respond to stimuli; an aspect of consciousness

_____ Includes observation of the size and shape of the head, spontaneous activity, postural reflex activity, sensory responses, symmetry of movement

_____ Depressed cerebral function; the inability to respond to sensory stimuli and have subjective experiences

_____ Provide information regarding the adequacy of circulation and the possible underlying cause of altered consciousness

_____ The aspect of consciousness that includes the ability to process stimuli and produce verbal and motor responsiveness

_____ The continuum of diminished alertness as a result of pathologic conditions

_____ Provides essential information about neurologic function; developmental tests used to determine this element of the neurologic assessment

_____ Often elevated in head injury; sometimes extreme and unresponsive to therapeutic measures

_____ Consists of a three-part assessment; created to meet a clinical need of experienced nurses for objective criteria for the consciousness level; the most popular scale that attempts to standardize the description and interpretation of depressed consciousness

_____ A sign of increased intracranial pressure observed in the eyes

_____ The total cessation of brainstem and cortical brain function

_____ A sign of dysfunction at the level of the midbrain; characterized by rigid extension and pronation of the arms and legs

_____ Most intensively disturbed in deep coma and in brainstem lesions

_____ Blinking of the eyelids when the cornea is touched with a wisp of cotton; used to test the integrity of the ophthalmic division of cranial nerve

_____ The fashion in which neurologic examination should be documented; enables the comparison of baseline, previous, and current findings; allows the observer to detect subtle changes in the neurologic status that might not otherwise be evident

_____ Child's head rotated quickly to one side and then the other; normally eyes will move in the direction opposite the head rotation

_____ A state of unconsciousness from which the patient cannot be aroused, even with powerful stimuli

_____ Oculovestibular response; elicited by irrigating the external auditory canal with ice water; causes movement of the eyes toward the side of the stimulation

_____ Seen with severe dysfunction of the cerebral cortex; includes adduction of the arms and shoulders; arms flexed on the chest; wrists flexed; hands fisted; lower extremities extended and adducted

3. The following terms are related to head injury. Match each term with its description.

a. Acceleration/ deceleration
b. Deformation
c. Coup
d. Contrecoup
e. Shearing stresses
f. Localized injuries
g. Generalized injuries

h. Concussion
i. Contusion/laceration
j. Linear fractures
k. Depressed fractures
l. Compound fractures
m. Basilar fracture
n. Diastatic fracture

o. Acute subdural hematoma
p. Chronic subdural hematoma
q. Postconcussion syndrome
r. Posttraumatic seizures
s. Structural complications

_____ A fracture in which the bone is locally broken, usually into several irregular fragments that are pushed inward, causing pressure on the brain

_____ Bruising at the point of impact

_____ Physical forces that act on the head when the stationary head receives a blow; the circumstances responsible for most head injuries; when the head receives a blow

_____ A common sequella to brain injury; common in children under 1 year of age; occurs within minutes to an hour after a head injury; the child sweats, becomes pale, irritable, sleepy, and may vomit

_____ Caused by hemorrhage; associated with contusions or lacerations and develops within minutes or hours of injury

_____ Involve the basilar portion of the frontal, ethmoid, sphenoid, temporal, or occipital bones

_____ Actual bruising and tearing of cerebral tissue

_____ An effect of brain movement that is caused by unequal movement or different rates of acceleration at various levels of the brain; may tear small arteries; the most serious effects are often in the area of the brainstem

_____ Distortion and cavitation that occur as the brain changes shape in response to the force transmitted from impact to the brain

_____ Occur in a number of children who survive a head injury; more common in children than in adults; more likely to occur with severe head injury; usually occur within the first few days after injury; associated with long-term epilepsy when they occur within a few seconds of the trauma

_____ Traumatic separation of the cranial sutures

_____ A head injury in which the force is spent on a local area of both the skull and underlying tissue

_____ Bruising at a distance from the point of impact

_____ A head injury in which the force is transmitted to the entire skull causing widespread movement, distortion, and damage

_____ Occur as a result of head injuries; include hydrocephalus and motor deficits

_____ The most common head injury; a transient and reversible neuronal dysfunction with instantaneous loss of awareness and responsiveness from trauma to the head that persists for a relatively short time

_____ Consists of a skin laceration that extends to the site of the bony fracture

_____ Comprise about 75% of childhood skull fractures

_____ Caused by hemorrhage; associated with contusions or lacerations, symptoms are delayed; more commonly seen in children with open fontanels and sutures

4. The following terms are related to intracranial infections. Match each term with its description.

a. Meningitis

b. Encephalitis

c. Human diploid cell rabies vaccine

d. Bacterial meningitis

e. Viral meningitis

f. Tuberculous meningitis

g. *Haemophilus influenzae* meningitis

h. Meningococcal sepsis

i. Waterhouse-Fredericksen syndrome

j. Hydrophobia

_____ The sudden, severe, and fulminating onset of meningococcemia

_____ Inflammatory process that affects the brain

_____ The term used to describe the symptoms of rabies; severe spasm of respiratory muscles resulting in apnea, cyanosis, and anoxia

_____ Pyogenic inflammation caused by pus-forming organisms, especially meningococcus, pneumococcus, and influenza bacillus

_____ Vaccine administered to confer active immunity after a rabid animal bite; administered with immune globulin and followed with injections at 3, 7, 14, and 28 days after the first dose.

_____ Aseptic meningitis

_____ Has decreased in incidence since the use of conjugate vaccines in 1990

_____ Inflammatory process that affects the meninges

_____ Meningococcemia; one of the most dramatic and serious complications associated with meningococcal infection

_____ Meningitis caused by the tuberculin bacillus

5. Match each structure of the brain with its corresponding function.

a. Parietal lobes

b. Temporal lobes

c. Cerebrum

d. Thalamus

e. Mesencephalon (midbrain)

f. Medulla

g. Cerebellum

h. Frontal lobes

i. Occipital lobe

j. Diencephalon

k. Hypothalamus

l. Pons

_____ Receive/interpret stimuli for the all of the senses

_____ Contains the vasomotor cranial nerves

_____ Contains pneumotaxic center and controls respiration

_____ Necessary for coordination and balance

_____ Vital control center of involuntary functions (temperature regulation)

_____ Center for consciousness, thought, memory, sensory input, and motor activity

_____ Receives stimuli for vision and spatial orientation

_____ Connects the forebrain to the hindbrain

_____ A major relay station for sensory impulses to the cerebral cortex

_____ Controls motor activity, social interaction, and abstract thinking

_____ Contains fibers that compose the reticular activation system

_____ Important for interpretation of sensation

6. Cerebral blood flow, oxygen consumption, and brain growth are all:
   a. less in adults than in children.
   b. greater in adults than in children.
   c. greater in adults than in infants.
   d. less in infants than in children.

7. Match each seizure term with its description.

   a. Idiopathic seizures
   b. Acquired seizures
   c. Epileptogenic focus
   d. Ictal state
   e. Postictal state
   f. Simple partial seizures with motor signs
   g. Aversive seizure
   h. Rolandic (Sylvian) seizure
   i. Jacksonian march
   j. Simple partial seizures with sensory signs

   k. Partial seizures
   l. Generalized seizures
   m. Unclassified epileptic seizures
   n. Psychomotor seizures
   o. Aura
   p. Deja vu
   q. Impaired consciousness
   r. Automatism
   s. Tonic phase
   t. Clonic phase
   u. Status epilepticus

   v. Drop attacks
   w. Infantile spasms
   x. Salaam seizure
   y. Lennox-Gastaut syndrome
   z. Idiopathic Lennox-Gastaut syndrome
   aa. Symptomatic Lennox-Gastaut syndrome
   bb. Resective surgery
   cc. Callosotomy
   dd. Multiple subpial transection

   _____ Occur as a result of brain injury during prenatal, perinatal, or postnatal periods; may be caused by trauma, hypoxia, infections, exogenous or endogenous toxins, and a variety of other factors

   _____ Simple motor seizure; consists of orderly, sequential progression of clonic movements that begin in a foot, hand, or face and, as electric impulses spread from the irritable focus to contiguous regions of the cortex, move body parts activated by these cerebral regions

   _____ Cause unknown; higher incidence of seizures among relatives of these children

   _____ Formerly called focal seizures; limited to a particular local area of the brain

   _____ A period of the seizure where there is a rolling of the eyes upward and immediate loss of consciousness

   _____ A feeling of familiarity in a strange environment

   _____ All seizures that cannot be classified

   _____ Arise from the area of the brain that controls muscle movement

   _____ Tonic-clonic movements involving the face, salivation, and arrested speech; most common during sleep

   _____ Horizontal fibers of the motor cortex divided to reduce seizures; vertical fibers spared to allow for function

   _____ A group of hyperexcitable cells that initiate the spontaneous electric discharge that produces a seizure

   _____ The period during the time the seizure is occurring

   _____ The period following a seizure

   _____ Characterized by various sensations, including numbness, tingling, prickling, paresthesia, or pain that originates in one area and spreads to other parts of the body

   _____ Seizures that involve both hemispheres of the brain

   _____ Partial seizures with complex symptoms

   _____ A characteristic of the complex partial seizure; repeated activities without purpose and carried out in a dreamy state such as smacking, chewing, drooling, or swallowing

_____ The period in the seizure where there are intense jerking movements as the trunk and extremities undergo rhythmic contraction and relaxation

_____ Atonic seizures; manifested as a sudden, momentary loss of muscle tone

_____ A common motor seizure in children; the eye(s) and head turn away from the side of the focus

_____ A rare disorder that has an onset within the first 6 to 8 months of life; also known as *infantile myoclonus, West syndrome*

_____ Separation of the connections between the two hemispheres of the brain; used to treat some generalized seizures

_____ A characteristic of the complex partial seizure; child may appear dazed and confused and be unable to respond when spoken to or to follow instruction

_____ Also known as *jackknife seizures*; observed as sudden, brief, symmetric muscular contractions by which the head is flexed, the arms extended, and the legs drawn up; the seizure observed in infantile spasms

_____ Focal area of seizure activity excised with the expectation that serious deficits will not be produced and that existing deficits will not be increased

_____ A seizure that lasts 30 minutes or longer or a series of seizures at intervals too brief to allow the child to regain consciousness between each seizure; requires emergency intervention

_____ Also called *cryptogenic Lennox-Gastaut syndrome*; appears in children with normal psychomotor development and no history of epilepsy or evidence of brain damage; may occur after infectious illness, vaccination, or febrile episodes

_____ Lennox-Gastaut syndrome with a history of encephalopathy and mental retardation or epilepsy; poorer prognosis than in the cryptogenic type

_____ Sensation or sensory phenomenon that reflects the complicated connections and integrative functions of that area of the brain

_____ A syndrome that develops in about 30% of children with infantile spasms

8. The blood-brain barrier in an infant is:
   a. less permeable than in the adult.
   b. impermeable to protein.
   c. impermeable to glucose.
   d. permeable to large molecules.

9. Which one of the following signs is used to evaluate increased intracranial pressure in the infant but not in the older child?
   a. Projectile vomiting
   b. Headache
   c. Nonpulsating fontanel
   d. Pulsating fontanel

10. Which of the following indicators is *best* to use to determine the depth of the comatose state?
    a. Motor activity
    b. Level of consciousness
    c. Reflexes
    d. Vital signs

11. Define the term *persistent vegetative state*.

12. The guidelines for establishing brain death in children:
    a. differ from age to age.
    b. are the same as in the adult.
    c. all require an observation period of at least 7 days.
    d. all require an observation period of at least 48 hours.

13. Of the following neurologic conditions, the one that is most associated with hypothermia is:
    a. intracranial bleeding.
    b. barbituate ingestion.
    c. heat stroke.
    d. serious infection.

14. A child in a very deep comatose state would exhibit:
    a. hyperkinetic activity.
    b. purposeless plucking movements.
    c. few spontaneous movements.
    d. combative behavior.

15. After a seizure in a child over 3 years of age, the Babinski reflex often:
    a. remains positive.
    b. changes from positive to negative.
    c. changes from negative to positive.
    d. remains negative.

16. Of the following reflex patterns, the one that would be considered *most* healthy in young infants is a:
    a. negative Moro reflex and a positive tonic neck reflex.
    b. negative Moro reflex and a negative tonic neck reflex.
    c. positive Moro reflex and a positive withdrawal reflex.
    d. positive Moro reflex and a negative withdrawal reflex.

17. If the patient has an increase in intracranial pressure, one test that should not be performed is the:
    a. lumbar puncture.
    b. subdural tap.
    c. computed tomography.
    d. digital subtraction angiography.

18. The diagnostic procedure that is usually noninvasive and permits visualization of the neurologic structures using radio frequency emissions from elements is called:
    a. digital subtraction angiography.
    b. positron emission tomography.
    c. magnetic resonance imaging.
    d. computed tomography scan.

19. The factor that is likely to have the greatest impact on the outcome and recovery of the unconscious child is the:
    a. gradual reduction in intracranial pressure.
    b. level of nursing care and observation skills.
    c. emotional response of the parents.
    d. level of discomfort the child experiences.

20. The nurse should suspect pain in the comatose child if the child exhibits:
    a. increased flaccidity.
    b. increased oxygen saturation.
    c. decreased blood pressure.
    d. increased agitation.

21. Intracranial pressure monitoring has been found to be useful in pediatric critical care to:
    a. provide quick and effective relief of increased pressure.
    b. evaluate children with Glasgow Coma Scale scores less than 7.
    c. maintain $PaCO_2$ at 25–30 mm Hg.
    d. prevent herniation.

22. Of the following activities, the one that has been shown to increase intracranial pressure is:
    a. using earplugs to eliminate noise.
    b. range-of-motion exercises.
    c. suctioning.
    d. osmotherapy.

23. The medications that are controversial in the management of increased intracranial pressure are:
    a. barbiturates.
    b. paralyzing agents.
    c. sedatives.
    d. antiepileptics.

24. If a child is permanently unconscious, it would be *inappropriate* for the nurse to:
    a. permit the parents to bring a child's favorite toy.
    b. provide guidance and clarify information that the physician has already given.
    c. suggest the parents plan for periodic relief from the continual care of their child.
    d. use reflexive muscle contractions as a sign of hope for recovery.

25. Because of the ability of the cranium to expand, very young children may tolerate which one of the following neurologic conditions better than an adult?
    a. Cerebral edema
    b. Hypoxic brain damage
    c. Cerebral edema
    d. Subdural hemorrhage

26. Head injury that causes the brain to be forced though the tentorial opening is usually referred to as:
    a. contrecoup.
    b. concussion.
    c. uncal herniation.
    d. deformation.

27. Of the following symptoms, the one that would *not* be considered a hallmark of concussion in a child is:
    a. alteration of mental status.
    b. amnesia.
    c. loss of consciousness.
    d. confusion.

28. Epidural hemorrhage is less common in children under 2 years of age than in adults because:
    a. the middle meningeal artery is embedded in the bone surface of the skull until approximately 2 years of age.
    b. fractures are less likely to lacerate the middle meningeal artery in children under 2 years of age.
    c. separation of the dura from bleeding is more likely to occur in children than in adults.
    d. there is an increased tendency for the skull to fracture in children under 2 years of age.

29. Which one of the following features is usually associated with subdural hematoma?
    a. Arterial hemorrhage
    b. Low mortality
    c. High mortality
    d. Age greater than 2 years

30. The goal in the management of a child with a head injury is to:
    a. eliminate ischemic brain damage.
    b. eliminate original primary insult.
    c. care for the secondary brain injuries.
    d. carry out all of the above.

31. Emergency treatment of a child with a head injury would generally *not* include:
    a. administering analgesics.
    b. checking pupils' reaction to light.
    c. stabilizing the neck and spine.
    d. checking level of consciousness.

32. The clinical manifestation that indicates a progression from minor head injury to severe head injury is:
    a. confusion.
    b. mounting agitation.
    c. an episode of vomiting.
    d. pallor.

33. Compared to adults after craniocerebral trauma, children usually have a:
    a. lower incidence of psychologic disturbances.
    b. higher mortality rate.
    c. less favorable prognosis.
    d. higher incidence of psychologic disturbances.

34. Family support for the child who has suffered head injury includes all of the following *except* to encourage the parents to:
    a. hold and cuddle the child.
    b. bring familiar belongings into the child's room.
    c. make a tape recording of familiar voices/sounds.
    d. search for clues that the child is recovering.

35. Identify three factors that contribute to accident risk in children.

36. A higher resistance to asphyxia and anoxia from submersion in water would be most likely found in:
    a. toddlers.
    b. preschool children.
    c. school-age children.
    d. adolescents.

37. Of the following factors, the *best* predictor of outcome in near-drowning victims is:
    a. respiratory rate.
    b. degree of acidosis upon admission.
    c. level of consciousness.
    d. length of time the child was submerged.

38. The etiology of bacterial meningitis has changed in recent years because of the:
    a. increased surveillance of tuberculosis.
    b. increased awareness of rubella vaccines.
    c. routine use of *H. influenzae* type B vaccine.
    d. routine use of hepatitis B vaccine.

39. The *most* common mode of transmission for bacterial meningitis is:
    a. vascular dissemination of a respiratory tract infection.
    b. direct implantation from an invasive procedure.
    c. direct extension from an infection in the mastoid sinuses.
    d. direct extension from an infection in the nasal sinuses.

40. A child who is ill and develops a purpuric or petechial rash may possibly have developed:
    a. aseptic meningitis.
    b. Waterhouse-Fredericksen syndrome.
    c. citobacter diversus meningitis.
    d. herpes simplex encephalitis.

41. Secondary problems from bacterial meningitis are *most* likely to occur in the:
    a. child with meningococcal meningitis.
    b. infant under 2 months of age.
    c. infant over 2 months of age.
    d. child with *H. influenzae* type B meningitis.

42. Which one of the following types of meningitis is self-limiting and least serious?
    a. Meningococcal meningitis
    b. Tuberculous meningitis
    c. *H. influenzae* meningitis
    d. Nonbacterial (aseptic) meningitis

43. The type of encephalitis that occurs in children one-third of the time is caused by:
    a. herpes simplex.
    b. measles.
    c. mumps.
    d. rubella.

44. The domestic animal that should be the target of a community rabies vaccination program is the:
    a. dog.
    b. hamster.
    c. cat.
    d. parakeet.

45. The recommended postexposure treatment for rabies includes:
    a. mass immunization using human rabies immune globulin.
    b. administration of human diploid cell rabies vaccine according to schedule for 3 months after the exposure.
    c. mass immunization using human diploid cell rabies vaccine.
    d. administration of human rabies immune globulin 90 days after the exposure.

46. The decrease in the incidence of Reye syndrome is widely believed to be linked to:
    a. improved definitive diagnosis using liver biopsy as a criterion.
    b. earlier diagnosis and more aggressive therapy.
    c. alerting the public about the potential hazard of using aspirin for the treatment of children with varicella or influenza.
    d. mass immunization programs.

47. Symptoms that are similar to those of Reye syndrome have occurred during viral illnesses when the child was given an:
    a. antiemetic drug.
    b. analgesic drug.
    c. antiepileptic drug.
    d. antiarrhythmic drug.

48. The drug that reduces the chance that the HIV-infected pregnant mother will infect her infant is called:
    a. valproate.
    b. zidovudine.
    c. nitrazepam.
    d. felbamate.

49. Name two factors that contribute to childhood seizures.

50. A child having a complex partial seizure rather than a simple partial seizure is *more* likely to exhibit:
    a. impaired consciousness.
    b. clonic movements.
    c. a seizure duration of less than 1 minute.
    d. all of the above.

51. One strategy that may provide a clue to the origin of a seizure is:
    a. to attempt to place an airway in the mouth.
    b. to gently open the eyes to observe their movement.
    c. to provide a clear description of the seizure.
    d. all of the above.

52. Which one of the following types of seizures is *most* common in children between the ages of 4 and 12 years?
    a. Generalized seizures
    b. Absence seizures
    c. Atonic seizures
    d. Jackknife seizures

53. The therapy for infantile spasms is likely to include:
    a. adrenocorticotropic hormone.
    b. valproic acid.
    c. ethosuximide.
    d. felbamate.

54. The drug of choice for the treatment of Lennox-Gastaut syndrome (LGS) is:
    a. nitrazepam.
    b. clonazepam.
    c. felbamate.
    d. valproate.

55. Therapy for epilepsy should begin with:
    a. short-term drug therapy.
    b. combination drug therapy.
    c. only one drug, if possible.
    d. drugs that correct the brain wave pattern.

56. The intravenous medication that is used to treat seizures and may be given in either saline or glucose is:
    a. fosphenytoin.
    b. phenytoin.
    c. valproic acid.
    d. felbamate.

57. A simple, effective, and safe treatment for home or prehospital management of status epilepticus is:
    a. rectal diazepam.
    b. intravenous valproic acid.
    c. intravenous phenytoin.
    d. rectal fosphenytoin.

58. A poor prognosis for the child with status epilepticus is associated with:
    a. previous developmental delays.
    b. previous neurologic abnormalities.
    c. concurrent serious illness.
    d. all of the above.

59. Nursing intervention for a child during a tonic-clonic seizure should include attempts to:
    a. halt the seizure as soon as it begins.
    b. restrain the child.
    c. remain calm and observe the child.
    d. place an oral airway in the child's mouth.

60. Emergency care of the child during a seizure includes:
    a. giving ice chips slowly.
    b. restraining the child.
    c. putting a tongue blade in the child's mouth.
    d. loosening restrictive clothing.

61. To prevent submersion injuries in children with epilepsy, the child should be instructed to:
    a. never go swimming.
    b. take showers.
    c. wear a bicycle helmet.
    d. follow all of the above.

62. In most children who have a febrile seizure, the factor that triggers the seizure tends to be:
    a. rapidity of the temperature elevation.
    b. duration of the temperature elevation.
    c. height of the temperature elevation.
    d. any of the above.

63. When a child has a febrile seizure, it is important for the parents to know that the child will:
    a. probably not develop epilepsy.
    b. most likely develop epilepsy.
    c. most likely develop neurologic damage.
    d. usually need tepid sponge baths to control fever.

64. In most cases, chronic recurrent headaches of childhood represent:
    a. tension.
    b. seizures.
    c. intracranial disease.
    d. migraine.

65. Treatment for migraine headaches in children may include:
    a. ergots.
    b. opioids.
    c. sumatriptan.
    d. all of the above.

Critical Thinking—Case Study

Jackson was riding his bike in the street by his house when he was hit by a car. He is 9 years old. He was not wearing a helmet at the time. He has been unconscious since the accident 8 hours ago. His mother and father both work full-time, and there are five other siblings at home ranging in ages from 7 years old to 19 years old.

66. Based on the preceding information, which of the following nursing diagnoses would have the highest priority?
    a. High risk for impaired skin integrity related to immobility
    b. Self-care deficit related to inability to feed himself
    c. Altered family process related to a permanent disability
    d. High risk for aspiration related to impaired motor function

67. In order to effectively deal with the altered family process related to the hospitalization, the nurse should:
    a. provide information about bicycle safety helmets.
    b. encourage expression of feelings.
    c. encourage the family to provide Jackson's hygiene needs.
    d. provide auditory stimulation for Jackson.

68. In order to help Jackson receive appropriate sensory stimulation, the nurse should:
    a. hang a black-and-white mobile above his bed.
    b. hang a calendar at the foot of his bed.
    c. encourage the family to bring a tape of his favorite music.
    d. administer pain medications as needed.

69. Jackson's parents visit him every day but never together. The nurse should be concerned about:
    a. marital problems that usually occur during stressful times like this.
    b. whether Jackson's parents are able to receive adequate support for each other with this arrangement.
    c. whether Jackson's siblings are being adequately cared for.
    d. all of the above.

CHAPTER 38

The Child with Endocrine Dysfunction

1. The following terms are related to hormones. Match each term with its description.

   a. Cell
   b. End organ
   c. Environment
   d. Local hormones
   e. General hormones
   f. Target tissues

   g. Anterior pituitary
   h. Tropic hormones
   i. Releasing/inhibitory hormones
   j. Neuroendocrine system

   k. Autonomic nervous system
   l. Parasympathetic system
   m. Sympathetic system
   n. Neurotransmitting substances

   _____ The master gland

   _____ Complex chemical substances produced and secreted into body fluids by a cell or group of cells that exert a physiologic controlling effect on other cells; produced in one organ or part of the body and carried through the bloodstream to a distant part, or parts, of the body, where they initiate or regulate physiologic activity of an organ or group of cells—e.g., thyroid

   _____ The component of the endocrine system that sends a chemical message by means of a hormone

   _____ Acetylcholine and norepinephrine

   _____ Secreted by the anterior pituitary to regulate the secretion of hormones from various target organs

   _____ The component of the endocrine system through which the chemical is transported (blood, lymph, extracellular fluid) from the site of synthesis to the site of cellular action

   _____ Consists of the sympathetic and parasympathetic systems; controls nonvoluntary functions, specifically of the smooth muscle myocardium and glands

   _____ Specific tissues on which hormones produce their effect; e.g., the pituitary hormones stimulating the adrenal glands to secrete adrenocorticotropin

   _____ Secreted by the hypothalamus and transported by way of the pituitary portal system to the anterior pituitary, where they stimulate the secretion of tropic hormones

   _____ Target cell; the component of the endocrine system that receives the chemical message

   _____ The system that maintains homeostasis through interaction between endocrine glands and the nervous system

   _____ Primarily involved in regulating digestive processes

   _____ Complex chemical substances produced and secreted into body fluids by a cell or group of cells that exert a physiologic controlling effect on other cells near the point of secretion—e.g., acetylcholine

   _____ Functions to maintain homeostasis during stress

2. The following terms are related to pituitary disorders. Match each term with its description.

a. Idiopathic hypopituitarism
b. Familial short stature
c. Constitutional growth delay
d. Creutzfeldt-Jakob disease (CJD)
e. biosynthetic growth hormone
f. Human Growth Foundation
g. Acromegaly
h. Hypothalamic-pituitary-gonadal axis
i. Central precocious puberty
j. Peripheral precocious puberty
k. Desmopressin acetate (DDAVP)
l. Premature thelarche
m. Premature pubarche
n. Premature menarche
o. Luteinizing hormone-releasing hormone (LHRH)
p. Neurogenic diabetes insipidus
q. Vasopressin

_____ Early puberty resulting from hormones other than hypothalamic Gn-RN–stimulated pituitary gonadotropic releasers

_____ Hormone that will alleviate the polyuria and polydipsia associated with neurogenic diabetes insipidus

_____ Refers to individuals (usually boys) with delayed linear growth and skeletal and sexual maturation that is behind that of peers

_____ Premature adrenarche; early development of sexual hair

_____ Prepared by recombinant DNA technology

_____ Regulates pituitary secretions; a synthetic analog is used to manage precocious puberty of central origin

_____ An organization that provides support and education for professionals and for families of a child with growth defects

_____ The sequence of events that stimulates the secretion of gonadotropic hormones from the anterior pituitary at the time of puberty

_____ Growth failure; usually related to growth hormone (GH) deficiency

_____ Results from premature activation of the hypothalamic-pituitary-gonadal axis, which produces early maturation and development of the gonads with secretion of sex hormones, development of secondary sex characteristics, and occassional production of mature sperm or ova; more common among girls

_____ A rare and fatal neurodegenerative condition that has been iatrogenically transmitted through human tissue from cadaver-derived growth hormone

_____ A long-acting analog of arginine vasopressin used to treat diabetes insipidus

_____ The condition that is produced when hypersecretion of growth hormone occurs after epiphyseal closure; growth occurs in transverse direction

_____ Development of breasts in prepubertal females

_____ Isolated menses without other evidence of sexual development

_____ Hyposecretion of antidiuretic hormone/vasopressin; produces a state of uncontrolled diuresis

_____ Refers to otherwise healthy children who have ancestors with adult height in the lower percentiles and whose height during childhood is appropriate for genetic background

3. The following terms are related to endocrine disorders. Match each term with its description.

a. Thyroid hormone
b. Thyrocalcitonin
c. Thyroid-stimulating hormone (TSH)
d. Hashimoto disease
e. Exophthalmos
f. Parathormone (PTH)
g. Vitamin D therapy
h. Hyperparathyroidism

i. Adrenal cortex
j. Glucocorticoids
k. Mineralocorticoids
l. Sex steroids
m. Corticotropin-releasing factor (CRF)
n. Adrenocorticotropic hormone (ACTH)

o. Aldosterone
p. Renin
q. Adrenal crisis
r. Waterhouse-Friderichsen syndrome
s. 21-hydroxylase deficiency
t. 11-hydroxylase deficiency
u. Ambiguous genitalia

_____ Most pronounced in the female with masculinization of the external genitalia; the term to use for any infant with hypospadias or micropenis and no palpable gonads

_____ The thyroid gland secretes this type of hormine in addition to thyroid hormone (T_3 and T_4); one of the two types of hormones secreted by the thyroid gland

_____ Juvenile autoimmune thyroiditis; lymphocytic thyroiditis; the most common cause of thyroid disease in children and adolescents; accounts for the largest percentage of juvenile hypothyroidism

_____ Produced by the anterior pituitary; controls the secretion of thyroid hormones

_____ Protruding eyeballs; observed in many children with Hashimoto disease; accompanied by a wide-eyed staring expression, increased blinking, lid lag, lack of convergence, and absence of wrinkling of the forehead when looking upward

_____ Treatment used in hypoparathyroidism

_____ Secreted by the parathyroid glands; maintains serum calcium levels

_____ The mineralocorticoid that promotes sodium retention and potassium excretion in the renal tubules

_____ Androgens, estrogens, and progestins

_____ Causes the pituitary gland to produce adrenocorticotropic hormone (ACTH)

_____ Disorder with clinical manifestations of hypercalcemia, elevated calcium, and decreased phosphorus; rare in childhood

_____ Cortisol and corticosterone

_____ The acute form of adrenocortical insufficiency

_____ Secretes the steroid hormones, catecholamines (epinephrine), and norepinephrine

_____ Aldosterone; one of the three groups of hormone secreted by the adrenal cortex

_____ Stimulates the adrenal glands to synthesize glucocorticoids

_____ Converts angiotensinogen to angiotensin I and then to angiotensin II, stimulating the adrenal cortex to secrete aldosterone, which preserves sodium, retains water, and increases the blood pressure

_____ The presentation of generalized hemorrhagic manifestations in adrenocortical insufficiency

_____ The most common biochemical defect associated with congenital adrenogenital hyperplasia (CAH)

_____ A type of hormone secreted by the thyroid gland; consists of the hormones thyroxine (T_4) and triiodothyronine (T_3)

_____ The form of adrenal hyperplasia in which there is an increase in the mineralocorticoid that leads to hypertension

4. The following terms are related to diabetes. Match each term with its description.

a. Type 1 diabetes
b. Immune-mediated diabetes mellitus
c. Idiopathic type 1 diabetes
d. Type 2 diabetes
e. Maturity onset diabetes in the young (MODY)
f. Insulin
g. Hyperglycemia
h. Glycosuria

i. Polyuria
j. Polydipsia
k. Glucogenesis
l. Polyphagia
m. Ketonuria
n. Acetone breath
o. Ketonemia
p. Ketoacidosis
q. Ketones

r. Kussmaul respirations
s. Nephropathy/retinopathy/ neuropathy
t. Glycosylation
u. Hyperglycemic
v. Ketotic
w. Diabetic ketoacidosis (DKA)

_____ Excessive thirst

_____ The rare form of type 1 diabetes that has no known cause

_____ Increased concentration of glucose

_____ The form of diabetes that results from an autoimmune destruction of beta cells; typically starts in slim children or young adults

_____ Organic acids that readily produce excessive quantities of free hydrogen ions

_____ Arises from insulin resistance with a relative insulin deficiency or insulin resistance with insulin secretion deficiency; typically occurs in individuals over the age of 45 who are over-weight, sedentary, or with a family history of diabetes

_____ Presence of β-hydroxybutyric acid, acetoacetic acid, and acetone in the urine

_____ Elimination of ketones through the lungs

_____ The metabolic hormone that supports the metabolism of carbohydrates, fats and proteins

_____ Osmotic diversion of water, a cardinal sign of diabetes

_____ Associated with monogenetic defects in beta-cell function; characterized by impaired insulin secretion with minimal defects in insulin action; inherited with an autosomal-dominant pattern, with the onset of hyperglycemia occurring at an early age; onset generally before age 25 years

_____ Process where protein is broken down and converted to glucose by the liver

_____ Dehydration electrolyte imbalance and acidosis from diabetes

_____ Characterized by the destruction of the pancreatic beta cells that produce insulin; usually leads to absolute insulin deficiency

_____ The lowering of the serum pH; results from ketone bodies in the blood

_____ Glucose in the urine

_____ Proteins from the blood become deposited in the walls of small vessels, where they become trapped by glucose compounds; causes narrowing of the microvascular vessels over time

_____ Increased food intake

_____ Term used to express that ketones are measurable in the blood and urine

_____ Long-term complications of diabetes that involve the microvasculature

_____ β-hydroxybutyric acid, acetoacetic acid, and acetone in the blood

_____ Hyperventilation characteristic of metabolic acidosis

_____ Elevated blood glucose and glucose in the urine

5. The following terms are related to the therapeutic management of diabetes. Match each term with its description.

a. Regular insulin
b. NPH/Lente insulin
c. Multiple daily injection (MDI)
d. Insulin pump
e. Islet cell/whole pancreas transplant
f. Self-monitoring of blood glucose (SMBG)
g. Insulin reaction
h. Glucagon
i. Somogyi effect
j. Injectease
k. NovoPen
l. Adrenergic symptoms
m. Neuroglycopenic symptoms

_____ Has been shown to reduce microvascular complication of diabetes in young, healthy patients who have type 1 diabetes

_____ An intermediate-acting drug

_____ An electromechanical device designed to deliver fixed amounts of a diluted solution of regular insulin continuously; more closely imitates the release of insulin

_____ A rapid-acting drug

_____ Has improved diabetes management; diabetes management depends on these values

_____ Used in persons who have serious diabetes complications, particularly those who require renal transplantation with immunosuppressive therapy

_____ Later signs of hypoglycemia; brain hypoglycemia; difficulty with balance, memory, attention, slurred speech

_____ Releases stored glycogen from the liver; prescribed for home treatment of hypoglycemia

_____ A syringe-loaded injector for use by children who do not wish to give themselves injections

_____ Often the most feared aspect of diabetes because severe brain symptoms may develop

_____ Rebound hyperglycemia

_____ Early signs of hypoglycemia; help to raise the blood glucose level; sweating, trembling

_____ A self-contained, compact device resembling a fountain pen, which eliminates conventional vials and syringes

6. For each of the following hormones, write the name of the target tissue or gland in the blank following the hormone. Then match each hormone and gland with their corresponding effect.

a. Thyroid-stimulating hormone _____
b. Luteinizing hormone _____
c. Somatotropic hormone _____
d. Gonadotropin _____
e. Melanocyte-stimulating hormone _____
f. Adrenocorticotropic hormone _____
g. Antidiuretic hormone _____
h. Follicle-stimulating hormone _____
i. Oxytocin _____
j. Prolactin _____

_____ Increases reabsorption of water
_____ Promotes growth of bone and soft tissue
_____ Stimulates the secretion of glucocorticoids
_____ Initiates spermatogenesis
_____ Regulates metabolic rate
_____ Maintains corpus luteum during pregnancy
_____ Promotes pigmentation of the skin
_____ Causes the let-down reflex
_____ Produces sex hormones
_____ Stimulates the secretion of testosterone in the male

7. A hormone that produces its effect on a specific tissue would be classified as a

   _____ hormone.

8. Match each hormone or gland with its corresponding effect.

   a. Parathyroid   e. Androgen   i. Insulin
   b. Cortisol   f. Glucagon   j. Estrogen
   c. Aldosterone   g. Epinephrine   k. Testosterone
   d. Thyroid   h. Progesterone

   _____ Prepares uterus for fertilized ovum
   _____ Influences development of secondary sex characteristics
   _____ Promotes breast development during puberty
   _____ Inhibits the secretion of insulin
   _____ Promotes normal fat, protein, and carbohydrate metabolism
   _____ Produces vasoconstriction and raises blood pressure
   _____ Stimulates renal tubules to reabsorb sodium
   _____ Stimulates testes to produce spermatozoa
   _____ Regulates metabolic rate
   _____ Promotes glucose transport into the cells
   _____ Promotes reabsorption of calcium and excretion of phosphorous

9. The difference between panhypopituitarism and idiopathic hypopituitarism is that:
   a. panhypopituitarism is often caused by a tumor.
   b. the incidence of idiopathic hypopituitarism is higher in girls.
   c. idiopathic hypopituitarism usually has a cause that is unknown.
   d. panhypopituitarism is the cause of short stature in most children whose height is in the lower percentiles.

10. A child with growth hormone deficiency will exhibit the signs of:
    a. retarded height and weight.
    b. abnormal skeletal proportions.
    c. malnutrition.
    d. retarded height but not necessarily retarded weight.

11. In a child with hypopituitarism, the growth hormone levels would usually be:
    a. elevated after 20 minutes of strenuous exercise.
    b. elevated 45 to 90 minutes after the onset of sleep.
    c. lower than normal or not measurable at all.
    d. rapidly increased in response to insulin.

12. Treatment of choice for the child with idiopathic hypopituitarism may include:
    a. biosynthetic growth hormone.
    b. human growth hormone.
    c. chemotherapy to shrink the tumor.
    d. any of the above.

13. It is true that in the child with idiopathic hypopituitarism, growth hormone replacement therapy:
    a. will continue for life.
    b. will not result in achievement of a normal familial height.
    c. requires subcutaneous injection.
    d. requires intramuscular injection.

14. Provocative testing for diagnosis of hypopituitarism may require that the nurse monitor the child's:
    a. calcium levels.
    b. phosphorous levels.
    c. glucose levels.
    d. hemoglobin levels.

    p. 1710

15. Explain the difference between acromegaly and the pituitary hyperfunction that is not considered to be acromegaly.

16. Parents of the child with precocious puberty need to know that:
    a. dress and activities should be aligned with the child's sexual development.
    b. heterosexual interest will usually be advanced.
    c. the child's mental age is congruent with the chronologic age.
    d. overt manifestations of affection represent sexual advances.

17. Desmopressin acetate may be administered:
    a. by mouth.
    b. intranasally.
    c. topically.
    d. by all of the above.

18. The immediate management of syndrome of inappropriate antidiuretic hormone (SIADH) consists of:
    a. increasing fluids.
    b. administering antibiotics.
    c. restricting fluids.
    d. administering vasopressin.

19. The *most* common cause of thyroid disease in children and adolescents is:
    a. Hashimoto disease.
    b. Graves disease.
    c. goiter.
    d. thyrotoxicosis.

20. The initial treatment for the child with hyperthyroidism would *most* likely be:
    a. subtotal thyroidectomy.
    b. total thyroidectomy.
    c. ablation with radioactive iodide.
    d. administration of antithyroid medication.

21. When a thyroidectomy is planned, the nurse should explain to the child that:
    a. iodine preparations will be mixed with flavored foods and then eaten.
    b. he or she will need to hyperextend the neck postoperatively.
    c. the skin, not the throat, will be cut.
    d. laryngospasm can be a life-threatening complication.

22. The child with long-standing hypoparathyroidism will usually exhibit:
    a. short, stubby fingers.
    b. dimpling of the skin over the knuckles.
    c. skeletal growth retardation.
    d. a short, thick neck.

23. A common cause of secondary hyperparathyroidism is:
    a. maternal hyperparathyroidism.
    b. chronic renal disease.
    c. maternal diabetes mellitus.
    d. adenoma of the parathyroid gland.

24. Hyperfunction of the adrenal medulla results in:
    a. release of epinephrine and norepinephrine from the sympathetic nervous system.
    b. pheochromocytoma.
    c. adrenal crisis.
    d. myxedema.

25. Diagnosis of acute adrenocortical insufficiency is made based on:
    a. elevated plasma cortisol levels.
    b. the history and physical exam.
    c. depressed plasma cortisol levels.
    d. depressed aldosterone levels.

26. Parents of a child who has Addison's disease should be instructed to:
    a. use extra hydrocortisone only when signs of crisis are present.
    b. discontinue the child's cortisone if side effects develop.
    c. decrease the cortisone dose during times of stress.
    d. report signs of Cushing's syndrome to the physician.

27. Which one of the following tests is particularly useful in diagnosing congenital adrenogenital hyperplasia?
    a. Chromosomal typing
    b. Pelvic ultrasound
    c. Pelvic x-ray
    d. Testosterone levels

28. The temporary treatment for hyperaldosteronism prior to surgery would usually involve administration of:
    a. spironolactone.
    b. phentolamine.
    c. furosemide.
    d. phenoxybenzamine.

29. Definitive treatment for pheochromocytoma consists of:
    a. surgical removal of the thyroid.
    b. administration of potassium.
    c. surgical removal of the tumor.
    d. administration of beta blockers.

30. Most children with diabetes mellitus tend to exhibit characteristics of:
    a. maturity-onset diabetes of youth.
    b. gestational diabetes.
    c. type 2 diabetes.
    d. type 1 diabetes.

31. The currently accepted etiology of type 1 diabetes mellitus takes into account:
    a. genetic factors.
    b. autoimmune mechanisms.
    c. environmental factors.
    d. all of the above.

32. An early sign of type 1 diabetes mellitus in the adolescent would be:
    a. a vaginal candida infection.
    b. obesity.
    c. Kussmaul respirations.
    d. all of the above.

33. Of the following blood glucose levels, the value that most certainly indicates a diagnosis of diabetes would be a:
    a. fasting blood glucose of 120 mg/dl.
    b. random blood glucose of 140 mg/dl.
    c. fasting blood glucose of 160 mg/dl.
    d. glucose tolerance test (oral) value of 160 mg/dl for the 2-hour sample.

34. State the goal of insulin replacement therapy.

35. Glycosolated hemoglobin is an acceptable method to use to:
    a. diagnose diabetes mellitus.
    b. assess the control of diabetes.
    c. assess oxygen saturation of the hemoglobin.
    d. determine blood glucose levels most accurately.

36. Even with good glucose control, a child with type 1 diabetes mellitus may frequently encounter the acute complication of:
    a. retinopathy.
    b. ketoacidosis.
    c. hypoglycemia.
    d. hyperosmolar nonketotic coma.

37. Describe the treatment for a mild hypoglycemic episode in a young child with diabetes mellitus.

38. Principles of managing diabetes during illness include all of the following *except*:
    a. monitoring blood glucose every 4 hours.
    b. using a sliding scale of regular insulin.
    c. omitting insulin when excessive vomiting occurs.
    d. using simple sugars as carbohydrate exchanges.

39. Diabetic ketoacidosis in children with diabetes mellitus:
    a. is the most common chronic complication.
    b. is a result of too much insulin.
    c. is a life-threatening complication.
    d. rarely requires hospitalization.

40. Which one of the following cardiac wave patterns is indicative of hypokalemia?
    a. Widening of the Q-T interval with a flattened T wave
    b. Shortening of the Q-T interval with an elevated T wave
    c. Shortening of the Q-T interval with a flattened T wave
    d. Widening of the Q-T interval with an elevated T wave

41. The *best* time to effectively teach a child and his or her family the complex concepts of the home management of diabetes mellitus is:
    a. a day or so after diagnosis.
    b. the first 3 or 4 days after diagnosis.
    c. 2 weeks after diagnosis.
    d. a month after diagnosis.

42. The child with diabetes mellitus is taught to weigh and measure food in order to:
    a. receive the nutrients prescribed.
    b. prevent hypoglycemia.
    c. learn to estimate food portions.
    d. prevent hyperglycemia.

43. In regard to meal planning for the child with diabetes mellitus, parents should be aware that:
    a. fast foods must be eliminated.
    b. foods must be always be weighed and measured.
    c. the exchange list is limited to one type of food.
    d. foods with sorbitol may be metabolized into glucose.

44. The most efficient rotation pattern for insulin injections involves giving injections in:
    a. one area of the body one inch apart.
    b. different areas of the body each day.

45. In regard to insulin administration:
    a. insulin should never be premixed.
    b. insulin syringes should never be reused.
    c. insulin doses under 2 units should be diluted.
    d. an air bubble in the syringe is insignificant.

46. The child with diabetes mellitus needs to test his or her urine:
    a. for ketones every day.
    b. for ketones at times of illness.
    c. for glucose every day.
    d. for glucose at times of illness.

47. Exercise for the child with diabetes mellitus may:
    a. be restricted to noncontact sports.
    b. require a decreased intake of food.
    c. necessitate an increased insulin dose.
    d. require an increased intake of food.

48. Problems with the child adjusting to the self-management of diabetes are most likely to occur when diabetes is diagnosed in:
    a. infancy.
    b. adolescence.
    c. the toddler years.
    d. the school-age years.

49. Describe the feelings that parents may have when they are raising a child with diabetes mellitus.

Critical Thinking—Case Study

Rebecca Bennett is an 8-year-old who has recently been diagnosed with diabetes mellitus. She is hospitalized with diabetic ketoacidosis, and she is beginning to learn about the disease process. Her parents are with her continuously. She has an identical twin sister who is staying with her maternal grandparents.

50. Mrs. Bennett is concerned that Rebecca's sister will also develop diabetes. Based on the preceding information, an acceptable response for the nurse to make would be to:
    a. reassure the parents that the disease is not contagious.
    b. discuss the hereditary and viral factors of type 1 diabetes.
    c. discuss the hereditary factors of type 1 diabetes.
    d. discuss the viral factors of type 1 diabetes.

51. Which one of the following nursing diagnoses is *most* likely to become a priority after the first few days of Rebecca's hospitalization?
    a. Fluid volume deficit related to uncontrolled diabetes
    b. Fluid volume excess related to hormonal disturbances
    c. Deficient knowledge related to newly diagnosed type 1 diabetes mellitus
    d. Impaired respiratory function related to fluid imbalance

52. In preparing the Bennett family for discharge, the nurse should plan to teach:
    a. only Rebecca how to inject insulin.
    b. only Rebecca's parents how to inject insulin.
    c. both Rebecca and her parents how to inject insulin.
    d. the family how to administer oral hypoglycemics.

53. To evaluate Rebecca's progress in relation to her diabetes self-management, the *best* measure would be Rebecca's:
    a. parents' verbalizations about the disease process.
    b. blood glucose levels.
    c. glycosolated hemoglobin values.
    d. demonstration of her insulin injection technique.

CHAPTER 39

The Child with Musculoskeletal or Articular Dysfunction

1. What eight topics does the nurse include in the educational plan to promote injury prevention among community children?

2. The nurse is suspicious for child abuse when:
   i.   there is a delay in seeking medical assistance for the injury.
   ii. the parent's history of the injury is not congruent with the actual injury.
   iii. x-rays demonstrate previous fractures in different stages of healing.
   iv. the child is crying and fearful of separation from the parent.

   a. i, ii, iii, and iv
   b. i, ii, and iii
   c. ii and iii
   d. ii, iii, and iv

3. The nurse neighbor of Jimmy, age 5, discovers him lying in the street next to his bicycle. The nurse sends another witness to activate the emergency medical system (EMS) while the nurse begins a primary assessment of Jimmy. Which one of the following *best* describes the primary assessment and its correct sequence?
   a. Body inspection, head-to-toe survey, and airway patency
   b. Airway patency, respiratory effectiveness, circulatory status
   c. Open airway, head-to-toe assessment for injuries, and chest compressions
   d. Weight estimation, symptom analysis, blood pressure measurement

4. The nurse suspects Jimmy (question 3) has a spinal cord injury. Describe immobilization technique.

5. Major consequences of immobilization in the pediatric patient include which one of the following?
   a. Bone demineralization leading to osteoporosis
   b. Orthostatic hypertension
   c. Dependent edema in the lower extremities
   d. Decrease in the metabolic rate

6. What are the three major cardiovascular consequences of immobility?

7. Symptoms of neurologic impairment that should be immediately evaluated are _____,

_____, _____ and _____.

8. Nursing interventions aimed at preventing problems associated with immobilization include which one of the following?
   a. Encouragement in self-care and allowing patients to do as much for themselves as they are able
   b. Fluid restrictions with strict intake and output
   c. Limitation of active range-of-motion exercises to once per day
   d. Decreased sensory stimulation to allow adequate rest

9. The fabrication and fitting of braces is termed _____.

   The fabrication and fitting of artificial limbs is termed _____.

10. Which one of the following is a complication of immobility that is easily prevented by an appropriate nursing intervention?
    a. Disuse atrophy and loss of muscle mass
    b. Constipation
    c. Hypocalcemia
    d. Pain

11. Which one of the following is *not* included in the teaching plan of a child with a brace or prosthesis?
    a. Frequent assessment of all areas in contact with the brace for signs of skin irritation
    b. Assessment of the stump area before application of the prosthesis
    c. Removal of the prosthesis limited to bedtime unless skin breakage occurs
    d. Use of protective clothing under the brace

12. List five effects that prolonged immobilization or disability of the child may have on the family.

13. Bone healing is characteristically more rapid in children because:
    a. children have less constant muscle contraction associated with the fracture.
    b. children's fractures are less severe than adult's.
    c. children have an active growth plate that helps speed repair with less likelihood of deformity.
    d. children have thickened periosteum and a more generous blood supply.

14. The method of fracture reduction is *not* determined by which of the following?
    a. The age of the child
    b. The manner in which the fracture occurred
    c. The degree of displacement
    d. The amount of edema

15. Match each term with its description.

a. Diaphysis   g. Simple or closed fracture   m. Bend fracture
b. Epiphysis   h. Open or compound fracture   n. Osteopenia
c. Epiphyseal plate   i. Complicated fracture   o. Ossification
d. Complete fracture   j. Comminuted fracture   p. Periosteum
e. Incomplete fracture   k. Greenstick fracture   q. Oblique
f. Transverse fracture   l. Buckle or torus fracture   r. Spiral

_____ Fracture with an open wound from which the bone has protruded
_____ Major portion of the long bone
_____ Fracture in which fracture fragments are separated
_____ Fracture in which fracture fragments remain attached
_____ Located at the ends of the long bones
_____ Also called the *growth plate* because it plays a major role in the longitudinal growth of the developing child
_____ Fracture that is crosswise, at right angles to the long axis of the bone
_____ Conversion of cartilage to bony structure
_____ Membrane covering all bone; contains blood vessels to nourish bone
_____ Fracture in which small fragments of bone are broken from the fractured shaft and lie in surrounding tissue
_____ Fracture in which bone fragments cause damage to surrounding organs or tissue
_____ Fracture that is slanting and circular, twisting around bone shaft
_____ Demineralization of the bone
_____ Appears as a raising or bulging at the site of the fracture
_____ Occurs more commonly in the ulna and fibula and can produce some deformity
_____ Occurs when a bone is angulated beyond the limits of bending
_____ Fracture has not produced a break in the skin
_____ Fracture that is slanting but straight, between a horizontal and a perpendicular direction

16. What are the five "Ps" of ischemia that are included when assessing fractures in order to rule out vascular injury?

17. Emergency treatment for the child with a fracture includes:
    a. moving the child to allow removal of clothing from the area of injury.
    b. immobilization of the limb, including joints above and below the injury site.
    c. pushing the protruding bone under the skin.
    d. keeping the area of injury in a dependent position.

18. What are the four goals of fracture management?

19. An appropriate nursing intervention for the care of a child with an extremity in a new cast is:
    a. keeping the cast covered with a sheet.
    b. using the fingertips when handling the cast to prevent pressure areas.
    c. using heated fans or dryers to circulate air and speed the cast-drying process.
    d. turning the child at least every 2 hours to help dry the cast evenly.

20. To reduce anxiety in the child undergoing cast removal, which of the following nursing interventions would the nurse expect to be *least* effective?
    a. Demonstrate how the cast cutter works to the child before beginning the procedure.
    b. Use the analogy of having fingernails or hair cut.
    c. Explain that it will take only a few minutes.
    d. Continue to reassure that all is going well and that their behavior is accepted during the removal process.

21. Julie, age 10, has been placed in a long leg cast for an open fracture. The nurse immediately notifies the physician if assessment findings include which of the following?
    a. Appearance of blood-stained area the size of a quarter on the cast
    b. 2+ pedal pulse
    c. Inability to move the toes
    d. Ability of the nurse to insert one finger under the edge of the cast

22. The three primary purposes of traction for reduction of fractures are:

23. The nurse is caring for 7-year-old Charles after insertion of skeletal traction. Which of the following is *contraindicated*?
    a. Gently massage over pressure areas to stimulate circulation.
    b. Release the traction when repositioning Charles in bed.
    c. Inspect pin sites for bleeding or infection.
    d. Assess for alterations in neurovascular status.

24. Nursing intervention for the child with an Ilizarov external fixator device includes:
    a. teaching the child to walk with crutches.
    b. observing for the common problem of infection.
    c. allowing full weight bearing once the fixation device has been applied.
    d. allowing full weight bearing following removal of the device.

25. The nurse is assessing Carol, age 8, for complications related to her recent fracture and the application of a flexion cast to her forearm and elbow. Carol is crying with pain, the nurse is unable to locate pulses in the affected extremity, and there is lack of sensitivity to the area as well as some edema. Which of the following would the nurse suspect as *most* likely to be occurring?
    a. Normal occurrence for the first few hours following application of traction
    b. Volkmann contracture
    c. Nerve compression syndrome
    d. Epiphyseal damage

26. Johnny, a 12-year-old with fracture of the femur, has developed chest pain and shortness of breath. The priority nursing action is:
    a. elevate the affected extremity.
    b. administer oxygen.
    c. administer pain medication.
    d. start an IV infusion of heparin.

27. Match each type of traction with its best description.

    a. Dunlop traction
    b. Bryant traction
    c. Buck extension
    d. Russell traction
    e. 90°-90° traction

    f. Balance suspension traction
    g. Thomas splint
    h. Pearson attachment
    i. Cervical traction
    j. Manual traction

    k. Skin traction
    l. Skeletal traction
    m. Distraction
    n. Osteomyelitis

    _____ Insertion of a wire or pin into the bone
    _____ Used to realign bone fragments for cast application
    _____ Applied when there is minimum displacement and little muscle spasticity but contraindicated when there is associated skin damage
    _____ Treatment of fractures of the humerus when the arm is suspended horizontally
    _____ A type of running traction where the pull is only in one direction
    _____ Infection of the bone
    _____ Uses skin traction on the lower leg and a padded sling under the knee
    _____ A type of skin traction with the leg in an extended position; used primarily for short-term immobilization
    _____ Skeletal traction where the lower leg is put in a boot cast or supported in a sling and a pin is placed in the distal fragment of the femur
    _____ Used with or without skin or skeletal traction; suspends the leg in a flexed position to relax the hip and hamstring muscles
    _____ Process of separating opposing bone to regenerate new bone in the created space
    _____ Accomplished by insertion of Crutchfield tongs through burr holes
    _____ Supports the lower leg
    _____ Extends from the groin to midair above the foot

28. Nursing interventions for the child following surgical amputation of a lower extremity include:
    a. applying special elastic bandaging to the stump, using a circular pattern to decrease stump edema.
    b. keeping the stump elevated for at least 72 hours postsurgery.
    c. encouraging the child to lie prone at least three times a day, increasing the time prone to tolerance of an hour at a time.
    d. recognizing that the child is only trying to gain the nurse's attention when the child says there is pain in the missing limb.

29. Jeff has accidentally amputated the distal one-third of his thumb. The camp nurse knows that the amputated thumb part should be:
    a. placed directly in ice water and transported to the emergency department with Jeff.
    b. immediately rinsed with water to remove dirt, placed back on the injury site, secured with a sterile gauze dressing, and transported with Jeff to the emergency department.
    c. rinsed in normal saline, wrapped in a sterile dressing, placed in a watertight bag in iced solution without freezing, and transported with Jeff to the emergency department.
    d. placed in a sterile dressing into a cold milk solution and transported with Jeff to the emergency department.

30. When matching children to participate in sports competition, which of the following is the *least* important consideration?
    a. Age
    b. Height and weight
    c. Physical fitness
    d. Physical skills

31. Match the term with its description.

    a. Contusion
    b. Ecchymosis
    c. Dislocation
    d. Strain
    e. Sprain

    _____ Occurs when the force of stress on the ligament is so great that it displaces the normal position of the opposing bone ends or the bone end to its socket

    _____ Damage to the soft tissue, subcutaneous structures, and muscle

    _____ Occurs when trauma to a joint is so severe that a ligament is either stretched or partially or completely torn by the force created as a joint is twisted or wrenched

    _____ Escape of blood into the tissues

    _____ Microscopic tear to the musculotendinous unit

32. Which of the following statements about "nursemaid's" elbow is correct?
    a. This most common partial dislocation of the radial head of the elbow, is usually found in children age 1 to 5 years.
    b. This condition is caused by a sudden pull at the wrist while the arm is fully extended and the forearm is pronated.
    c. The longer the dislocation is present, the longer it takes the child to recover mobility after treatment.
    d. All of the above statements are correct.

33. Immediate treatment of sprains and strains includes:
    a. rest and cold application.
    b. disregarding the pain and "working out" the sprain or strain.
    c. rest, elevation, and pain medication.
    d. compression of the area and heat application.

34. Major sprains or tears to the ligamentous tissues rarely occur in growing children because the

    _____ are stronger than bone. The _____ and the

    _____ _____ are the weakest parts of the bone and the usual sites of injury.

35. Identify the following as either true or false.

    _____ Athletes who run can experience shin splints, a ligament tear away from the tibial shaft.

    _____ Achilles tendonitis is caused by repeated, forcible traction on the short tendon.

    _____ Jumper's knee is caused by epiphysitis of the calcaneus.

    _____ Osgood-Schlatter disease may present with pain and tenderness over the tibial tubercle and an overprominence of involved tubercle.

    _____ Little league elbow presents with pain in the elbow, aggravated by use, and is caused from repetitive strain on lateral epicondylitis.

    _____ Children are less vulnerable to heat injury than adults because of their greater ratio of surface area to body mass and reduced production of metabolic heat for body mass.

    _____ Heat cramps are caused by calcium depletion during vigorous exercise in a hot environment.

    _____ Heat exhaustion occurs from excessive loss of fluids during exercise in a hot environment. Symptoms include thirst, headache, fatigue, dizziness, anxiety, or nausea and vomiting.

_____ The child with heat exhaustion should have external cooling applied with cold towels immediately.

_____ Heatstroke represents a failure of normal thermoregulatory mechanisms. Onset is rapid and disorientation is present, along with a temperature in excess of 104° F.

_____ Salt tablets are rarely needed during exercise and may actually do harm by increasing dehydration.

_____ The recommended dietary energy intake for adolescents involved in sports is 55% to 60% of total energy from carbohydrates, 12% to 15% from protein, and 25% to 30% from fat.

_____ It is not necessary to counsel female athletes about pregnancy prevention, because they have delayed menarche.

_____ Drug misuse by athletes most often includes psychomotor stimulants and anabolic steroids.

_____ Idiopathic hypertrophic subaortic stenosis as a medical cause of sudden death during a sports activity has a typical triad of severe chest pain with dizziness, prominent pulses, and a murmur at the left lower sternal border.

36. Sixteen-year-old Ben has been brought to the school nurse's office for heatstroke. He has a temperature of 104° F and is awake but disoriented. Which of the following is *contraindicated*?
    a. Immediate removal of clothing and application of cool water to the skin
    b. Administration of antipyretics
    c. Use of fans directed at Ben
    d. Activation of EMS system for transport to hospital

37. Zac, a 16-year-old football star at the local high school, is at the school nurse practitioner's office for acne that is not clearing. During the physical exam it is noted that Zac has achieved a marked increase in muscle and strength in a very short time. Which of the following would the nurse suspect caused these changes?
    a. Use of ergogenic aid, anabolic steroids
    b. More frequent and/or more strenuous workouts in the gym
    c. Increased protein and vitamins in the diet
    d. Use of Ritalin or Preludin

38. The condition recognized in the infant with limited neck motion, where the neck is flexed and turned to the affected side as a result of shortening of the sterocleidomastodid muscle, is:
    a. torticollis.
    b. paralysis of the brachial nerve.
    c. Legg-Calvé-Perthes disease.
    d. a self-limiting injury.

39. Bob, age 7, is diagnosed with Legg-Calvé-Perthes disease. Which of the following manifestations is *not* consistent with this diagnosis?
    a. Intermittent appearance of a limp on the affected side
    b. Hip soreness, ache, or stiffness that can be constant or intermittent
    c. Pain and limp most evident on arising and at the end of a long day of activities
    d. Specific history of injury to the area

40. Slipped femoral capital epiphysis is suspected when:
    a. an adolescent or preadolescent begins to limp and complains of continuous or intermittant pain in the hip.
    b. an exam reveals no restriction on internal rotation or adduction but restriction on external rotation.
    c. referred pain goes into the sacral and lumbar areas.
    d. all of the above occur.

41. An accentuation of the lumbar curvature beyond physiologic limits is termed _____.
An abnormally increased convex angulation in the curvature of the thoracic spine is termed

_____. _____ is the forward slipping of one vertebral body onto another, usually L5 and S1.

42. Diagnostic evaluation is important for early recognition of scoliosis. Which of the following is the correct procedure for the school nurse conducting this examination?
a. View the child, who is standing and walking fully clothed, to look for uneven hanging of clothing.
b. View all children from the left and right side to look mainly for asymmetry of the hip height.
c. Completely undress all children before the exam.
d. View the child, who is wearing underpants, from behind and when the child bends forward.

43. The surgical technique for the correction of scoliosis consists of:

44. Marilyn, age 13, has been diagnosed with scoliosis and placed in a Milwaukee brace. Marilyn asks the nurse about the brace and how long she has to wear it. What is the *best* response?
a. "The brace will need to be worn only until you have corrective surgery."
b. "The brace will need to be worn between 16 and 23 hours a day to halt or slow the progression of the curvature."
c. "The brace will not need to be worn to school, only at home, and you will need to sleep in the brace."
d. "You will need to get specific information about your schedule from your doctor."

45. Nursing implementation directed toward nonsurgical management in a teenager with scoliosis primarily includes:
a. promoting self-esteem and positive body image.
b. preventing immobility.
c. promoting adequate nutrition.
d. preventing infection.

46. Osteomyelitis resulting from a blood-borne bacterium that could have developed from an infected lesion is termed:
a. acute hematogenous osteomyelitis.
b. exogenous osteomyelitis.
c. subacute osteomyelitis.
d. any of the above.

47. The plan of care for the child during the acute phase of osteomyelitis always includes:
a. performing wound irrigations.
b. maintaining the IV infusion site.
c. isolating the child.
d. incorporating passive range-of-motion exercises for the affected area.

48. Which of the following statements about septic arthritis is true?
a. The most common causative agent in children under 2 years of age is *H. influenzae*.
b. Knees, hips, ankles, hands, and feet are the most common joints affected.
c. Early radiographic findings show soft tissue swelling and erosions of the bone.
d. IV antibiotic use is based on Gram stain and clinical presentation.

49. The most common sites for tubercular infection of the bones in older children are:
    a. carpals and phalanges and corresponding bones of the feet.
    b. vertebrae.
    c. long bones of the legs.
    d. all of the above.

50. Nursing considerations for the patient diagnosed with osteogenesis imperfecta include:
    a. preventing fractures by careful handling.
    b. providing nonjudgmental support while parents are dealing with accusations of child abuse.
    c. providing guidelines to the parents in planning suitable activities that promote optimum development.
    d. all of the above.

51. Which of the following nursing goals is *most* appropriate for the child with juvenile rheumatoid arthritis?
    a. Child will exhibit signs of reduced joint inflammation and adequate joint function.
    b. Child will exhibit no signs of impaired skin integrity due to rash.
    c. Child will exhibit normal weight and nutritional status.
    d. Child will exhibit no alteration in respiratory patterns or respiratory infection.

52. What should the nurse teach the patient and family of the child diagnosed with SLE regarding each of the following topics?

    a. NSAIDs

    b. Diet

    c. Sun exposure

    d. Birth control medication

53. What are the two goals of therapeutic management for SLE?

54. The principal drugs used in SLE to control inflammation are the _____.

55. What are the two primary nursing goals for the nurse caring for the child with SLE?

Critical Thinking—Case Study

Sandy, age 10, has developed joint and leg pain, some joint swelling, fever, malaise, and pleuritis. The physician has ordered laboratory testing to include sedimentation rate, rheumatoid factor, and a complete blood count. Tentative diagnosis has been established as juvenile arthritis, systemic onset.

56. If the diagnosis is correct, which of the following would represent the expected laboratory results?
    a. Leukocytosis
    b. Elevated sedimentation rate
    c. Negative rheumatoid factor
    d. All of the above

57. The primary group of drugs prescribed for juvenile arthritis is nonsteroidal anti-inflammatory drugs. Education regarding the use of these drugs should include which of the following?
    a. They produce excellent analgesic and anti-inflammatory effects but little antipyretic effect.
    b. They are administered in the lowest effective dose and given on alternate days rather than daily.
    c. Antiinflammatory effect occurs 3 to 4 weeks after therapy is begun.
    d. Because there is a narrow margin between effective and toxic dosage, levels need to be monitored regularly until therapeutic dosage is established.

58. Which of the following is the *most* appropriate nursing intervention to promote adequate joint function in the child with juvenile rheumatoid arthritis?
    a. Incorporate therapeutic exercises in play activities.
    b. Provide heat to affected joints by use of tub baths.
    c. Provide written information for all treatments ordered.
    d. Explore and develop activities in which the child can succeed.

59. An expected outcome for the nursing diagnosis of high risk for body image disturbance related to the disease process of juvenile arthritis is:
    a. the patient and family members are able to explain the disease process.
    b. the patient is accepted by peers.
    c. the patient will express feelings and concerns.
    d. the child will understand and use effective communication techniques.

60. What laboratory monitoring is required if Sandy is started on methotrexate?

61. The nutritional goal for Sandy includes:

CHAPTER 40

The Child with Neuromuscular or Muscular Dysfunction

1. Identify the following as true or false.

   _____ Upper motor neuron lesions produce weakness associated with spasticity, increased deep tendon reflexes, and abnormal superficial reflexes.

   _____ The primary disorder of lower motor neuron dysfunction is cerebral palsy.

   _____ Lower motor neuron lesions interrupt the reflex arc, causing weakness and atrophy of the skeletal muscles involved with associated hypotonia or flaccidity, with final progression to varying degrees of contracture.

   _____ Lower motor neuron involvement is most often asymmetric.

   _____ In most instances the sudden appearance of flaccid paralysis in a previously healthy child can be attributed to an infectious process.

   _____ Hereditary factors and metabolic disease are more often responsible for muscular weakness and atrophy of gradual onset.

   _____ The most useful classification of neuromuscular disorders defines the source of the lesion: cerebral cortex, anterior horn cells of the spinal cord, peripheral nerves, myoneural junction, and muscle.

   _____ Deep tendon reflexes are briskly active in upper motor neuron disease and diminished or absent in lower motor neuron disease.

2. Match each diagnostic tool with its description.

   a. Electromyogram (EMG)   d. CPK
   b. Nerve conduction velocity   e. Aldolase
   c. Muscle biopsy

   _____ Elevated in skeletal muscle disease; most specific test
   _____ Present in skeletal and heart muscle
   _____ Ketamine used to decrease the pain with this procedure
   _____ Measures electric impulse conduction along motor nerves
   _____ Measures electric potential of individual muscle

3. The nurse knows that the etiology of cerebral palsy is *most* commonly related to which of the following?
   a. Existing prenatal brain abnormalities
   b. Maternal asphyxia
   c. Childhood meningitis
   d. Preeclampsia

4. The nurse is preparing the long-term care plan for a child with cerebral palsy. Which of the following is included in the plan?
   a. No delay in gross motor development is expected.
   b. The illness is not progressively degenerative.
   c. There will be no persistence of primitive infantile reflexes.
   d. All children will need genetic counseling as they get older before planning for a family.

5. Match each term with its description.

a. hemiparesis   e. Triplegia   i. Dyskinetic cerebral palsy

b. Quadriparesis   f. Paraplegia   j. Ataxic cerebral palsy

c. Diplegia   g. Parietal lobe syndrome   k. Mixed-type cerebral palsy

d. Monoplegia   h. Spastic cerebral palsy

_____ Pure cerebral paraplegia of lower extremities

_____ Involving three extremities

_____ Involves only one extremity

_____ Similar parts of both sides of the body involved

_____ Most common form of spastic cerebral palsy; motor deficit greater in upper extremity; one side of the body affected

_____ Cortical sensory function impairment and therefore impaired two-point discrimination and position sense

_____ All four extremities equally affected

_____ Characterized by abnormal involuntary movement, such as athetosis—slow, worm-like, writhing movements that usually involve the extremities, trunk, neck, facial muscles, and tongue

_____ Characterized by wide-based gait; rapid, repetitive movements performed poorly; disintegration of movements of the upper extremities when the child reaches for objects

_____ Combination of spasticity and athetosis

_____ May involve one or both sides; hypertonicity with poor control of posture, balance, and coordinated motion; impairment of fine and gross motor skills; abnormal postures and overflow of movement to other parts of the body, increased by active attempts at motion

6. Children with cerebral palsy often have manifestations including alterations of muscle tone. Which of the following is an example of a finding in a child with altered muscle tone?
   a. Demonstrate increased or decreased resistance to passive movements
   b. Develops hand dominance by the age of 5 months
   c. Has an asymmetric crawl
   d. When placed in prone position, maintains hips higher than trunk, with legs and arms flexed or drawn under the body

7. Associated disabilities and problems related to the child with cerebral palsy include which of the following?
   a. All children with cerebral palsy will have intelligence testing in the abnormal range.
   b. There are a large number of eye cataracts associated with cerebral palsy, which will need surgical correction.
   c. Seizures are a common occurrence among children with athetosis and diplegia.
   d. Coughing and choking, especially while eating, predispose children with cerebral palsy to aspiration.

8. The nurse is completing a physical exam on 6-month-old Brian. Which of the following would be an abnormal finding suggestive of cerebral palsy?
   a. Brian is able to hold onto the nurse's hands while being pulled to a sitting position.
   b. Brian has no moro reflex.
   c. Brian has no tonic neck reflex.
   d. Brian has an obligatory tonic neck reflex.

9. The goal of therapeutic management for the child with cerebral palsy is:
   a. assisting with motor control of voluntary muscle.
   b. maximizing the capabilities of the child.
   c. delaying the development of sensory deprivation.
   d. surgically correcting deformities.

10. Which of the following would be expected in the infant presenting with hypotonia?
    a. When held in horizontal suspension, the infant will respond by slightly raising the head.
    b. When pulled to a sitting position, the infant will demonstrate head lag that is quickly corrected to a normal position.
    c. When placed in horizontal suspension position, the infant's head droops over the examiner's supporting hand and the infant's extremities hang loosely.
    d. The infant presents with a slower weight gain but has a good sucking reflex.

11. The major diagnostic test in diagnosing the infant with hypotonia is _____.

12. The disease inherited only as an autosomal-recessive trait and characterized by progressive weakness and wasting of skeletal muscles caused by degeneration of anterior horn cells is:
    a. Werdnig-Hoffmann disease.
    b. cerebral palsy.
    c. Kugelberg-Welander disease.
    d. Guillain-Barré syndrome.

13. Nursing considerations for the infant with Werdnig-Hoffmann disease should include which of the following for normal growth and development?
    a. Feeding by nasogastric tube
    b. Using an infant walker to develop muscle strength
    c. Incorporating verbal, tactile, and auditory stimulation
    d. Encouraging the parents to seek genetic counseling

14. a. What are the predominant features associated with juvenile spinal muscular atrophy?

    b. Describe the management and nursing considerations when treating the child with juvenile spinal muscular atrophy.

15. Which of the following is a true statement about Guillain-Barré syndrome?
    a. GBS is an autosomal-recessive inherited disease.
    b. GBS is more likely to affect children than adults, with children under the age of 4 years having the higher susceptibility.
    c. GBS is an acute demyelinating polyneuropathy with a progressive, usually ascending, flaccid paralysis.
    d. GBS is an autoimmune disorder associated with the attack of circulating antibodies on the acetylcholine receptors.

16. Diagnostic evaluation for the patient with Guillain-Barré syndrome would include which of the following results?
    a. CBC elevated
    b. Cerebrospinal fluid high in protein
    c. CPK elevated
    d. Sensory nerve conduction time increased

17. The priority nursing consideration for the child in the acute phase of Guillain-Barré syndrome is:
    a. careful observation for difficulty in swallowing and respiratory involvement.
    b. prevention of contractures.
    c. prevention of bowel and bladder complications.
    d. prevention of sensory impairment.

18. What are the characteristic symptoms of generalized tetanus?

19. a. Where are the spores of tetanus normally found?

    b. What is the incubation period for tetanus?

20. Terry, age 10 years, received his last tetanus toxoid immunization at the age of 4 years. He now presents to the clinic with a minor laceration sustained while working on his model airplanes. Is a dose of tetanus toxoid booster necessary at this time?
    a. Yes
    b. No

21. Maria, age 5, was born in a South American country and has been in the United States less than 1 year. While outside playing in the garden, she suffers a minor cut. Since Maria's mother does not think that Maria has ever received immunizations, which of the following actions would be most appropriate at this time to prevent tetanus?
    a. Have Maria go to the clinic tomorrow for the start of administration of all her needed immunizations.
    b. Administer tetanus immune globulin now.
    c. Administer first injection of tetanus toxoid now.
    d. Administer both tetanus immune globulin and tetanus toxoid now.

22. Primary nursing implementations for the child with tetanus include:
    i.   controlling or eliminating stimulation from sound, light, and touch.
    ii. maintaining body alignment.
    iii. arranging for the child not to be left alone since these children are mentally alert.
    iv. realizing that pancuronium bromide (Pavulon) does not cause total paralysis.
    v.   encouraging high intake of fluid.

    a. i, ii, and iii
    b. ii, iv, and v
    c. i and ii
    d. i and iii

23. Risk factors for infant botulism include:
    a. ingestion of honey.
    b. infants with diarrhea before the age of 3 months.
    c. infants living in urban areas.
    d. infants diagnosed with hypertonicity.

24. Infant botulism usually presents with symptoms of:
    a. diarrhea and vomiting.
    b. constipation and generalized weakness.
    c. high fever and decrease in spontaneous movement.
    d. failure to thrive.

25. What is the diagnosis of botulism based on?

26. Nursing considerations for the pediatric patient with botulism include:
    a. teaching the parents the importance of administering enemas and cathartics for bowel function.
    b. preparing the parents for the fact that the child will have muscular disability after the illness.
    c. using honey as a formula sweetener to increase oral intake.
    d. teaching parents that boiling is not an adequate prevention.

27. Tammy, age 13, is diagnosed with myasthenia gravis. The nurse, in preparing a teaching plan for the family, includes which of the following as a priority?
    a. Watching for signs of overmedication of anticholinesterase drugs, which include respiratory distress, choking, and aspiration
    b. Encouraging strenuous activity
    c. Suggesting to Tammy and her parents to limit Tammy's scholastic accomplishments in school in order to allow for adequate rest
    d. Reducing Tammy's weight to reduce symptom occurrence

28. Spinal cord injury causes three stages of response. The second stage is characterized by which of the following?
    a. Spinal shock syndrome
    b. Loss of temperature and vasomotor control
    c. Replacement of flaccid paralysis by spinal reflex activity, which results in spastic paralysis
    d. Development of scoliosis

29. Diagnostic evaluation of the child who presents with a spinal injury includes a complete neurologic exam. Motor system evaluation is done by:
    a. stimulating peripheral receptors by eliciting reflexes such as the patellar.
    b. observation of gait, noting balance maintenance and the ability to lift, flex, and extend extremities.
    c. testing all 12 cranial nerves.
    d. using the blunt end of a safety pin and the sharp point to test each dermatome.

30. What is the general guideline used when determining whether the paraplegic has the capacity to be self-helped to walk?

31. Management during the first stage of spinal cord injury may include:
    a. steroid administration.
    b. maximization of potential for self-help.
    c. observation for hypotension and hyponatremia.
    d. rehabilitation.

32. Discuss the benefits of functional electrical stimulation (FES) for the child with SCI.

33. Children with neurogenic bladder should be taught:
    a. to keep urine alkaline.
    b. how to perform the Credé maneuver to express urine.
    c. that the bladder that empties periodically by reflex action will not need intermittent catheterization.
    d. the importance of cranberry juice therapy to decrease urinary tract infections.

34. In discussing sexuality with the teenager that has a spinal injury, the nurse correctly includes which of the following in the discussion?
    a. Development of secondary sex characteristics will be delayed.
    b. Well-motivated young people can look forward to successful participation in marital and family activities.
    c. If injury occurs before onset of menstruation, ovulation and conception are not possible.
    d. Females can easily experience vaginal or clitoral orgasms.

35. Clinical manifestations of dermatomyositis include:
    i.   proximal limb and trunk muscle weakness.
    ii. stiff and sore muscles.
    iii. decreased muscle strength and reflex response.
    iv. red, indurated skin lesions over the malar areas and nose.
    v.   erythematous, scaly, atopic skin over extensor muscle surfaces

    a. i, ii, and iii
    b. i, ii, iv, and v
    c. iii, iv, and v
    d. ii, iii, and iv

36. Match each type of major muscular dystrophy with its characteristics. (Dystrophies may be used more than once.)

    a.   Pseudohypertrophic (Duchenne/Becker)

    b.   Limb-girdle

    c.   Facioscapulohumeral (Landouzy-Déjerine)

    _____   Lack of facial mobility; forward shoulder slope

    _____   Weakness of proximal muscles of both pelvic and shoulder girdles

    _____   Lordosis; waddling gait; difficulty in rising from floor and climbing stairs

    _____   Onset in late childhood; autosomal-recessive

    _____   Very slow progression and may have periods with no progression

    _____   Onset ages 3-5 years, early childhood

37. What are the major complications of muscular dystrophy?

38. Major goals in the nursing care of children with muscular dystrophy include which of the following?
    a. Promoting strenuous activity and exercise
    b. Promoting large caloric intake
    c. Preventing respiratory tract infection
    d. Preventing mental retardation

39. Diagnostic evaluation of muscular dystrophy includes serum levels of CPK, aldolase, and SGOT. When there is severe muscle wasting and incapacitation related to the disease process, the nurse would expect these serum levels to be:
    a. elevated.
    b. decreased.
    c. normal.
    d. unable to accurately be determined with muscle wasting and incapacitation.

Critical Thinking—Case Study

Kevin, age 4, has a history of premature delivery with cerebral palsy being diagnosed shortly after birth. Assessment findings include quadriplegia and deficient verbal communication skills but apparently normal level of intelligence. Kevin has been hospitalized several times in the past because of respiratory infection and gastric reflux. During Kevin's regular follow-up visit, his mother tells the nurse it is becoming harder to care for Kevin because of his needs. Because of Kevin's recent admission to the hospital for pneumonia, she worries that she is not giving Kevin the care he needs.

40. The nurse should explain to Kevin's mother that one of the complications associated with cerebral palsy is respiratory problems. Which of the following assessment findings could *most* help explain why Kevin is having these problems?
    a. Constant drooling, which contributes to wet clothing and chilling
    b. Dietary imbalance with poor nutritional intake
    c. The presence of nystagmus and amblyopia
    d. Coughing and choking, especially while eating, and history of gastric reflux

41. Kevin's mother asks the nurse how she can improve Kevin's communication skills, and a diagnosis of "impaired verbal communication" is developed. Which of the following plans would be *most* appropriate for Kevin at this time to improve his communication skills?
    a. Purchase an electric typewriter or computer to facilitate communication skills.
    b. Enlist the services of a speech therapist.
    c. Teach Kevin the use of nonverbal communications skills like sign language.
    d. Use audio tapes with Kevin to improve his speech abilities.

42. The nurse recognizes that an additional diagnosis is altered family processes related to a child with a lifelong disability. Which of the following implementations should the nurse recognize as being important to include in the plan of care?
    a. Explore potential for additional caregiving support.
    b. Refer the family to a support group of other parents of children with cerebral palsy.
    c. Refer parents to social services for additional suggestions.
    d. All of the above are important.

43. Based on the information given about Kevin, identify the nursing goals that would assist him and his family.

44. While Kevin is in the hospital, the nurse should plan appropriate play activities that include:
    a. minimized speaking, since Kevin has difficulty with his speech.
    b. solitary play to allow Kevin's parents to be away from Kevin so that they could rest.
    c. those that help Kevin relax muscles that are tense.
    d. those that require little intellectual functioning.

Answers

CHAPTER 1

1. hh (p. 13), r (p. 6), p (p. 4), n (p. 3), g (p. 2), b (p. 1), y (p. 7), ff (p. 13), f (p. 2), c (p. 1), i (p. 2), gg (p. 13), a (p. 1), l (p. 3), k (p. 3), u (p. 6), m (p. 3), s (p. 6), w (p. 7), o (p. 4), x (p. 7), d (p. 2), bb (p. 11), v (p. 6), ee (p. 13), cc (p. 13), t (p. 6), aa (p. 10), q (p. 6), z (p. 10), dd (p. 13), h (p. 2), j (p. 2), e (p. 2)
2. b (p. 13), e (p. 14), a (p. 13), u (p. 21), f (p. 15), y (p. 22), c (p. 14), i (p. 16), d (p. 14), dd (p. 23), k (p. 16), g (p. 16), m (p. 16), h (p. 15), o (p. 18), aa (p. 23), p (p. 19), t (p. 20), r (p. 20), l (p. 16), q (p. 20), j (p. 16), n (p. 16), s (p. 20), v (p. 21), bb (p. 23), z (p. 23), w (p. 21), x (p. 21), cc (p. 23), ee (p. 22)
3. d (p. 25), m (p. 28), b (p. 25), f (p. 26), a (p. 24), g (p. 27), n (p. 28), c (p. 25), h (p. 27), k (p. 27), e (p. 26), i (p. 27), l (p. 27), j (p. 27)
4. b (p. 2)
5. c (pp. 2, 3)
6. a (p. 3)
7. d (p. 4; Table 1-4)
8. Folic acid (p. 3)
9. b (p. 4)
10. d (p. 4; Table 1-4)
11. b (pp. 4, 5)
12. c (pp. 4, 5; Tables 1-3 and 1-4)
13. b (p. 6)
14. d (p. 6)
15. *Possible answers:* Respiratory illnesses, infection, acute illness (p. 6)
16. *Possible answers:* Homelessness; poverty; low birth weight; chronic illnesses; adoption; daycare centers (p. 6)
17. c (p. 6)
18. a (p. 6)
19. b (pp. 7, 8)
20. d (pp. 9, 10)
21. Active: a, c, d, e, g, i, j, l, m, o, p
    Passive: b, f, h, k, n (p. 10)
22. b (pp. 10, 11)
23. Anticipatory guidance (p. 10)
24. Modern: a, b, d, e, g, h, j, k, m, n, o, q, r, t, u, v, x, y, aa, bb, dd, ee, ff, hh, jj, kk, ll, mm, oo, qq
    Colonial: c, f, i, l, p, s, w, z, cc, gg, ii, nn, pp (pp. 11, 12)
25. e, g, h, c, b, i, d, a, f, j (pp. 12, 13)
26. *Financial*—no insurance; insurance that does not cover certain services; inability to pay for services
    System—need to travel great distances; state-to-state variations in benefits
    Information—lack of knowledge about prenatal or child health supervision; being unaware of available services (p. 13)
27. *Diagnosis-related groups*—a prospective payment system that allows for pretreatment billing for hospitals reimbursed by Medicare
    Health maintenance organizations—health services that use a network of specific providers for a set fee
    Managed care—a way to efficiently coordinate delivery of health services with the intent to provide an integrated approach to health care delivery (p. 13)

28. a (p. 14)
29. c (p. 14)
30. c (p. 15)
31. Case management (p. 15)
32. c (p. 15)
33. e, j, b, g, f, i, d, c, h, a (pp. 19-22)
34. c (p. 25)
35. a (p. 26)
36. d (pp. 25, 26)
37. c (p. 27)
38. b (p. 27)
39. a (p. 27)

CHAPTER 2

1. j (p. 32), c (p. 31), a (p. 30), d (p. 31), g (p. 31), p (p. 41), f (p. 31), n (p. 40), k (p. 34), i (p. 32), b (p. 31), h (p. 32), l (p. 40), o (p. 39), r (p. 62), m (p. 40), q (p. 41), e (p. 31), s (p. 41)
2. d (p. 35), b (p. 35), e (p. 35), c (p. 35), i (p. 33), k (p. 34), f (p. 35), h (p. 33), m (p. 43), g (p. 33), l (p. 32), j (p. 34), a (p. 38)
3. f (p. 44), h (p. 47), c (p. 44), e (p. 44), a (p. 44), l (p. 48), g (pp. 47, 52), n (p. 48), d (p. 44,) k (p. 48), o (p. 48), i (pp. 48, 52), b (p. 44), m (pp. 48, 52), j (pp. 48, 52)
4. e, g, c, b, d, a, f (p. 49)
5. b (p. 31)
6. a (p. 32)
7. d (p. 33)
8. g (p. 35), k (p. 38), e (p. 41), i (p. 37), a (p. 34), d (p. 40), b (p. 34), f (p. 42), h (p. 57), c (p. 35), j (p. 37)
9. d (p. 32)
10. a (p. 35)
11. b (p. 35)
12. a (p. 34)
13. b (pp. 33, 44)
14. a (p. 49)
15. d (p. 51)
16. f, i, e, a, d, g, h, c, b (p. 56; Table 2-3)
17. c (p. 56; Table 2-3)
18. b (p. 36)
19. d (p. 39)
20. c (p. 35)
21. a (p. 43)
22. d, e, b, a, c (pp. 43, 44)
23. c (p. 45)
24. a (p. 46; Table 2-1)
25. f, c, e, b, d, a (pp. 45, 46; Table 2-1)
26. d (p. 47)
27. a (p. 47)
28. d (p. 49)
29. a (p. 48)
30. b (p. 50)
31. c (p. 51)
32. a (p. 51)
33. b (p. 51)
34. b (p. 48)
35. d (p. 45)
36. a (p. 60; Table 2-4)
37. a (pp. 52-54)

CHAPTER 3

1. f, j, m, a, c, e, h, d, n, b, g, o, i, p, k, l, q (pp. 65, 66, 68, 70, 72, 73, 83, 85, 86, 87, 89)
2. c (p. 65)
3. b, a, a, b, c, c, d (pp. 65-69)
4. b (p. 69)
5. c (pp. 70-73)
6. Caregiving; nurturing; training (p. 73)
7. Poverty; lack of family structure and parenting resources; increased isolation from neighbors and extended families; living in neighborhoods with drugs, violence and decreased services (p. 74)
8. d (p. 74)
9. T, F, T, T, F (pp. 75, 76)
10. d (p. 76)
11. Birth order (p. 77)
12. c (p. 77)
13. a (p. 77)
14. c (p. 79)
15. b (p. 80)
16. c (pp. 81-82)
17. a (p. 81)
18. Survival—by promoting health of child
    Economic—so that child can provide for economic self-maintenance as an adult
    Self-actualization—to maximize cultural values and beliefs (p. 82)
19. b (p. 84)
20. F, T, F, F (pp. 82-83)
21. b, a, c (p. 84)
22. a (pp. 85-86)
23. a (pp. 86-87)
24. a (p. 87)
25. b (pp. 86-88)
26. d (pp. 89-91)
27. c (pp. 94-96)
28. F, T, F, T, T, T (p. 94)
29. c (p. 96)
30. Crisis phase that usually lasts for a year or longer and is characterized by an emotional upheaval, affecting the relationship with the parent granted custody; adjustment phase characterized by the child settling down and beginning to adapt to life in a single-parent home (p. 96)
31. a, c, b (pp. 97-99)
32. d (p. 68)
33. a (pp. 68, 69, 82-83)
34. b (pp. 81-83)
35. d (pp. 65, 66, 67, 83-84)
36. Establish a healthy family unit. Seek support from extended family; seek parenting instruction. Attend support group for parents with twins. Identify community resources available for the family. (pp. 73-74)
37. a. Occurs without any intervention; effective only when the consequences are meaningful; e.g., forgetting ballet slippers results in the child having to dance in stocking feet
    b. Directly related to the rule; e.g., not permitted to visit a friend's house for one day after coming home late from that friend's house
    c. Those that are imposed deliberately; e.g., no watching TV until homework is finished (p. 87)
38. It usually takes the form of spanking and causes a dramatic short-term decrease in the behavior. However, the flaws include the following:
    a. It teaches children that violence is acceptable.
    b. The spanking is often a result of parental anger.
    c. The spanking may physically harm the child.
    d. Children become accustomed to spanking.

e. More severe corporal punishment may be needed each time.
f. Parents may resort to using paddles or other objects.
g. The punishment may interfere with effective parent-child interactions.
h. Child learns what they should *not* do, not what they *should* do.
i. Misbehavior is likely to occur when the parent is not around.
j. Punishment may interfere with the child's development of moral reasoning. (p. 88)

CHAPTER 4

1. g, c, a, d, b, f, e (pp. 103, 104)
2. b (p. 104), m (p. 105), d (p. 104), i (p. 105), e (p. 105), c (p. 104), q (p. 106), g (p. 105), k (p. 105), h (p. 105), l (p. 105), f (p. 105), j (p. 105), p (p. 106), o (p. 106), n (p. 105), a (p. 104)
3. c, f, a, e, g, b, d (pp. 106, 107)
4. d (p. 103)
5. A healthy community "practices ongoing dialogue, generates leadership, shapes its future, embraces diversity, knows itself, connects people and resources, and creates a sense of community." (p. 103)
6. b (p.104)
7. d (p.104)
8. a (p.104)
9. c (p.104)
10. b (p.104)
11. c (p.105)
12. d (p.106)
13. c (p.106)
14. b (p.106)
15. c (p.106)
16. d (p.106)
17. d (p.106)
18. a (p.107)
19. Health and social services, communication, recreation, physical environment, education, safety and transportation, politics and government, and economics (p. 107)
20. b (p.107)
21. c, a, b (p. 108)
22. c, a, a, b, c, b, c, b, a (p. 105)
23. c (pp. 107, 108)
24. b (pp. 107, 108)
25. a (pp. 107, 108)
26. d (pp. 107, 108)

CHAPTER 5

1. c (p. 113), e (p. 113), a (p. 111), f (p. 113), b (p. 111), g (p. 111), d (p. 113), i (p. 113), k (p. 113), h (p. 113), j (p. 113), p (p. 114), r (p. 116), n (p. 114), v (p. 120), m (p. 113), t (p. 116), l (p. 113), o (p. 114), q (p. 114), x (p. 121), s (p. 116), z (p. 121), u (p. 117), w (p. 121), y (p. 121), bb (p. 122), aa (p. 122), ii (p. 124), cc (p. 122), gg (p. 123), ee (p. 118), dd (p. 122), ff (p. 123), hh (p. 123), jj (p. 124)
2. b (p. 127), d (p. 128), p (p. 133), e (p. 128), g (p. 130), i (p. 130), c (p. 127), a (p. 126), f (p. 129), h (p. 130), m (p. 131), j (p. 130), q (p. 136), o (p. 131), l (p. 131), k (p. 130), n (p. 131), r (p. 136)
3. d (p. 116)
4. c (pp. 116, 117)
5. a (p. 117)
6. b, b, a, a, c, b, c, c, b, a, b, b, b, a, a, a, b, b (p. 119)
7. d (p. 124)
8. c (p. 124)
9. a (p. 124)

10. a (p. 124)
11. b (p. 127)
12. b (p. 127)
13. c (pp. 125-127)
14. c, b, d, a (pp. 128-130)
15. d (p. 130)
16. a (pp. 130-132)
17. d (p. 131)
18. a (p. 131)
19. b (p. 132)
20. c (p. 132; Box 5-5)
21. d (p. 132)
22. b (p. 134)
23. d (p. 136)
24. b (p. 128)
25. a (p. 138)
26. a (p. 131)
27. c (p. 131)

CHAPTER 6

1. d, n, h, c, k, i, b, l, j, a, m, e, f, g (pp. 139, 140, 142, 160, 168)
2. c (p. 140)
3. b (p. 141)
4. Parent is more likely to reveal personal information about the child and family. Helps to identify child's and family's concerns and ways to deal with problem. Education of the health consumer about the advanced role of nurses. (p. 141)
5. b (p. 141)
6. d (pp. 143-144)
7. d (p. 142)
8. b (p. 145)
9. d (p. 147)
10. F, T, T, T, F (pp. 147-148)
11. d (p. 146)
12. b, a, b, b, c, c, d (pp. 148-150)
13. d (p. 150)
14. a. Storytelling
    b. "I" messages
    c. Bibliotherapy
    d. Drawing
    e. Directed play (pp. 151-152)
15. Identifying information; chief complaint; present illness; past history; family medical history; psychosocial history; sexual history; family history; nutritional assessment; review of systems (p. 153)
16. b (p. 154)
17. c (p. 154)
18. a (p. 154)
19. Approximate weight at 6 months, 1 year, 2 years, and 5 years of age; approximate length at 1 and 4 years; dentition, including age of onset, number of teeth, and symptoms during teething (p. 156)
20. Age of holding up head steadily; age of sitting alone without support; age of walking without assistance; and age of saying first words with meaning (p. 156)
21. d (p. 158)
22. Type, location, severity, duration, and influencing factors (p. 154)
23. Genogram; pedigree (pp. 160, 162)
24. a (p. 160)
25. c (p. 160)

26. b (p. 162)
27. Family composition; home and community environment; occupation and education of family members; cultural and religious traditions (p. 160)
28. c (p. 162)
29. d (pp. 143-145)
30. a (p. 154)
31. c (p. 164)
32. a (p. 167)
33. d (p. 153)
34. Including the parent in the problem-solving process helps the nurse to identify and eliminate solutions previously attempted. In addition, a parent who is included in the problem-solving process is more apt to follow through with a course of action. (pp. 145-146)

CHAPTER 7

1. b (p. 171)
2. a (pp. 172-174)
3. d (pp. 172-174)
4. Body mass index for age, 3rd and 97th smoother percentiles on all charts, 85th percentile for the weight-for-stature (p. 174)
5. a (p. 175)
6. With the child in a supine position, fully extend the body by holding the head in midline position, grasping the knees together gently, and pushing down on the knees until the legs are fully extended and flat against the table. Mark the end points of the tip of the head and the heel of the feet, and measure between the two spots. (pp. 175-176)
7. T, F, T, T, F (pp. 175, 177)
8. b (p. 175)
9. b (pp. 177-178)
10. Apical; 1 full minute; abdominal; 1 full minute (p. 179)
11. c (p. 178)
12. c (p. 184)
13. d (p. 186)
14. a, d, b, c, d, e, f, k, l, m, i, j, g, h, o, n (pp. 188-191, 224)
15. d (p. 189)
16. c (p. 190)
17. a (pp. 190-191)
18. Maxillary; ethmoid (p. 191)
19. Pupils equal, round, react to light and accommodation (p. 194)
20. d, e, h, i, m, a, c, n, k, g, f, b, j, l (pp. 192-195)
21. b (pp. 194-195)
22. a, b, c (p.197)
23. d (p. 198)
24. d (p. 202)
25. d (p. 205)
26. b (p. 206)
27. a (pp. 207-208)
28. a (p. 209)
29. d (p. 212)
30. b (p. 213)
31. a (p. 215)
32. c (p. 215)
33. a (p. 216)
34. d (p. 217)
35. b (p. 221)
36. c (p. 223)

37. Position child supine and flex the child's head; if this causes pain or causes the knees and hips to flex involuntarily, sign is positive; meningeal irritation (p. 226)
38. b, a, c (p. 238)
39. Preconventional; conventional; postconventional (pp. 232-233)
40. a (p. 235)
41. a (p. 236)
42. b (p. 173)
43. d (pp. 217-220)
44. d (p. 217)
45. c (p. 172)
46. b (p. 219)
47. Corneal light reflex test—When light is shined directly into eyes from 16 inches, it is not reflected symmetrically within each pupil.
    Cover test—The uncovered eye moves. (pp. 195, 196)
48. S_1, apex; S_2, base (p. 215)
49. d (p. 215)

CHAPTER 8

1. Low oxygen; high carbon dioxide; low pH (p. 241)
2. The sudden chilling of the infant as the infant enters a cooler environment from the warmer environment (p. 241)
3. c (p. 241)
4. b (p. 241)
5. a (p. 241)
6. T, F, T, F, T, F, F, T, F, F, F, T (pp. 241-243)
7. Rate of fluid exchange is 7 times greater in infant; infant's rate of metabolism is twice as great in relation to body weight; infant's immature kidneys cannot sufficiently concentrate urine to conserve body water. (p. 242)
8. b, a, c (p. 242)
9. Maternal circulation; breast milk (p. 243)
10. d (p. 243)
11. a. 8 inches
    b. Yellow; green; pink; geometric shapes and checkerboards
    c. Low; high (pp. 243-244)
12. c (p. 244)
13. a, b, c (p. 245)
14. b (p. 245)
15. a (p. 249)
16. c (pp. 251-252)
17. g, a, c, i, b, d, j, e, h, f, l, k (pp. 243, 251, 252, 257)
18. b (p. 255)
19. a (pp. 256-257)
20. Increased intracranial pressure; dehydration (p. 258)
21. a (p. 291)
22. d (pp. 258-259)
23. Making a sharp, loud noise close to the infant's head should produce a startle reflex or other reaction, such as twitching of the eyelids. (p. 259)
24. Obligatory nose breathers and are unable to breathe orally (p. 259)
25. c (pp. 251-254)
26. c, d, e, a, g, b, f (pp. 260, 261, 262, 263)
27. a. Radiation
    b. Conduction
    c. Convection
    d. Evaporation (p. 265)
28. d (p. 265)

29. a. Silver nitrate, erythromycin, or tetracycline ophthalmic drops or ointment
    b. Vitamin K
    c. Hepatitis B vaccine (pp. 265, 266, 267)
30. a (p. 267)
31. a (pp. 268-269)
32. The medical benefits of male newborn circumcision are not sufficient to recommend it as a routine procedure. The policy stresses the need for parents to determine what is best for their child after they have been given accurate and unbiased information about the risks and benefits and alternatives to this elective procedure. It also advises that procedural analgesia be given to the infant during circumcision. (p. 270)
33. d (pp. 273-274)
34. All statements are true. (pp. 277-280)
35. d (p. 278)
36. d (pp. 283-284)
37. c (p. 244)
38. Posture—full flexion of the arms and legs; square window—full flexion, hand lies flat on ventral surface of forearm; arm recoil—quick return to full flexion after arms released from full extension; popliteal angle—less angle/degree behind knee, less than 90 degrees; scarf sign—elbow does not reach midline with infant's arm pulled across the shoulder so that infant's hand touches shoulder; heel to ear—knees flexed with a popliteal angle of less than 10 degrees when the infant's foot is pulled as far as possible up toward ear (pp. 248, 250)
39. a (pp. 244, 245, 250, 251, 255, 256, 265, 266)
40. Infant will maintain a patent airway. Infant will maintain a stable body temperature. Infant will experience no infection or injury. Infant will receive optimum nutrition. (p. 263)
41. Vital signs; daily weights; stool patterns; voiding patterns; feeding patterns and intake; cord condition and care (p. 289)
42. c (pp. 274-277)
43. c (p. 287)
44. Wet diapers—six to ten per day; stools—at least two to three per day with breastfeeding; activity—has four to five wakeful periods per day; cord—keep above diaper line, nonodorous, drying; position for sleep—side or back (p. 287)
45. d (p. 259)
46. Adherent patches on the tongue and/or palate that cannot be wiped off may indicate an abnormal condition called "thrush" (candidiasis). If the patches can be wiped off, it is a normal finding, probably from the milk. (p. 252)
47. a. Wash hands before working with each infant and between infants.
    b. Avoid use of artificial and long fingernails and contaminated hand lotions.
    c. Use standard precautions of wearing gloves when handling infant until the blood and amniotic fluid are removed by bathing. (pp. 265, 268)

CHAPTER 9

1. d, g, a, h, c, i, b, j, f, e (pp. 295, 298, 300, 301, 303, 304, 306, 308)
2. c (p. 295)
3. c (p. 296)
4. d (p. 296)
5. c, b, a (p. 296)
6. a (p. 296)
7. b, a, a, c, b, a, b, a (pp. 298-300)
8. c (p. 300)
9. T, T, F, T, F, T, F, F (pp. 300-301)
10. d (p. 301)
11. a. Port-wine
    b. Strawberry hemangioma
    c. Café-au-lait spots (pp. 301-302)

12. d (pp. 302-303)
13. Hyperbilirubinemia; jaundice (p. 303)
14. Heme; globin; unconjugated bilirubin; conjugated bilirubin (p. 304)
15. c (p. 304)
16. a (p. 305)
17. a (p. 305)
18. c (p. 305)
19. a (pp. 305, 307)
20. b (pp. 304, 305)
21. a (p. 305)
22. Especially suited for home phototherapy, permits more infant-parent interaction, provides better temperature control, eliminates use of eye patches (p. 306)
23. b (p. 308)
24. a. Rh incompatibility
    b. Rh-negative, Rh-positive; O, A, B
    c. Indirect Coombs; direct Coombs
    d. 72 hours; 26-28; intramuscular (pp. 310, 312, 314)
25. Documentation of blood volumes exchanged, the amount of blood withdrawn and infused, the time of each procedure, and the cumulative record of the total volume exchanged; vital signs monitored and evaluated frequently and correlated with the removal and infusion of blood; observation for signs of transfusion reaction and side effects (p. 315)
26. a (p. 316)
27. c (p. 317)
28. b (p. 317)
29. a (p. 316)
30. 125 mg/dl; 150 mg/dl (p. 317)
31. d (p. 318)
32. b (p. 318)
33. d (p. 319)
34. Administer 0.5 to 1 mg into the vastus lateralis muscle or ventrogluteal muscle. (p. 319)
35. d (p. 321)
36. d (p.323)
37. d (pp. 323, 324)
38. a (p. 325)
39. b (p. 321)
40. *T*oxoplasmosis
    *O*ther agents such as hepatitis, parovirus, varicella zoster, measles, mumps
    *R*ubella
    *C*ytomegalovirus
    *H*erpes simplex viruses (p. 326)
41. d (p. 330)
42. Transplacentally, during vaginal delivery, through breast milk (p. 321)
43. c (p. 303)
44. a (p. 305)
45. c (pp. 307, 313)
46. d (p. 308)
47. d (p. 313)
48. Time phototherapy was started and stopped, proper shielding of eyes, type of fluorescent lamp by manufacturer, number of lamps, distance between lamp and infant (no less than 18 inches), used in combination with incubator or open bassinet, photometer measurement of light intensity, and occurrence of side effects (p. 308)
49. There is often an increase in the serum bilirubin level called "rebound effect"; this often resolves without resuming therapy. (p. 308)

CHAPTER 10

1. a. Low-birth-weight infant
   b. Extremely-low-birth-weight infant
   c. Small-for-gestational-age infant
   d. Large-for-gestational-age infant
   e. Premature (preterm) infant
   f. Full-term infant
   g. Postmature (postterm) infant
   h. Fetal death
   i. Neonatal death
   j. Perinatal mortality
   k. Thermal stability
   l. Neutral thermal environment
   m. Convective heat loss
   n. Radiant heat loss
   o. Conductive heat loss (p. 334)
2. d (p. 334)
3. c (p. 335)
4. c (p. 335)
5. Feeding behavior; activity; color; vital signs (p. 336)
6. a (p. 335)
7. T, F, F, T, T, F, F (p. 337)
8. Infant will exhibit adequate oxygen; infant will maintain stable body temperature (p. 338)
9. Nonshivering thermogenesis (p. 338)
10. a (p. 338)
11. Hypoxia; metabolic acidosis; hypoglycemia (p. 339)
12. a, b, d, c, f, e (pp. 329-340)
13. b (pp. 339-340)
14. Determine respiratory rate and regularity. Auscultate and describe breath sounds. Observe for accessory muscle use and nasal flaring. Observe for substernal, intercostal, or subclavicular retractions. Determine whether suctioning is needed. Inspect shape of the chest, symmetry, presence of incisions, chest tube. Assess cry if not intubated. Determine ambient oxygen and method of delivery. If intubated, note the size of the tube and determine whether the ventilator settings and tube secured correctly. Determine oxygen saturation if on pulse oximeter and determine partial pressure of oxygen and carbon dioxide by transcutaneous oxygen and transcutaneous carbon dioxide. (p. 336)
15. a (p. 341)
16. a. Peripheral veins on the dorsal surfaces of the hands or feet
    b. Percutaneous central venous catheter (PCVC), also called the *peripherally inserted central venous catheter (PICC)*
    c. Redness, edema, or color change at site; blanching at site (p. 342)
17. b (p. 342)
18. c (p. 343)
19. F, T, F, T, T, T, F, F (p. 344)
20. a (pp. 344-346)
21. b (p. 346)
22. d (p. 347)
23. c (p. 348)
24. Nonnutritive sucking (p. 348)
25. d (pp. 349-350)
26. d (pp. 349-351)
27. b (p. 352)
28. T, T, F, T, F, T, F, T, T, T, F, T (pp. 358, 360-365)
29. Supine (p. 366)
30. Morphine, fentanyl (p. 357)

31. a (p. 368)
32. Vulnerable child syndrome (p. 369)
33. a (pp. 368-369)
34. c (pp. 369-370)
35. b (p. 376)
36. d (p. 378)
37. c (p. 379)
38. b (p. 378)
39. a (p. 381)
40. a (p. 387)
41. Deficient surfactant production causes unequal inflation of alveoli on inspirations and the collapse of alveoli on end expiration; infants are unable to keep their lungs inflated and therefore exert a great deal of effort to reexpand the alveoli with each breath. (p. 380)
42. c, d, a, e, b, g, f, h , i (pp. 381-384)
43. b (p. 388)
44. d (p. 390)
45. a (p. 392)
46. Because of the infant's poor response to pathogenic agents, there is often no local inflammatory response at the portal of entry to indicate an infection. (p. 393)
47. d (p. 394)
48. d (p. 395)
49. c (p. 397)
50. b (p. 397)
51. c (pp. 397-398)
52. a (p. 398)
53. Hematocrit of 65% or greater; the small-for-gestational-age infant (p. 399)
54. Cryotherapy, laser therapy (p. 400)
55. Infant may be stuporous or comatose; seizures may begin after 6-12 hours and become more frequent and severe. Between 24-72 hours, deterioration in the level of consciousness may occur, with stupor and disturbances of sucking and swallowing. Muscular weakness of the hips and shoulders in the full-term infant and lower limb weakness in the premature infant occur. Apneic episodes may occur. (p. 407)
56. d (p. 402)
57. c (pp. 403-404)
58. b (p. 405)
59. c (p. 406)
60. c (p. 334)
61. b (pp. 379-380)
62. b (p. 371)
63. c (pp. 366-368)
64. a (p. 371)
65. Number of apneic spells; the appearance of the infant during and after attacks, whether the infant self-recovers or whether tactile stimulation is needed to restore breathing (p. 379)
66. Strong, vigorous suck; coordination of sucking and swallowing; a gag reflex; sucking on the gavage tube, hands, or pacifier; rooting and wakefulness before and sleeping after feedings (pp. 345, 347)
67. Prone; supine (pp. 363, 371)

CHAPTER 11

1. f, g, e, a, b, c, d (p. 416)
2. b (p. 416)
3. c (pp. 419-420)
4. d (p. 419)
5. All are true. (p. 423)
6. d (p. 420)
7. b (p. 425)

8. a (pp. 424, 430)

9. c, d, a, b, i, g, f, j, h, e (pp. 424-426, 437, 446)

10. Urinary tract infection; meningitis (p. 427)

11. a. Ultrasound of the uterus and elevated maternal concentrations of alpha-fetoprotein (AFP)

  b. 16-18 weeks gestation (p. 427)

12. b (p. 427)

13. a. Preserve renal function

  b. Preserve renal function and achieve maximal urinary continence (p. 428)

14. d (p. 429)

15. c (p. 431)

16. b (p. 431)

17. c (p. 433)

18. Congenital; acquired: bulging fontanels with or without head enlargement; headaches on awakening with improvement after emesis or when in upright position, papilledema, strabismus, and ataxia (pp. 437-438)

19. a (p. 440)

20. c (p. 442)

21. Infection; malfunction (p. 440)

22. 2 months; 18 months; 10 to 12 months (p. 443)

23. F, T, T, F, T, T (p. 444)

24. c (p. 445)

25. a (p. 445)

26. d (pp. 445-446)

27. Rotate the side of the head on which the infant sleeps and place the infant prone while awake and being observed (p. 446)

28. Involves use of a helmet to fit the largest diameter of the head. The helmet is worn 23 hours a day, usually for 3 months, and is most effective up to 9 months of age. (p. 446)

29. b, a, c (p. 446)

30. b (p. 448)

31. c, a, b (p. 450)

32. It worsens hip development by promoting hip extension. (p. 450)

33. c, e, a, d, f, b, k, i, h, g, j (p. 447)

34. b, a, c, d (p. 452)

35. d (p. 452)

36. d, b, a, c, e (pp. 453-454)

37. c (p. 455)

38. Speech impairments that require speech therapy; improper drainage from the middle ear, resulting in recurrent otitis media, which can led to hearing impairment and insertion of PE tubes for prevention; extensive malposition of teeth and maxillary arches, requiring extensive orthodontics and dental prosthesis; social adjustment problems with cognitive and motor delays, posing higher threats to self-image (p. 458)

39. c (p. 459)

40. d (p. 460)

41. b (p. 463)

42. c (p. 461)

43. a (p. 463)

44. Look for physical findings of an absent anal opening; identify infants not passing stool within the first 24 hours after birth or infants who have meconium that appears at a location other than the anal opening; watch for other symptoms, including abdominal distention, vomiting, flat perineum, and absence of midline intergluteal groove (pp. 468, 470)

45. b (p. 470)

46. Incarcerated (p. 474)

47. All are true. (p. 474)

48. d (pp. 475-476)

49. c, b, a, j, d, e, l, i, f, g, h, k (pp. 472-473, 477-481, 484)

50. Evaluation of prenatal and postnatal influences, karyotype, anatomic features, surgical possibilities, future fertility, and sexual function (pp. 489-490)
51. c (pp. 430-431)
52. b (p. 430)
53. b (p. 434)
54. Infant will not experience complications. Infant will not receive damage to the spinal lesion/surgical site. Family will receive support and education. (p. 431)
55. c (p. 431)
56. Urine retention (p. 432)
57. a (p. 432)

CHAPTER 12

1. i (p. 496), b (p. 495), t (p. 497), d (p. 496), f (p. 496), a (p. 495), g (p. 496), c (p. 495), h (p. 496), e (p. 496), j (p. 496), p (p. 496), n (p. 496), bb (p. 500), l (p. 496), k (p. 496), m (p. 496), o (p. 496), r (p. 497), z (p. 498), q (p. 496), x (p. 497), v (p. 497), s (p. 497), w (p. 497), aa (p. 500), u (p. 497), y (p. 497)
2. l (p. 503), a (p. 501), u (p. 524), c (p. 502), b (p. 502), e (p. 502), i (p. 502), d (p. 502), g (p. 502), f (p. 502), k (p. 502), h (p. 502), j (p. 502), p (p. 503), m (p. 503), r (p. 507), n (p. 503), t (p. 516), o (p. 503), q (p. 505), v (p. 526), s (p. 507), w (p. 527)
3. e (p. 516), c (p. 516), a (p. 516), d (p. 516), b (p. 516)
4. c (p. 529), e (p. 528), a (p. 528), d (p. 533), f (p. 534), h (p. 528), g (p. 528), j (p. 541), i (p. 541), b (p. 529)
5. g (p. 545), e (p. 544), a (p. 543), c (p. 544), b (p. 544), i (p. 546), d (p. 544), h (p. 545), f (p. 544)
6. c (p. 494)
7. b (p. 494)
8. a (p. 494)
9. Expected behavioral responses: f, d, c, e, b, a (p. 494)
   Ages of appearance: d, c, a, e, f, b (p. 494)
10. d (p. 494)
11. c (p. 495)
12. b (p. 496)
13. c (p. 595; Box 12-3)
14. a (p. 496)
15. d (p. 496)
16. Liver (p. 496)
17. a (p. 496)
18. a (p. 497)
19. b (p. 497)
20. b (p. 497)
21. a (p. 497)
22. d (p. 497)
23. 1.000 to 1.010 (p. 497)
24. c (p. 497)
25. b (p. 498)
26. d (p. 498)
27. b (pp. 498-501)
28. a (pp. 498-501)
29. a (p. 501)
30. b (pp. 502-504)
31. c (p. 504)
32. b (p. 504)
33. b (pp. 505, 506)
34. c (p. 505)
35. d (pp. 507-508; Table 12-2)

36. c (p. 509)
37. b (p. 516)
38. d (p. 516)
39. b (p. 516)
40. c (p. 516)
41. b (pp. 518-519)
42. c (p. 519)
43. a (p. 520)
44. d (p. 520)
45. c (p. 521)
46. b (p. 521; Table 12-4)
47. c (p. 522)
48. c (p. 523)
49. a (p. 522)
50. b (p. 523)
51. d (p. 525)
52. A culturally sensitive approach may consider the weaning process as beginning in utero, with the transmission of food flavors via amniotic fluid, and extending through childhood as the infant becomes accustomed to culturally indigenous foods introduced by the parents. (p. 525)
53. c (p. 527)
54. c, e, b, d, a (p. 526; Table 12-5)
55. c (p. 537; Table 12-14)
56. c (p. 537; Table 12-14)
57. a (p. 539)
58. b (p. 544)
59. c (p. 544)
60. c (p. 545)
61. a (p. 545)
62. d (p. 546)
63. a (p. 544)
64. Nutrition, sleep and activity, number and condition of teeth, immunization status, safety precautions used in the home (pp. 493-550)
65. c (p. 541)
66. b (p. 550)
67. d (p. 550)

CHAPTER 13

1. g (p. 560), c (p. 554), f (p. 560), a (p. 554), d (p. 555), b (p. 554), k (p. 564), m (p. 566), h (p. 560), e (p. 560), i (p. 564), l (p. 566), j (p. 564), r (p. 580), n (p. 568), v (p. 570), o (p. 568), s (p. 570), w (p. 571), p (p. 568), x (p. 571), q (p. 568), t (p. 570), y (p. 576), u (p. 570)
2. c (p. 583), e (p. 576), a (p. 577), d (p. 580), b (pp. 585, 586)
3. b (p. 555)
4. b (pp. 555, 556)
5. c (pp. 555, 556)
6. a (p. 555)
7. c, d, a, b, e (p. 560)
8. Protein (p. 560)
9. Estimated average requirements, tolerable upper-limit nutrient intakes, nutrient intakes associated with a low risk for adverse effects, adequate intakes (p. 564)
10. c (p. 564)
11. c (pp. 565, 566)
12. b (p. 566)
13. d (p. 566)
14. c (p. 567)

15. c (p. 567)
16. d (p. 568; Box 13-3)
17. d (p. 569; Box 13-4)
18. c (p. 569)
19. c (pp. 569, 570)
20. b (p. 570)
21. a (p. 570)
22. c (p. 570)
23. b (pp. 570, 571)
24. a (p. 572)
25. a (p. 572)
26. c (p. 574)
27. b, a, c (p. 574)
28. Possible responses: Poverty, health beliefs, inadequate nutritional knowledge, family stress, feeding resistance, insufficient breast milk (p. 574)
29. Growth delay or growth failure (p. 575)
30. a (p. 574)
31. c (p. 576)
32. c (p. 577)
33. b (p. 578)
34. d (p. 579)
35. a (p. 581)
36. c (p. 581)
37. F, T, T, F, T (pp. 582, 583)
38. d (pp. 569-577)
39. a (pp. 568-571)
40. c (p. 569)
41. b (p. 570)

CHAPTER 14

1. n (p. 596), c (p. 592), a (p. 591), e (p. 592), g (p. 594), b (p. 592), f (p. 594), h (p. 594), j (p. 594), l (p. 595), i (p. 594), k (p. 594), d (p. 592), m (p. 596), o (p. 596), q (p. 596), u (p. 597), p (p. 596), x (p. 598), w (p. 598), y (p. 600), r (p. 596), aa (p. 605), cc (p. 609), t (p. 597), bb (p. 609), s (p. 596), z (p. 602), v (p. 597), dd (p. 609)
2. p (p. 618), m (p. 618), o (p. 618), n (p. 618), i (p. 615), k (p. 618), g (p. 613), j (p. 616), h (p. 613), e (p. 611), l (p. 618), c (p. 611), f (p. 612), d (p. 611), a (p. 611), b (p. 611)
3. c (p. 592)
4. a (p. 593)
5. b (p. 593)
6. c (p. 593)
7. c (p. 594)
8. a (p. 595)
9. b (pp. 596, 597)
10. d, a, f, e, b, h, g, c (p. 597)
11. d (p. 598)
12. c (p. 598)
13. b (p. 599)
14. c (p. 599)
15. c (p. 599)
16. a (p. 600)
17. Physical—voluntary control of anal and urethral sphincters; ability to stay dry for 2 hours; regular bowel movements; gross motor skills of sitting, walking, and squatting; fine motor skills to remove clothing

Mental—recognizes urge to defecate or urinate; communicative skills to indicate needs; cognitive skills to imitate behavior and follow directions

Psychological—expresses willingness to please parent; able to sit for 5 to 10 minutes; demonstrates curiosity about toilet habits; impatient with soiled or wet diapers (pp. 603-605)

18. a (pp. 603-605)
19. a (p. 605)
20. c (p. 606)
21. d (p. 607)
22. c (p. 608)
23. d (p. 608)
24. Negativism—toddlers do not like to take orders; regression—they fear losing new skills; rigidity—upset when rituals are disrupted; self-centeredness—believe the world revolves around them; stranger anxiety; toilet training; security object lost; overstimulation; fears (p. 608; Box 14-2)
25. d (p. 609)
26. b (p. 609)
27. a (p. 609)
28. c (p. 609)
29. d (p. 609)
30. b (p. 610)
31. c (p. 610)
32. b (p. 611)
33. a (p. 611)
34. a (p. 611)
35. b (p. 612)
36. d (p. 612)
37. c (p. 613)
38. b (p. 613)
39. d (p. 613)
40. c (p. 615)
41. d, e, c, f, a, b (p. 617; Table 14-8)
42. Motor vehicle (p. 616)
43. a (pp. 616, 618, 619)
44. c (pp. 619, 620)
45. b (pp. 617, 620)
46. b (p. 620)
47. b (p. 620)
48. a (p. 621)
49. b (p. 622)
50. c (p. 623)
51. Foods—hot dogs, nuts, dried beans, pits from fruit, bones, gum
    Play objects—anything with small parts
    Household objects—drawstring jackets or hoods, thumbtacks, nails, screws, coins, jewelry, old refrigerators, storage chests
    Electric—outlets, garage doors, car windows (p. 623)
52. Temperament, psychosocial development, nutrition, sleep and activity, dental health, injury prevention (p. 591, Chapter Outline, 624)
53. a (p. 624)
54. d (pp. 605-607)
55. b (pp. 607, 624)

CHAPTER 15

1. m (p. 630), i (p. 630), a (p. 628), k (p. 630), c (p. p.629), q (p. 631), j (p. 630), b (p.629), e (p. p.629), n (p. 631), f (p. 630), l (p. 631), g (p. 630), p (p. 631), h (p. 630), o (p. 631), d (p. 629)
2. ee (p. 635), h (p. 632), x (p. 642), k (p. 633), g (p. 632), c (p. 631), e (p. 631), a (p. 631), f (p. 631), b (p. 631), i (p. 632), l (p. 634), d (p. 631), r (p. 641), u (p. 641), m (p. 635), v (p. 642), n (p. 636), cc (p. 643), p (p. 640), y (p. 642), w (p. 642), aa (p. 642), o (p. 640), j (p. 633), s (p. 641), z (p. 642), bb (p. 643), q (p. 640), t (p. 641), ff (p. 642), dd (p. 642)
3. 3; 5 (p. 628)
4. 5 (p. 628)
5. b (p. 629)
6. d (p. 630)
7. c (p. 632)
8. a (p. 631)
9. b (p. 631)
10. c (p. 631)
11. d (p. 632)
12. c (p. 632)
13. c (p. 632)
14. a (p. 633)
15. c (p. 633)
16. d (p. 633)
17. b (p. 634)
18. b (p. 636)
19. Present ideas as exciting, talk to the child about activities they will be involved with, behave confidently on the first day (p. 637)
20. b (p. 637)
21. a (p. 638)
22. c (p. 640, 641; Box 15-1)
23. d (p. 641)
24. b (p. 642)
25. c (p. 643; Box 15-2)
26. d (p. 643)
27. b (p. 643)
28. F, T, F, F (p. 645; Box 15-3)
29. d (pp. 646, 647)
30. a (pp. 636, 637)
31. c (pp. 636, 637)
32. b (pp. 636, 637)
33. d (pp. 636, 637)

CHAPTER 16

1. f, g, h, a, c, b, e, d, i, j, l, k, q, o, m, p, n (p. 650)
2. Child will not spread infection to others; child will not experience complications; child will have minimal discomfort; child and family will receive adequate emotional support. (p. 650)
3. c, a, b, d, g, f, e, h, j, i (pp. 652-654)
4. d (p. 650)
5. a (p. 650)
6. d (p. 651)
7. b (p. 651)
8. Varicella (chickenpox) and zoster (herpes zoster or shingles) (p. 651)
9. Warn parents about recent outbreaks of communicable diseases to prevent exposure of high-risk children. (p. 660)
10. a (p. 660)

11. c (p. 660)
12. c (p. 661)
13. d (p. 661)
14. a (p. 663)
15. d (p. 663)
16. T, T, T, T, F, F, F (pp. 664-665)
17. c (p. 667)
18. a (p. 667)
19. d (p. 668)
20. a (p. 667)
21. d (p. 668)
22. d (pp. 668-669)
23. b (p. 669)
24. c (p. 669)
25. Inducing vomiting; counteracting the toxin with activated charcoal; performing gastric lavage; increasing bowel motility; administering an antidote (p. 670)
26. Assessment; supportive measures; gastric decontamination; family support; prevention of recurrence (pp. 669-673, 696)
27. a (p. 671)
28. b (p. 672)
29. Lead; mercury; iron (p. 675)
30. c (p. 676)
31. T, T, T, F, T, F, T, T (pp. 676-679)
32. d (p. 681)
33. a (p. 679)
34. d (p. 681)
35. d, c, b, a, e, f (pp. 683-684)
36. a (pp. 684-685)
37. b (p. 685)
38. a (p. 685)
39. e, d, a, b, f, c (pp. 685-687)
40. c (p. 687)
41. d (pp. 686-687, 690)
42. a (p. 664)
43. b (p. 662)
44. b (p. 662)
45. a (p. 663)
46. b (p. 663)
47. a (p. 662)
48. c (p. 668

CHAPTER 17

1. c (p. 698)
2. Begins with shedding of the first deciduous tooth; ends at puberty with the acquisition of final permanent teeth (p. 698)
3. a (p. 699)
4. T, F, T, F, T, F, T, F, T, T (pp. 699-700)
5. b (p. 700)
6. b (p. 700)
7. d (p. 700)
8. d (p. 700)
9. a (p. 702)
10. c (p. 700)
11. 10 years; 12 years (p. 700)

12. a (pp. 700-701)
13. c (p. 702)
14. b (p. 702)
15. c (p. 702)
16. f, g, e, c, d, b, a, h, j, i (pp. 703-704, 706)
17. c (pp. 704, 705)
18. b (p. 705)
19. b (pp. 706-707)
20. d (p. 706)
21. d (p. 708)
22. c (p. 708)
23. Their own self-assessment and what they interpret as the opinion of family members and outside social contacts (pp. 708, 709)
24. a (p. 710)
25. Information is given in simple, accurate terms and includes how virus is transmitted, the effects of the virus on the body, and the resource personnel in the school who can answer children's questions about AIDS. (p. 710)
26. Children learn to subordinate personal goals to group goals. Children learn that division of labor is an effective strategy for the attainment of a goal. Children learn about the nature of competition and importance of winning. (p. 711)
27. d (p. 712)
28. F, T, T, T, F, T, F, T, T, F, T (pp. 714-716, 718)
29. c (p. 716)
30. To help the child interrupt or inhibit forbidden actions; to help child identify an acceptable form of behavior so that he or she can identify what is right in future situations; to provide understandable reasons as to why one action is appropriate and another action is not; to stimulate child's ability to empathize with the victim (p. 716)
31. a (p. 717)
32. b (pp. 718, 719)
33. b (pp. 719-720)
34. Children in elementary school who are left to care for themselves without adult supervision before or after school (p. 720)
35. Hygiene; nutrition; exercise; recreation; sleep; safety (p. 720)
36. Amount of food eaten and physical activity should be in balance to maintain appropriate weight; diet should include a variety of foods, especially adequate grain products, vegetables, and fruits; diet should be low in fat, including saturated fats and cholesterol; diet should include a moderate intake of sodium and sugar (p. 723)
37. a (p. 723)
38. c (p. 724)
39. T, F, F, F, T, T, T, T (pp. 724, 727, 728)
40. Health appraisal; emergency care and safety; communicable disease control; counseling and guidance (p. 728)
41. c (p. 732)
42. c (pp. 699, 700, 702, 706, 714, 720, 721, 724)
43. a (pp. 724, 725)
44. a (p. 721)
45. b (pp. 700, 707, 708)
46. b (pp. 721, 722)

CHAPTER 18

1. d (p. 740)
2. Epidermis; dermis; subcutaneous tissue (pp. 740-741)
3. e, f, g, h, i, j, k, a, c, b, d (pp. 742, 743)
4. f, h, a, b, d, c, e, i, g (p. 745)
5. d (p. 743)
6. f, g, i, k, a, c, b, l, j, h, e, d (pp. 743, 744, 745)
7. c, e, a, b, d (p. 746)
8. c (p. 747)
9. a (p. 747)
10. c (p. 748)
11. c (p. 749)
12. a (p. 749)
13. b (p. 749)
14. c (p. 751)
15. Increased erytherma, especially beyond the wound margin; edema; purulent exudate; increased temperature (p. 751)
16. b (p. 752)
17. c (p. 755)
18. b (p. 755)
19. a (p. 759)
20. c (p. 759)
21. a (p. 759)
22. d (pp. 760-761)
23. Observation of the white eggs (nits) firmly attached to the hair shafts that do not dislodge easily when removal is attempted; scratch marks and/or inflammatory papules caused by secondary infection may be found on the scalp. (pp. 761-762)
24. a (p. 762)
25. b (pp. 761, 762, 763)
26. d (p. 761)
27. b (p. 764)
28. d (pp. 765-766)
29. e, d, f, a, c, b (pp. 764, 765)
30. b (p. 766)
31. a (p. 766)
32. d (p. 768)
33. a (p. 770)
34. c (p. 770)
35. d, c, f, e, b, a, g (pp. 769-771)
36. b (p. 771)
37. b (p. 773)
38. d (pp. 773-774)
39. c (p. 772)
40. a (p. 774)
41. b (pp. 775-776)
42. a (p. 778)
43. b (p. 778)
44. b (p. 778)
45. c (p. 779)
46. d (pp. 779-780)
47. c (p. 781)
48. d (p. 782)
49. b (p. 785)
50. d (p. 786)

51. a (pp. 789-790)
52. T, F, T, F (p. 791)
53. c (p. 792)
54. d (p. 793)
55. T, F, F, T, T, T, T, T, F, T, T (pp. 794-796)
56. b (p. 751)
57. c (p. 768)
58. a (p. 756)
59. d (pp. 753, 756)
60. b (p. 768)

CHAPTER 19

1. d (p. 803)
2. a (p. 805)
3. T, T, T, F, T, F, F, T (pp. 804, 805, 807)
4. f, d, a, e, b, c, g (pp. 803-806)
5. c (p. 805)
6. Pubertal delay (p. 805)
7. b (p. 806)
8. a (p. 807)
9. Growth spurt (p. 807)
10. b (p. 807)
11. d (p. 808)
12. b (p. 808)
13. 2; 8; 15; 55; 4; 12; 15; 65 (p. 808)
14. c (p. 809)
15. d (p. 810)
16. b (p. 810)
17. b (p. 810)
18. b (p. 811)
19. c (p. 811)
20. c (p. 811)
21. a (p. 812)
22. d (p. 812)
23. d (pp. 814-815)
24. c (p. 814)
25. Realization of romantic or erotic attractions; erotic day dreaming; romantic partners or dates without sexual activity; sexual activity with others; self-identification of the orientation that best fits one's current circumstances and understanding; publicly self-identifying sexual orientation; intimate committed sexual relationship (p. 815)
26. b (p. 816)
27. a (p. 817)
28. d (p. 817)
29. Parental expectations of mature behavior on the part of the adolescent and setting and enforcing reasonable limits for behavior; related to greater psychosocial maturity and school performance and less substance abuse among adolescents (p. 817)
30. a (p. 818)
31. d (p. 811)
32. a (p. 818)
33. b (p. 819)
34. d (p. 819)
35. Injuries; homicide; suicide (p. 820)
36. a (p. 820)
37. c (p. 821)

38. d (p. 821)
39. T, T, F, T, T, F, T, T, F, F, F, T, T, T, T, F, T, T, T (pp. 815, 819, 820, 823, 825, 826, 830, 831, 832, 833)
40. Accessible; appropriate (p. 824)
41. Giving adolescents written materials during "teachable moments"; directing the adolescent to health resources in the community and on the Internet; teaching adolescents how the health care system works and how to keep their own personal health information (p. 824)
42. Active listening; responding to an adolescent's emotions; ensuring confidentiality and privacy (p. 824)
43. c (p. 828)
44. b (p. 829)
45. c (p. 829)
46. d (p. 829)
47. b (p. 830)
48. Smoking; hypertension; obesity; elevated cholesterol and triglycerides (p. 833)
49. b (p. 831)
50. The adolescent has a specific plan. (p. 832)
51. c (p. 814)
52. c (pp. 830, 833, 834)
53. d (p. 804)
54. c (pp. 833-834)
55. c (p. 835)

CHAPTER 20

1. c (p. 840)
2. d (p. 840)
3. a (pp. 840-841)
4. d (p. 841)
5. c (p. 841)
6. d (p. 843)
7. c (p. 843)
8. a (p. 843)
9. d (p. 844)
10. d, a, d, b, c, b, c (pp. 843, 844)
11. Primary amenorrhea; secondary amenorrhea (p. 845)
12. Oral contraceptive pills will protect the endometrium and provide sufficient estrogen for bone density. Unopposed estrogen can lead to endometrial hyperplasia and risk for endometrial adenocarcinoma. (p. 846)
13. c (p. 847)
14. d (p. 845)
15. b, c, d, j, a, h, f, e, g, i (pp. 845, 846, 847, 848, 849)
16. c (p. 847)
17. Wipe from the front to the back after toileting. Avoid use of irritating substances in the perineal area, such as bubble bath, douches, and deodorant pads. Avoid foreign objects, especially unremoved tampons. Discuss sexual transmission of disease and use of condoms for prevention. (p. 849)
18. T, T, F, F, F, T, T, T, F, T (pp. 849, 850, 851, 853)
19. a (p. 850)
20. d (pp. 849, 850, 851)
21. c (p. 852)
22. b (p. 852)
23. a (p. 853)
24. d (p. 854)
25. c (p. 854)
26. d (p. 855)
27. c (p. 855)
28. a (p. 855)

29. Allowing adolescents to role-play refusal skills (for sexual activity) in a safe environment (p. 857)
30. d (p. 859)
31. a (p. 859)
32. F, F, T, T, T, T, F, F, T, T (pp. 860, 861, 862, 863)
33. d (p. 863)
34. b (p. 863)
35. Human papillomavirus; anogenital warts; cervical dysplasia; carcinoma (p. 864)
36. Types 16, 18, 31, 45, and 56; patient; provider (p. 864)
37. b (p. 865)
38. a (p. 865)
39. b (p. 840)
40. a (p. 840)
41. a (p. 840)
42. c (p. 840)
43. d (p. 852)
44. d (p. 852)
45. a (p. 849)

CHAPTER 21

1. T, T, F, F, F, T, T, T, T, T, T, T, T (pp. 870, 871, 872)
2. d (p. 872)
3. d (pp. 870-872, 875)
4. d (p. 872)
5. Age of onset of obesity, presence of emotional disturbances, and negative evaluation of obesity by others (p. 873)
6. Track a child within a percentile range over time and detect at an early age children who are showing signs of being at risk for overweight and obesity. (p. 873)
7. c (p. 874)
8. b (pp. 875, 876)
9. Reduce the quantity eaten; alter the quality consumed; alter situations by severing the association between eating and other stimuli (p. 875)
10. 10 to 25; emaciation as a result of self-inflicted starvation (p. 877)
11. A purging binge eater regularly engages in self-induced vomiting or misuse of laxatives, diuretics or enemas. A nonpurging binge eater uses other behaviors, such as fasting or excessive exercise, rather than self-induce vomiting. (pp. 882, 883)
12. d (p. 877)
13. c (pp. 878, 881)
14. a (p. 882)
15. d (p. 878)
16. Older adolescent girls and young women; male (p. 882)
17. c (p. 882)
18. d (p. 882)
19. b (pp. 882, 883)
20. Serotonin-reuptake inhibitors (p. 882)
21. d (pp. 883, 884)
22. T, T, F, F, T, F, T (pp. 884, 885, 890)
23. a (p. 885)
24. b (p. 887)
25. c (p. 888)
26. b (p. 887)
27. a (p. 889)
28. Cohesive family, strong attachment to parents, peer models for conventional behavior, church attendance or regular involvement in church activities, commitment to schooling, participation in school activities, belief in the generalized expectations and values of society, and the development of resiliency (p. 890)

29. b (p. 894)
30. a. Crack (or rock)
    b. Injection
    c. Antifatigue agent; long periods of sleep
    d. Constricted pupils, respiratory depressions and cyanosis, and needle marks can be seen on extremities of chronic users.
    e. Rohypnol
    f. Methamphetamine
    g. Rapid loss of consciousness, respiratory arrest, and asphyxiation (pp. 890, 892)
31. c (p. 895)
32. d (pp. 897, 898, 899)
33. d (pp. 899, 900)
34. a (p. 893)
35. c, f, d, b, g, a, e, h, i (pp. 870, 876, 882, 895, 896)
36. d (pp. 897-899)
37. c (pp. 901, 902)
38. a (pp. 901, 902)
39. c (pp. 901, 902)

CHAPTER 22

1. f (p. 906), b (p. 906), h (p. 906), a (p. 906), d (p. 906), i (p. 908), c (p. 906), j (p. 908), g (p. 906), e (p. 906)
2. b (p. 909), f (p. 913), c (p. 909), e (p. 909), a (p. 909), d (p. 909)
3. b (p. 915), n (p. 935), c (p. 921), a (p. 915), d (p. 931), f (p. 932), h (p. 934), o (p. 935), i (p. 934), l (p. 934), g (p. 932), j (p. 934), e (p. 931), k (p. 934), p (p. 939), m (p. 934)
4. a (p. 906)
5. d (p. 906, 907)
6. b (p. 907)
7. d (p. 908)
8. a (p. 909)
9. d (p. 910)
10. e, c, a, b, d (pp. 910-917; Table 22-1)
11. b (p. 918)
12. b (p. 918)
13. b (p. 919)
14. c (p. 920)
15. a (p. 921)
16. d (p. 922)
17. c (p. 922)
18. b (p. 922)
19. Possible responses: Share complete information. Share information in manageable doses. Be sensitive to parents' reactions. Listen carefully. Provide technical information in understandable terms. Offer to share information. Provide information about resources. (p. 923)
20. a (p. 924)
21. Home; school (p. 925)
22. a (pp. 926, 927)
23. c (p. 928)
24. d (p. 929)
25. b (p. 928)
26. False reassurance; assuring parents that the child will grow out of the problem when the parents are struggling to accept reality (p. 930)
27. Approach behaviors: a, c, e, f, g
    Avoidance behaviors: b, d (pp. 931, 932)
28. b (p. 932)
29. d (p. 932)

30. c (p. 933)
31. d (p. 933)
32. a (p. 933)
33. *Possible answers:* Facilitate support from professionals; encourage expression of emotions; describe the behavior; give evidence of understanding; give evidence of caring; help parents focus on feelings; facilitate parent-to-parent support (p. 936)
34. b (p. 933)
35. d (p. 934)
36. c (p. 934)
37. *Possible answers:* Makes many sacrifices; helps the child even when the child is capable; inconsistent discipline; dictatorial; hovers and overdoes praise; protects the child from every discomfort; restricts play; denies the child opportunities for growth; sets goals too high or too low; monopolizes the child's time (p. 935; Table 22-6)
38. a (pp. 937, 938)
39. d (p. 935)
40. d (p. 935)
41. a (p. 935)
42. a (p. 936)
43. b (p. 936)
44. a. Recipients of care
    b. Silent in care
    c. Manager of care
    d. Monitors of care (p. 938; Table 22-3)
45. a (p. 939)
46. c (p. 939)
47. a (p. 921; Table 22-2)
48. c (pp. 939-944; Nursing Care Plan)
49. c (p. 939; Nursing Care Plan)
50. b (p. 940; Nursing Care Plan)
51. a (p. 911; Table 22-1)

CHAPTER 23

1. b (p. 949), d (p. 957), e (p. 948), a (p. 949), c (p. 957), j (p. 973), f (p. 955), i (p. 973), g (pp. 950, 966), h (p. 971)
2. b (p. 948)
3. c (p. 949)
4. *Possible answers:* Listen for an "invitation" to talk about the situation; use open-ended, nonjudgmental questions to explore the family's wishes; answer questions honestly; address fantasies or misunderstandings; remain neutral. (p. 950; Box 23-2)
5. c (p. 951; Table 23-2)
6. d (p. 952; Table 23-2)
7. a (p. 952)
8. c (p. 954)
9. a (p. 953)
10. b (p. 953)
11. d (p. 954)
12. c (p. 954)
13. Children who are dying are allowed the opportunity to remain with those they love and with whom they feel secure. Many children who were thought to be in imminent danger of death have gone home and have lived longer than expected. Siblings can feel more involved in the care and often have a more positive perception of the death. Parental adaptation is often more favorable, as is shown by their perceptions of how the experience at home affected their marriage, social reorientation, religious beliefs, and views on the meaning of life and death. Parents who have used home hospice feel significantly less guilt after the child's death than those whose child died in the hospital. (p. 956)

14. d (p. 956)
15. b (p. 957)
16. d (p. 959; Table 23-4)
17. d (p. 959)
18. *Possible answers:* Loss of senses; confusion; muscle weakness; loss of bowel and bladder control; difficulty swallowing; change in respiratory pattern; weak, slow pulse (pp. 960-961; Box 23-6)
19. d (p. 960)
20. Possible responses: Recall events that were important with their family; draw pictures/leave messages for important friends and family; reassure parents and others that they are not afraid and are ready to die; experience visions of "angels"; mention that someone is waiting for them. (p. 961)
21. c (p. 968)
22. a (p. 960
23. a (pp. 964, 965)
24. F, F, F, F, F (pp. 966-967)
25. d (p. 967)
26. a (p. 967)
27. c (p. 969)
28. c (p. 969)
29. d (p. 968)
30. d (p. 968)
31. d (p. 971)
32. *Possible answers:* Denial, anger, depression, guilt, and ambivalence (p. 972)
33. b (p. 973)
34. a (p. 963)
35. c (p. 957)
36. d (p. 971)
37. a (p. 963)

CHAPTER 24

1. h (p. 979), a (p. 977), c (p. 978), b (p. 978), e (p. 978), d (p. 978), f (p. 978), i (p. 979), g (p. 979), m (p. 989), j (p. 981), l (p. 989), k (p. 989), n (p. 990), o (p. 993)
2. a (p. 994), c (p. 995), b (p. 994), f (p. 995), d (p. 995), e (p. 995), g (p. 995), k (p. 995), h (p. 995), m (p. 995), i (p. 995), j (p. 995), l (p. 995), n (p. 996), q (p. 998), o (p. 998), p (p. 997), r (p. 998)
3. g (p. 1000), n (p. 1004), j (p. 1003), c (p. 1000), e (p. 1000), l (p. 1004), f (p. 1000), h (p. 1002), p (p. 1006), b (p. 1000), i (p. 1003), d (p. 1000), k (p. 1004), m (p. 1004), r (p. 1006), o (p. 1004), a (p. 1000), q (p. 1006)
4. o (p. 1012), l (p. 1012), c (p. 1007), e (p. 1007), b (p. 1007), g (p. 1007), a (p. 1007), d (p. 1007), h (p. 1007), f (p. 1007), k (p. 1008), q (p. 1012), n (p. 1012), i (p. 1007), p (p. 1012), j (p. 1007), m (p. 1012)
5. b, d, c, a (p. 978; Table 24-1)
6. b (p. 977)
7. *Possible answers:* Nonresponsiveness to contact; poor eye contact during feeding; diminished spontaneous activity; decreased alertness to voice or movement; irritability; slow feeding (p. 979; Box 24-2)
8. a (p. 980)
9. *Fading* means to take the child physically through each sequence of the desired activity and gradually fade out physical assistance so that the child becomes more independent. (p. 981)
10. *Shaping* means to wait for the child to give a response that approximates the desired behavior, then reinforce the child by gestures of social approval, such as touching or talking to him or her. (p.982)
11. d (p. 982)
12. Pros: Marriage could help the couple achieve a mutually satisfying and supportive relationship, meaningful companionship, and a more normal social-sexual adjustment.
Cons: Concerns about suitable living accommodations, contraceptive methods to prevent pregnancy. Parenting would require specialized assistance to help couple learn to meet the needs of their offspring. (p. 982)

13. c (p. 982)
14. b (p. 982)
15. *Task analysis* means to break the process of a skill into its components. It is used when teaching a mentally retarded child to help the child master one part at a time, building on the parts that the child has mastered already. (p. 981)
16. d (p. 985)
17. The child should be able to sit quietly for 3 to 5 minutes; watch what he or she is doing while working on a task; follow physical gestures or cues; follow verbal commands; relate clothing with the appropriate body part; be willing to participate (p. 985)
18. b (p. 986)
19. c (p. 989)
20. b (p. 989)
21. *Possible answers:* Separated sagittal suture; oblique palpebral fissures (upward, outward slant); small nose; depressed nasal bridge (saddle nose); high, arched narrow palate; excess and lax neck skin; wide space between big and second toes; plantar crease between big and second toes; hyperflexibility; muscle weakness (p. 989; Box 24-5)
22. b (p. 991)
23. c (p. 992)
24. a (p. 993)
25. d (p. 993)
26. c (p. 994)
27. d (p. 995)
28. d (p. 995; Table 24-5)
29. b (pp. 996, 997; Box 24-8)
30. a (pp. 996-997)
31. d (p. 998)
32. d (p. 998)
33. a (p. 999)
34. b (pp. 1000-1001)
35. d (p. 1003)
36. f, d, b, a, e, c (p. 1002; Box 24-9)
37. *Possible answers:* Talk to the child about everything that is occurring. Emphasize aspects of procedures that are felt/heard. Approach the child with identifying information. Explain unfamiliar sounds. Encourage rooming-in for parents. Encourage parents to participate in the care. Bring familiar objects from home. Orient the child to the immediate surroundings. If the child has sight on admission, use this opportunity to point out significant aspects of the room and to practice ambulating with the eyes closed. (pp. 1004-1005)
38. b (p. 1005)
39. a (p. 1006)
40. b (p.1006)
41. b (p. 1008; Box 24-11)
42. c (pp. 1010, 1011)
43. a (p. 1007)
44. d (p. 1109; Box 24-12)
45. c (p. 1010)
46. b (p. 1011; Family Home Care Box)
47. A *situated approach* shifts the emphasis from repairing the disabilities to supporting those with disabilities so that they can achieve more. (p. 1008)
48. c (p. 1011)
49. c (pp. 1010, 1012, 1013)
50. a (p. 1013)
51. d (p. 990; Appendix B: Denver Developmental Screening Test)
52. d (pp. 990-991)
53. b (p. 988)
54. c (p. 988)

CHAPTER 25

1. j (p. 1022), i (pp. 1020, 1021), g (p. 1020), a (p. 1016), c (p. 1017), h (p. 1020), b (p. 1016), d (p. 1017), f (p. 1019), e (p. 1018)
2. Responses should include the following: Advances in medical technology, parents' desire, cost considerations, recognition of families' valuable contributions (pp. 1016, 1017)
3. c (p. 1017)
4. c (p. 1017)
5. d (p. 1017)
6. b (p. 1018)
7. The child's medical, nursing, education, and other therapeutic needs; family members' (including siblings') education and training, coping skills, and adjustment needs; community readiness in areas such as availability of equipment, appropriate nursing and other personnel, education and developmental services, respite care, and emergency plans; financial arrangements (p. 1018)
8. Fully trained pediatric staff; 24-hour availability; family-centered care; continuing education; certification; accreditation such as JCAHO/CHAP (p. 1018; Box 25-3)
9. c (p. 1019)
10. d (p. 1019)
11. d (p. 1020)
12. Facilitate timely access to services; promote continuity of care; provide family support; improve outcomes; maximize use of resources. (p. 1020)
13. a (p. 1020)
14. b (p. 1020)
15. c (p. 1021)
16. Responses should include the following: Encourage self-confidence and self-esteem; display respect for family; recognize family diversity; demonstrate ability to understand family's approach; share perspectives; support family members in their roles; exchange expertise; assist family members to see their worth; identity strengths; negotiate options; assist family to find meaning (p. 1022)
17. c (p. 1022)
18. c (p. 1023)
19. c (p. 1023)
20. d (p. 1024)
21. d (p. 1024)
22. b (p. 1025)
23. *Possible answers:* Respect the family's choices even when the nurse's approach is different from the family's. A parent's authority should be respected unless risk or harm is posed to the child or the written medical orders are not followed. Communicate honestly and respectfully. Document carefully. Use agency policy as a guide. Call on the case manager or nursing supervisor to help negotiate. (p. 1022)
24. b (p. 1027)
25. c (p. 1028)
26. c (p. 1028)
27. b (p. 1028)
28. a (p. 1028)
29. c (p. 1025)
30. b (p. 1027)
31. c (p. 1024)

CHAPTER 26

1. k (p. 1045), j (p. 1041, 1073), i (p. 1040), h (p. 1040), g (p. 1040), f (p. 1040), e (p. 1032), d (p. 1032), c (p. 1032), b (p. 1032), a (p. 1032)
2. d (p. 1050, 1068), o (p. 1062), a (p. 1047), i (p. 1061), f (p. 1050), b (p. 1050), j (p. 1057), g (p. 1057, 1058), e (p. 1049), c (p. 1050, 1068), h (p. 1061), k (p. 1162), s (p. 1066), q (p. 1063), m (p. 1061), y (p. 1067), t (p. 1066), r (p. 1066), p (p. 1062), v (p. 1067), l (p. 1060), n (p. 1062), w (p. 1067), aa (p. 1068), x (p. 1067), z (p. 1068), u (p. 1067)
3. b (p. 1071), e (p. 1096), a (p. 1071), d (p. 1093), c (p. 1084)
4. b (p. 1032)
5. b, c, a (p. 1032)
6. b (p. 1034)
7. a (p. 1034)
8. b (p. 1035)
9. c (p. 1036)
10. c (pp. 1036, 1037; Fig. 26-3)
11. d (p. 1038)
12. d (p. 1039)
13. c (p. 1040)
14. *Possible answers:* Presentation of opportunities for children to master stress and feel competent in their coping abilities; new socialization experiences; broadened interpersonal relationships (p. 1040)
15. b (p. 1041)
16. c (p. 1042)
17. *Possible answers:* Include family in care planning; observe for negative effects of continuous visiting by parents (encourage the parents to leave for brief periods; arrange for sleeping quarters on the unit but outside the child's room; plan a schedule of alternating visits with the other parent or with another family member); provide information; therapeutic presence; complement and augment the parents' caregiving responsibilities (pp. 1042, 1043)
18. c (p. 1043)
19. d (pp. 1043, 1044)
20. b (p. 1045, 1046)
21. b (p. 1046; Box 26-5)
22. c (p. 1046)
23. c (p. 1046)
24. b (p. 1046)
25. c (p. 1046)
26. *Q*uestion the child.
    *U*se pain rating scales.
    *E*valuate behavior and physiologic changes.
    *S*ecure parents' involvement.
    *T*ake cause of pain into account.
    *T*ake action and evaluate results. (pp. 1049, 1050)
27. b (p. 1049)
28. True: a, c, d, f, g, h, j, l, n, o, p, q, s, u
    False: b, e, i, k, m, r, t (pp. 1047, 1049; Box 26-7)
29. d (pp. 1051, 1052; Table 26-2)
30. b (p. 1052; Table 26-2)
31. a (pp. 1052, 1053; Table 26-2)
32. b (p. 1054)
33. c (p. 1054)
34. d (p. 1050)
35. d (p. 1056; Table 26-3)
36. b (p. 1057)
37. *Possible answers:* Distraction, relaxation, guided imagery, positive self-talk, thought stopping, cutaneous stimulation, behavioral contracting (pp. 1057, 1059)

38. a (p. 1055)
39. d (p. 1060)
40. b (p. 1061)
41. *Possible answers:* Patient-administered boluses; nurse-administered boluses; continuous basal infusion (p. 1063)
42. d (p. 1063)
43. c (p. 1065)
44. a (p. 1066)
45. a (p. 1066)
46. b (p. 1067)
47. d (p. 1067)
48. c (p. 1068)
49. *Possible answers:* Provides diversion; brings about relaxation; helps child feel secure; helps lessen stress; provides a means for tension release; encourages interaction; helps develop positive attitudes; acts as an expressive outlet; provides a means for accomplishing therapeutic goals; places child in active role; gives more control and choices to the child (p. 1069; Box 26-13)
50. a (p. 1070)
51. *Possible answers:* Allows for creative expression; allows nurse to assess adjustment and coping; serves as a springboard for discussion; provides distraction, diversion (p. 1071)
52. c (p. 1073)
53. c (p. 1084)
54. The child-life specialist is a health care professional with extensive knowledge of child growth and development and the special psychosocial needs of children who are hospitalized and their families. These professionals help prepare children for hospitalization, surgery, and procedures. It is a collaborative role that is designed to help ensure the best possible hospital experience for the child and family. (p. 1084)
55. d (p. 1086)
56. *Possible answers:* Encourage parents to stay with their child. Provide information about child's condition in understandable language. Establish a routine that maintains some similarity to daily events in child's life whenever possible. Schedule undisturbed times. Reduce stimulation. (p. 1094)
57. d (p. 1089; Box 26-14)
58. c (p. 1089; Box 26-14)
59. c (p. 1090)
60. d (p. 1091)
61. d (p. 1091, 1092)
62. c (p. 1092)
63. *Postvention* is the term used for counseling after an event has occurred. It is particularly therapeutic after emergency hospitalization. (p. 1093)
64. a (p. 1094)
65. c (p. 1095)
66. d (p. 1097)
67. a (p. 1075)
68. d (pp. 1076-1078)
69. d (p. 1078)
70. a (p. 1079)

CHAPTER 27

1. m (p. 1121), c (p. 1102), b (p. 1103), h (p. 1118), a (p.1103), l (p. 1120), f (p. 1109), d (p. 1108), k (p. 1120), g (p. 1113), n (p. 1121), j (p. 1120), e (p. 1108), i (p. 1118)
2. m (p. 1122), h (p. 1130), j (p. 1130), k (p. 1130), a (p. 1123), e (p. 1124), b (p. 1124), d (p. 1124), c (p. 1124), i (p. 1130), l (p. 1130), f (p. 1125), g (p. 1130)
3. l (p. 1148), e (p. 1133), f (p. 1134), b (p. 1133), i (p. 1144), a (p. 1132), g (p. 1134), c (p. 1133), h (p. 1134), j (p. 1144), m (p. 1148), k (p. 1147), d (p. 1133)

4. j (p. 1164), e (p. 1158), a (p. 1150), h (p. 1162), g (p. 1162), b (p. 1150), k (p. 1166), c (p. 1157), f (p. 1162), d (p. 1158), i (p. 1162)

5. d (p. 1102)

6. d (p. 1102)

7. c (p. 1103)

8. d (p. 1103)

9. b (pp. 1103, 1104)

10. c (p. 1107)

11. a (p. 1104)

12. b (p. 1108)

13. d (p. 1107)

14. *Possible answers:* Expect success. Have extra supplies handy. Involve the child. Provide distraction. Allow expression of feelings. Praise the child. Use play in preparation and postprocedure. (p. 1109)

15. Examples of appropriate responses:

    a. Ambulation: Give a toddler a push-pull toy.

    b. Range of motion: Touch or kick Mylar balloons.

    c. Injections: Make creative objects out of syringes.

    d. Deep breathing: Practice band instruments.

    e. Extending the environment: Move the patient's bed to the playroom.

    f. Soaks: Put marbles or coins at the bottom of bath container.

    g. Fluid intake: Make freezer pops using the child's favorite juice. (p. 1111; Box 27-1)

16. b (p. 1110)

17. c (p. 1110)

18. a (p. 1112)

19. b (p. 1112)

20. c (p. 1113)

21. c (p. 1113)

22. d (pp. 1113, 1117)

23. c (p. 1119)

24. c (p. 1120)

25. c (p. 1120)

26. c (p. 1122)

27. a (p. 1125)

28. b (pp. 1124, 1125)

29. d (p. 1126)

30. c (p. 1127)

31. a (p. 1128)

32. c (p. 1128)

33. a (p. 1129)

34. a (p. 1130)

35. d (pp. 1130, 1131)

36. a (p. 1131)

37. c (p. 1130; Box 27-3)

38. a (p. 1133)

39. d (p. 1134)

40. *Possible answers:* Horizontal position with the back supported and the thigh grasped firmly by the carrying arm; the football hold; the upright position with the buttocks on the nurse's forearm and the front of the body resting against the nurse chest; transport in bassinet, crib, stroller, wheeled feeding chair/table, wheelchair, wagon with raised sides, gurney with high sides up and safety belt in place (pp. 1136, 1137)

41. *Possible answers:* Remove and reapply restraints periodically. Secure restraints to the frame, *not* the side rails, of the bed or crib. Leave one fingerbreadth between skin and the device. Tie quick release knots. Ensure that the restraint does not tighten as the child moves. (p. 1138)

42. b (p. 1141; Fig. 27-11)

43. d (p. 1141; Fig. 27-14)

44. c (p. 1141)

45. d (p. 1142)
46. a (p. 1143)
47. b (p. 1147; Fig 27-17)
48. b (p. 1146)
49. b (p. 1146)
50. a (p. 1147)
51. c (pp. 1147, 1148)
52. b (p. 1148)
53. d (p. 1148)
54. a (p. 1150)
55. d (p. 1151)
56. b (pp. 1151, 1152; Fig. 27-21)
57. a (p. 1151)
58. c (p. 1154)
59. c (p. 1156; Table 27-7)
60. d (p. 1158)
61. a (p. 1159)
62. d (p. 1159)
63. a (p. 1159)
64. b (p. 1160)
65. c (p. 1162)
66. b (p. 1162)
67. a (p. 1164)
68. c (p. 1165)
69. a (p. 1166)
70. b (p. 1105)
71. b (pp. 1115-1117)
72. a (p. 1116)
73. d (p. 1116)

CHAPTER 28

1. c, b, a, f, g, d, e, k, l, m, p, i, n, j, o, h (pp. 1171, 1172)
2. d (pp. 1172, 1173)
3. a (p. 1173)
4. d (pp. 1173-1174)
5. Isotonic (p. 1176)
6. Hypotonic; less (p. 1177)
7. Hypertonic; loss; intake; greater (p. 1177)
8. b (p. 1178)
9. c (p. 1178)
10. c (p. 1179)
11. c (pp. 1180, 1183)
12. c (p. 1180)
13. b (p. 1180)
14. Anasarca (p. 1180)
15. b (p. 1180)
16. c (p. 1181)
17. d, c, a, b (pp. 1182, 1183, 1184)
18. a (p. 1185)
19. 1 g wet diaper weight equals 1 ml urine. (p. 1186)
20. b (p. 1183)
21. d (p. 1185)

22. Oral rehydration solution (containing 75-90 mmol sodium and 111-139 mmol glucose; Pedialyte RS, Rehydralyte) for the first 4 to 6 hours; if this is tolerated, then fluids (containing 30-60 mmol sodium and 111-139 mmol glucose; Pedialyte, Lytren, Resol, or Infalyte) for the next 18 to 24 hours at 1-2 ounces per pound divided into frequent feedings (p. 1186)
23. a (p. 1186)
24. a (p. 1188)
25. c (pp. 1189, 1192)
26. F, T, T, T, F, F, T, T, F, F, T, T, T (pp. 1189, 1190, 1191, 1197, 1198, 1201)
27. Infusions of systemic fluids with a large bore needle inserted into the medullary cavity of a long bone that provides a safe and rapid alternate route for administration of fluids; used when systemic access is vital and venous access cannot be obtained quickly (p. 1191)
28. b (p. 1192)
29. c (pp. 1195, 1196, 1197)
30. c (p. 1196)
31. a (p. 1197)
32. b (p. 1197)
33. b (p. 1197)
34. d, c, b, a, c (pp. 1198, 1202)
35. Line connections are taped to prevent accidental disconnection. Number of line openings for blood withdrawal and medication administration is minimized. Central dressing protocols are established, and only nurses specifically trained should do dressing changes. Return demonstration should be done by family members for home care of the lines. (p. 1201)
36. b (p. 1202)
37. d (p. 1203)
38. c (p. 1203)
39. Parents' ability to perform the procedure; existence of family support system; availability of a pharmacy that can prepare the solution; insurance coverage (p. 1204)
40. c (p. 1180)
41. c (p. 1184)
42. d (p. 1185)
43. d (pp. 1185-1186)
44. c (p. 1179)
45. c (p. 1179)
46. a (pp. 1182, 1184)
47. c (p. 1191)

CHAPTER 29

1. d, c, f, a, b, e (pp. 1207, 1208, 1216)
2. a (p. 1208)
3. T, T, T, F, F, F, T, T (pp. 1208, 1209, 1210, 1211, 1213, 1226)
4. b (p. 1211)
5. a. *Clostridium difficile*
   b. Bacterial gastroenteritis
   c. Sugar intolerance
   d. Fat malabsorption
   e. Parasitic infection or protein intolerance (p. 1211)
6. Assessment of fluid and electrolyte imbalance; rehydration; maintenance fluid therapy; reintroduction of adequate diet (p. 1211)
7. a (p. 1212)
8. d (p. 1213)
9. c (p. 1214)
10. Intractable diarrhea of infancy (p. 1216)
11. b (p. 1217)
12. d (p. 1218)

13. a. Hypovolemic
    b. Cardiogenic
    c. Vasogenic
    d. Anaphylactic
    e. Septic (p. 1219)
14. g, e, f, b, j, d, h, a, i, c, k (pp. 1220, 1221)
15. b (p. 1220)
16. c (p. 1222)
17. Ventilation, fluid administration, improvement of the pumping action of the heart (vasopressor support) (p. 1221)
18. c, a, b (p. 1222)
19. a (p. 1224)
20. d (p. 1226)
21. Wash hands before inserting the tampon; do not use a soiled or dropped tampon; insert carefully to avoid vaginal abrasion; alternate use with sanitary napkins (e.g., use tampons during the day and sanitary napkins during the night); do not use superabsorbent tampons; do not leave tampon in the body longer than 4-6 hours; remove the tampon immediately with development of sudden fever, rash, vomiting, diarrhea, muscle pain, dizziness, or feeling of near-fainting. (pp. 1226, 1227)
22. Thermal; electrical; chemical; radioactive (p. 1227)
23. Immersion in hot water and contact with hot objects such as cigarettes (p. 1227)
24. All are true. (pp. 1227, 1228, 1233)
25. a (p. 1228)
26. b (p. 1229)
27. d (p. 1229)
28. a (p. 1229)
29. c (p. 1230)
30. c (p. 1231)
31. b (p. 1230)
32. d (p. 1231)
33. b (p. 1232)
34. a (p. 1232)
35. d (p. 1232)
36. Airway compromise; shock; infection (p. 1233)
37. c (p. 1235)
38. c (p. 1236)
39. b (p. 1237)
40. a (p. 1237)
41. a (p. 1238)
42. a (p. 1240)
43. b (p. 1239)
44. b (p. 1242)
45. b (p. 1229)
46. a (pp. 1233, 1236)
47. b (pp. 1230, 1231)
48. c (p. 1250)
49. d (pp. 1234, 1245)
50. c (p. 1252)

CHAPTER 30

1. F, T, T, F, F, T, T, T, T, T, T, T, T, F (pp. 1255-1260, 1264, 1267)
2. a, n, a, a, n, n, a (p. 1261)
3. c, f, h, j, k, b, d, i, e, g, a, m, l, o, n, p (pp. 1258, 1260, 1262, 1272, 1274, 1275, 1283, 1293)
4. a (p. 1264)
5. d (p. 1263)

6. d (p. 1265)
7. d (p. 1266)
8. b (p. 1266)
9. a. Eliminate the current infection.
   b. Identify contributing factors to reduce the risk of recurrence.
   c. Prevent systemic spread of the infection.
   d. Preserve renal function. (p. 1267)
10. a (p. 1266)
11. d (p. 1266)
12. d (p. 1267)
13. b (p. 1268)
14. c (p. 1269)
15. b (p. 1271)
16. b (p. 1271)
17. Hypertensive encephalopathy; acute cardiac decompensation; acute renal failure (p. 1272)
18. b (p. 1273)
19. b (p. 1274)
20. a (pp. 1274-1275)
21. a (p. 1275)
22. c (p. 1277)
23. a (p. 1277)
24. F, T, T, T, F, T, T, F (pp. 1279, 1280, 1281, 1282)
25. c (p. 1281)
26. a (pp. 1281-1282)
27. a (p. 1283)
28. c (pp. 1283-1284)
29. b (p. 1284)
30. a (p. 1286)
31. c (p. 1286)
32. Monitoring and assessing fluid and electrolyte balance (p. 1287)
33. b (p. 1289)
34. b (p. 1290)
35. The child will receive encouragement in his or her normal growth and development, minimizing the impact of the disease process. The child will remain free of complications. The child and family will receive appropriate support, guidance, and education. (p. 1292)
36. a. Hemodialysis; peritoneal dialysis; hemofiltration
    b. Hemodialysis
    c. Protein loss
    d. Hemodialysis
    e. Peritonitis
    f. Growth rate; skeletal maturation; normal growth
    g. Fluid overload; surgical procedures (pp. 1293, 1297, 1298)
37. a (p. 1300)
38. b (p. 1275)
39. d (pp. 1276-1278)
40. c (p. 1278)
41. d (p. 1278)
42. Teach the family to recognize signs of relapse and to bring the child for treatment at the earliest indications of relapse; provide instruction about testing urine for albumin, administration of medications, side effects of medications, and prevention of infection; emphasize the importance of restricting salt— for example, no additional salt during relapse and steroid therapy, then a regular diet for the child in remission. (pp. 1278-1279)
43. Teach the family and Darlene about the disease, its implications and the therapeutic plan; the possible psychologic effects of the disease and the treatment; the technical aspects of the procedure, including possible complications and changes to observe for. (p. 1298)

44. Provide dietary instructions for foods that reduce excretory demands on kidneys and provide sufficient calories and protein for growth. Encourage intake of carbohydrates to provide calories for growth and foods high in calcium to prevent bone demineralization. Recommend foods that are rich in folic acid and iron because anemia is a complication of chronic renal failure. Arrange for renal dietitian to meet with Darlene and her family to help them understand dietary needs and to assist Darlene in independent formulation of dietary allowances when she is away from home. (pp. 1290, 1294)

CHAPTER 31

1. g (p. 1304), b (p. 1303), i (p. 1304), a (p. 1303), e (p. 1304), j (p. 1304), d (p. 1304), k (p. 1304), c (p. 1304), aa (p. 1306), l (p. 1305), t (p. 1305), m (p. 1305), x (p. 1305), u (p. 1305), n (p. 1305), h (p. 1304), w (p. 1304), v (p. 1305), o (p. 1305), f (p. 1304), y (p. 1306), p (p. 1305), q (p. 1305), z (p. 1306), r (p. 1305), s (p. 1305)
2. h (p. 1307), b (p. 1307), i (p. 1307), c (p. 1307), j (p. 1307), n (p. 1308), a (p. 1306), k (p. 1307), f (p. 1307), o (p. 1309), d (p. 1307), l (p. 1308), g (p. 1307), m (p. 1308), p (p. 1309), t (p. 1309), e (p. 1307), v (p. 1309), q (pp. 1309, 1315; Fig. 31-10), w (p. 1309), x (p. 1309), u (p. 1309), s (p. 1309), r (p. 1309)
3. f, a, e, g, d, b, h, c (p. 1310)
4. q (p. 1310), k (p. 1311), d (p. 1310), e (p. 1310), l (p. 1311), h (p. 1311), n (p. 1311), b (p. 1310), p (p. 1311), f (p. 1310), a (p.1310), c (p. 1310), g (p. 1310), o (p. 1311), i (p. 1311), m (p. 1311), j (p. 1311)
5. g (p. 1316), c (p. 1314), a (p. 1313), e (pp. 1314, 1315), f (p. 1316), b (p. 1313), d (p. 1314)
6. c (p. 1317), e (p. 1317), a (p. 1317), g (p. 1319), i (p. 1319), f (p. 1319), h (p. 1319), u (p. 1330), j (p. 1319), n (p. 1320), q (p. 1323), t (p. 1324), m (p. 1320), k (p. 1319), o (p. 1320), s (p. 1324), p (p. 1322), l (p. 1320), b (p. 1317), r (pp. 1323, 1324), d (p. 1317)
7. e (p. 1331), b (p. 1331), f (p. 1331), h (p. 1331), d (p. 1331), i (p. 1331), a (p. 1331), j (p. 1331), l (p. 1331), c (p. 1331), m (p. 1331), r (p. 1338), g (p. 1331), q (p. 1338), n (p. 1334; Fig. 31-25), s (p. 1341), o (p. 1334; Fig. 31-25), k (p. 1331), p (p. 1334; Fig. 31-25)
8. b (p. 1306)
9. a (p. 1304)
10. c (p. 1304)
11. b (p. 1304)
12. c (p. 1305)
13. Fewer number of alveoli; smaller size of the alveoli; more shallow air sacks; decreased surface area for gas exchange (p. 1306)
14. d (p. 1306)
15. b (p. 1307)
16. a (p. 1307)
17. c (p. 1307)
18. b (p. 1308)
19. d (p. 1309)
20. a (p. 1310)
21. c (p. 1312)
22. Capacities are combinations of two or more lung volumes. These include inspiratory capacity (IC), functional residual capacity (FRC), and vital capacity (VC). (p. 1312; Fig. 31-8)
23. b, c, a, c, b, a (p. 1313; Table 31-1)
24. b, f, a, e, d, c (pp. 1314, 1315)
25. c (p. 1313)
26. b (p. 1316)
27. a (p. 1317; Table 31-4)
28. b (p. 1317)
29. c (p. 1318)
30. b (p. 1318)
31. c (p. 1319)
32. b (p. 1319)

33. a (p. 1320)
34. d (p. 1320)
35. a (p. 1320)
36. c (p. 1320)
37. c (p. 1320)
38. b (p. 1323)
39. b (p. 1324)
40. d (p. 1325)
41. c (p. 1326)
42. a (p. 1326)
43. b (p. 1326)
44. c (p. 1328)
45. b (p. 1328)
46. Avoid toys, blankets, clothing, and pets that shed fine hair or lint. Avoid aerosols, powder, dust, and smoke. Toys with removable parts should be eliminated. Clothing should have loose-fitting collars that do not cover the tracheostomy tube opening. When the child is outside, the artificial nose or a thin cloth is used to prevent cold air, dust, dirt, or sand from entering the tube. Bathe the child in a tub filled with shallow water; no water or soap should enter the tube. (p. 1330)
47. a (p. 1330)
48. *Possible responses:* Obstructive lung disease—tracheomalacia; choanal atresia; vocal paralysis; meconium aspiration; aspiration of a foreign body, mucus, or vomitus; epiglottitis; pneumonia; pertussis; severe tonsillitis; tumors; anaphylaxis; laryngospasm
    Restrictive lung disease—respiratory distress syndrome; cystic fibrosis; pneumothorax; pulmonary edema; pleural effusion—abdominal distention; muscular dystrophy; paralytic conditions
    Respiratory center depression—cerebral trauma at birth; intracranial tumors; central nervous system infection; drug overdose (p. 1331)
49. d (p. 1332; Box 31-8)
50. b (p. 1332)
51. c (p. 1333)
52. b (p. 1334)
53. a (p. 1334)
54. a (p. 1338)
55. c (p. 1338)
56. i, h, c, b, e, f, g, d, a (p. 1339; Table 31-6)
57. d (p. 1341)
58. b (p. 1312)
59. c (p. 1312)
60. a (p. 1332; Box 31-8)
61. d (p. 1320)

CHAPTER 32

1. d (p. 1351), i (p. 1352), e (p. 1351), m (p. 1353), g (p. 1352), b (p. 1343), h (p. 1352), p (p. 1355), a (p. 1343), l (p. 1353), f (p. 1352), q (p. 1356), n (p. 1354), c (p. 1351), j (p. 1352), r (p. 1356), o (p. 1355), k (p. 1352)
2. j (p. 1358), o (p. 1358), b (p. 1357; Box 32-4), k (p. 1358), n (p. 1358), a (p. 1357; Box 32-4), g (p. 1358), l (p. 1358), e (p. 1357), i (p. 1358), m (p. 1358), d (p. 1357; Box 32-4), h (p. 1358), f (p. 1357), p (p. 1358), c (p. 1357; Box 32-4), q (p. 1361)
3. o (p. 1374), d (p. 1366), p (p. 1375), u (p. 1369; Box 32-8), b (p. 1364), g (p. 1370), a (p. 1361), q (p. 1365), h (p. 1372), t (p. 1369; Box 32-8), e (p. 1367), v (p. 1367), l (p. 1373), i (p. 1372), n (p. 1373), s (p. 1369; Box 32-8), f (p. 1367), c (p. 1366), r (p. 1369), j (p. 1372), m (p. 1373), k (p. 1372)
4. c (p. 1381), b (p. 1381), e (p. 1382), d (p. 1382), a (p. 1378)

5. o (p. 1407), f (p. 1391), i (p. 1398), a (p. 1390), j (p. 1398), c (p. 1390), k (p. 1401), e (p. 1391), b (p. 1390), h (p. 1395), l (p. 1406), q (p. 1408), p (p. 1408), g (p. 1394), n (p. 1406), d (p. 1391), s (p. 1409), m (p. 1406), r (p. 1408), w (p. 1391), aa (p. 1405), t (p. 1387), x (p. 1392), u (p. 1389), z (p. 1405), v (p. 1389), y (p. 1395), bb (p. 1405)
6. b (p. 1344)
7. c (p. 1344)
8. c (p. 1344; Box 32-1)
9. c (p. 1346)
10. b (p. 1346)
11. b (p. 1346)
12. a (p. 1350)
13. b (p. 1350)
14. c (p. 1351)
15. d (p. 1351)
16. b (p. 1352)
17. c (p. 1353)
18. c (p. 1353)
19. d (p. 1353)
20. c (p. 1353)
21. c (p. 1354)
22. a (p. 1354)
23. c (p. 1355)
24. c (p. 1355)
25. b (p. 1355)
26. a (p. 1356)
27. a (p. 1357; Box 32-5)
28. *Possible answers:* Tympanic membrane retraction; tympanosclerosis; tympanic perforation; adhesive otitis media; chronic suppurative otitis media; labyrinthitis; mastoiditis; meningitis; cholesteatoma (pp. 1357, 1358)
29. d (p. 1358)
30. c (p. 1358)
31. b (p. 1358)
32. a (p. 1359)
33. d (p. 1359)
34. b (p. 1360)
35. c (p. 1361)
36. c (p. 1362)
37. d (p. 1362)
38. c (p. 1362)
39. a (p. 1363)
40. b (p. 1363)
41. c (p. 1364; Box 32-6)
42. a (p. 1364)
43. b (p. 1365)
44. d (p. 1366)
45. a (p. 1367)
46. c (p. 1368)
47. c, a, b (p. 1369)
48. d (p. 1370)
49. *Possible answers:* Perform respiratory assessment; administer oxygen; administer antibiotics; institute isolation procedures; promote rest and conservation of energy; administer antitussives; administer fluids; use mist tent; prevent chilling; position the child comfortably; control fever; suction to maintain patent airway; promote postural drainage; involve the family (p. 1371)
50. c (pp. 1371-1372)
51. b (p. 1373)
52. d (p. 1374)

53. a (p. 1374; Box 32-12)
54. c (p. 1376
55. c (p. 1377)
56. a (p. 1377; Figs 31-25 and 31-26)
57. c (p. 1379)
58. *Possible answers:* Prevent infection. Treat precipitating disease. Maintain intravascular volume and hydration status. Monitor urinary output. Treat fever. Establish and maintain neutral thermal environment. Maintain tissue oxygenation (oxygen, positioning, mechanical ventilation, suctioning). Employ comfort measures and treat pain. Provide psychological and emotional support. Initiate pharmacological therapy. Provide nutritional support. (p. 1380)
59. c (p. 1380)
60. b (p. 1381)
61. Cotinine (p. 1382)
62. *Possible answers:* Allergic shiners, obligate mouth breathing, nasal crease, facial tics and mannerisms to avoid scratching the nose, open mouth caused by chronic nasal obstruction (allergic gape), extra wrinkles below the lower eyelids (Dennie lines) (p. 1383)
63. b (p. 1385)
64. c (p. 1386; Box 32-16)
65. c (p. 1386)
66. d (pp. 1386-1387)
67. b (p. 1388)
68. a (p. 1388)
69. b (pp. 1388-1389)
70. b (p. 1389)
71. d (p. 1390)
72. c (p. 1392)
73. c (p. 1398)
74. b (p. 1399)
75. c (pp. 1402, 1403)
76. d (p. 1400)
77. b (p. 1408)
78. c (p. 1408)
79. d (p. 1408)
80. b (p. 1409)
81. a (pp. 1412-1413)
82. d (p. 1411)

CHAPTER 33

1. b (p. 1416)
2. F, T, T, T, T, F (p.1417)
3. a. Digestion; absorption; metabolism
   b. Enzymes; hormones; hydrochloric acid; mucus; water and electrolytes
   c. Small intestine (pp.1417, 1418)
4. Measurement of intake and output; measurement of height; measurement of weight; abdominal examination; laboratory studies of urine and stool (p. 1419)
5. a (p. 1422)
6. n, j, f, g, h, m, a, l, o, d, e, b, i, k, c (pp. 1420, 1422, 1424)
7. b (p. 1423)
8. d (p. 1423)
9. "Although the blood test does determine whether you have antibodies to the *H. pylori* germ, it does not tell if you still have it or if it is an old infection. Looking into your stomach allows your doctor to actually view your stomach for signs of change from the disease and allows for biopsy of your stomach to determine if the germ is still present and active in your stomach." (p. 1421)
10. b (p. 1425)

11. d (p. 1426)
12. b (p. 1425)
13. d (p. 1426)
14. c (p. 1427)
15. d (p. 1427)
16. Absence of autonomic parasympathetic ganglion cells in the submucosal and myenteric plexuses in one or more segments of the colon, which produces the functional defect or absence of peristalsis in the affected section (p. 1426)
17. a (p. 1428)
18. d (p. 1429)
19. b (p. 1429)
20. Passive regurgitation or emesis (p. 1429)
21. b (pp. 1430, 1431)
22. a (p. 1432)
23. d (p. 1433)
24. a. McBurney point
    b. Located midway between the right anterosuperior iliac crest and the umbilicus
    c. Referred pain (p. 1433)
25. c (pp. 1435, 1437)
26. a (pp. 1437, 1439)
27. In CD the chronic inflammatory process may involve any part of the GI tract from the mouth to the anus but most commonly affects the terminal ileum. It can affect segments of the intestine with intact mucosa in between. CD involves all layers of the wall. The inflammation may result in ulcerations, fibrosis, adhesions, stiffening of the bowel wall, and obstruction. In UC the inflammation is limited to the colon and rectum, with the distal colon and rectum often the most severely affected. UC involves the mucosa and submucosa; it also involves continuous segments with varying degrees of ulceration, bleeding and edema. Long-standing UC can cause shortening of the colon and strictures. (pp. 1438, 1439)
28. c (p. 1440)
29. a (p. 1442)
30. c (p. 1443)
31. c (p. 1443)
32. Proton pump inhibitor (omeprazole, lamsoprazole), amoxicillin, clarithromycin (p. 1445)
33. b (p. 1445)
34. d (p. 1446)
35. b (p. 1446)
36. d (pp. 1447, 1448)
37. c (p. 1448)
38. a (p. 1448)
39. a (p. 1448)
40. The administration of air pressure to reduce intussusception is as successful as barium and more rapid-acting. Neither water-soluble contrast nor air pressure carries the risk for barium peritonitis. (p. 1449)
41. c (p. 1449)
42. Malrotation; volvulus (p. 1449)
43. a (p. 1450)
44. c (p. 1450)
45. d (p. 1451)
46. a (p. 1455)
47. a, a, e, a, d, c, b, b, f (pp. 1456, 1457)
48. a (p. 1459)
49. c (p. 1459)
50. Early detection; support and monitoring of the disease; recognition of chronic liver disease; and prevention of spread of the disease (p. 1459)
51. c (p. 1461)

52. Questions about the patient's pain: When did the pain start? Has it been constant or intermittent? What were you doing when the pain started? Where did the pain start and does the pain radiate or move to other areas? How would you describe the pain intensity and quality? What makes the pain better? What makes it worse? How have you tried to treat the pain? Has there been change in normal activities because of the pain?
    Questions about related symptoms or review of associated symptoms: Is there nausea or vomiting? If there is, did it start before or after the pain? Is there diarrhea or constipation? How would you describe the last stool? When did it occurr? Are there urinary tract signs and symptoms such as frequency, difficulty with flow, burning? Is there fever? If so, how much fever? How long has the fever been present? Have medications been taken for the fever? If so, when was the last dose taken? Is there hunger or lack of hunger?
    Questions about the reproductive system: For females—When was your last menstrual period? For males and females—Are you sexually active? Do you have any genital discharge? (pp. 1434, 1435)
53. b (p. 1433)
54. d (pp. 1434-1436)
55. A white blood cell count with a differential elevated to around 15,000 to 20,000 mm^3 with an elevated number of bands indicating a shift to the left (pp. 1433-1434)
56. a (p. 1436)
57. a (p. 1436)

CHAPTER 34

1. p, h, m, j, f, d, b, k, a, l, e, i, c, n, o, g (p. 1465)
2. d (p. 1465), k (p. 1466), a (p. 1465), l (p. 1466), c (p. 1465), j (p. 1465), n (p. 1466), e (p. 1465), b (p. 1465), h (p. 1465), g (p. 1465), i (p. 1465), m (p. 1466), f (p. 1465)
3. j (p. 1468), e (p. 1468), o (p. 1467), m (p. 1469), a (p. 1467), l (p. 1469), d (p. 1468), q (p. 1467), g (p. 1468), b (p. 1467), i (p. 1468), c (p. 1467), f (p. 1468), p (p. 1467), k (p. 1468), r (p. 1467), h (p. 1468), n (p. 1469)
4. d, a, e, b, f, c, (pp. 1469-1470; Figure 34-4)
5. t, v, q, g, u, f, l, b, i, m, d, j, o, s, n, a, e, h, r, c, k, p (all answers from pp. 1469-1472; Table 34-1)
6. f (p. 1476), d (p. 1476), b (p. 1475), e (p. 1476), a (p. 1475), g (p. 1476), c (p. 1475)
7. h, c, l, a, f, m, g, j, r, n, d, i, o, k, e, p, b, q (p. 1478)
8. f (p. 1480; Table 34-5), e (p. 1480; Table 34-5), b (p. 1479), g (p. 1480; Table 34-5), d (p. 1480; Table 34-5), h (p. 1480; Table 34-5), a (p. 1479), c (p. 1479)
9. m (p. 1488), i (p. 1487), f (p. 1486), b (p. 1484), l (p. 1488), d (p. 1484), j (p. 1487), a (p. 1484), g (p. 1486), k (p. 1487), e (p. 1486), c (p. 1484), h (p. 1487)
10. aa (p. 1521), p (p. 1519), h (pp. 1511, 1512), q (p. 1519), b (p. 1511), ee (p. 1523), i (p. 1514), c (p. 1511), r (p. 1520), k (p. 1517), d (p. 1511), dd (p. 1523), v (p. 1520), f (p. 1511), cc (p. 1522), a (p. 1511), g (p. 1511), n (p. 1519), w (p. 1520), s (p. 1520), j (p. 1516), e (p. 1511), t (p. 1520), l (p. 1517), m (p. 1518), bb (p. 1521), y (p. 1520), o (p. 1519), z (p. 1520), u (p. 1520), x (p. 1520)
11. e (p. 1507), j (p. 1507), g (p. 1507), a (p.1504), h (p. 1507), f (p. 1507), c (p. 1504), i (p. 1507), d (p. 1504), b (p. 1504)
12. g (p. 1525), o (p. 1526), c (p. 1525), d (p. 1524), j (p. 1525), k (p. 1525), e (p. 1524), h (p. 1526), l (p. 1525), f (p. 1524), a (p. 1524), i (p. 1526), m (p. 1525), n (p. 1526), b (p. 1525)
13. a (p. 1465)
14. a (p. 1465)
15. b (p. 1465)
16. c (p. 1466)
17. a (p. 1466)
18. b (p. 1468)
19. d (p. 1468)
20. a (p. 1469)
21. b (p. 1469)
22. c (p. 1471)
23. c (p. 1471)
24. b (p. 1472)

25. *Possible answers:* Loss of circulation to the affected extremity; dysrhythmias; hemorrhage; cardiac perforation; hematoma; hypovolemia and dehydration; hypoglycemia in infants; temperature and color of the affected extremity; vital signs (pp. 1473-1474)
26. d (p. 1473)
27. d (p. 1476)
28. c (p. 1478)
29. d (p. 1478)
30. b (p. 1478)
31. c (p. 1478)
32. a (p. 1479)
33. b (p. 1479)
34. c (p. 1480)
35. d (p. 1483)
36. c (p. 1483)
37. d (p. 1487)
38. b (p. 1487)
39. b (p. 1490)
40. a (p. 1490)
41. c, d, c, d, b, c, d, a, d, a, d, b, c, b, b (defects with increased pulmonary blood flow: pp. 1491-1494; obstructive defects: pp. 1494-1496; defects with decreased pulmonary blood flow: pp. 1496-1498; mixed defects: pp. 1498-1501)
42. c (pp. 1492, 1493, 1497, 1501)
43. d (pp. 1493, 1497, 1499, 1501)
44. b (pp. 1491-1501)
45. c (pp. 1491-1501)
46. a (p. 1501)
47. c (p. 1502)
48. d (pp. 1502-1503)
49. *Possible answers:* Signs of congestive heart failure; activity restrictions and/or guidance; nutritional guidelines; medications (p. 1503)
50. c (p. 1503)
51. a (pp. 1503, 1504)
52. a (p. 1504)
53. b (pp. 1504, 1505)
54. d (p. 1505)
55. *Possible answers:* Tachypnea; bradycardia; laryngospasm; dysrhythmias; use of accessory muscles; skin color of the face; the child's tolerance of the procedure (p. 1505)
56. d (p. 1505)
57. a (p. 1505)
58. a (pp. 1505, 1506)
59. b (p. 1505)
60. d (p. 1506)
61. d (p. 1506)
62. d (p. 1506)
63. b (p. 1506)
64. c (p. 1506)
65. Hematologic—hemolysis, clotting abnormalities, renal tubular necrosis, anemia, hemorrhage, fat emboli, thromboemboli, and infection
    Cardiac—heart failure, low cardiac output syndrome, decreased peripheral perfusion, dysrhythmias, hypokalemia, and cardiac tamponade
    Pulmonary—atelectasis, pneumothorax, pulmonary edema, and pleural effusion.
    Neurologic—cerebral edema, brain damage, and seizure activity
    Other—Bacterial endocarditis, postpericardiotomy syndrome (pp. 1507-1508)
66. c (p. 1508)
67. b (p. 1510)
68. a (p. 1510)

69. a (p. 1511)
70. d (p. 1512)
71. d (p. 1512)
72. b (p. 1514)
73. c (p. 1515)
74. a (p. 1515)
75. c (p. 1516)
76. b (p. 1517)
77. c (p. 1518)
78. d (pp. 1518-1519)
79. c (p. 1520)
80. b (p. 1521)
81. a (p. 1522)
82. b (p. 1526)
83. c (p. 1525)
84. c (p. 1485)
85. a (p. 1486)
86. d (p. 1508)

CHAPTER 35

1. F, F, F, T, T, T, T, F, T, F, T, F, T, F, T, T (pp. 1531-1535)
2. c (p. 1537)
3. Inadequate production of RBCs or RBC components, increased destruction of RBCs, excessive loss of RBCs (p. 1535)
4. Decrease in the oxygen-carrying capacity of blood and consequently a reduction in the amount of oxygen available to the cells (p. 1537)
5. k, h, f, j, l, i, o, p, q, b, c, a, g, n, m, d, e (pp. 1532-1535, 1537, 1546, 1561)
6. b (p. 1537)
7. b (pp. 1538-1539)
8. c (p. 1540)
9. b (p. 1541)
10. a (p. 1542)
11. a (pp. 1544-1545)
12. b (p. 1544)
13. d (p. 1545)
14. a (p. 1546)
15. "This is a normally expected change and usually means that an adequate dosage of iron has been reached." (p. 1546)
16. b (p. 1546)
17. d (p. 1547)
18. c (p. 1547)
19. Dehydration; acidosis; hypoxia; temperature elevations (p. 1547)
20. b (pp. 1547-1549)
21. c (p. 1549)
22. d (p. 1550)
23. d (pp. 1552-1553)
24. a (pp. 1552, 1556)
25. d (p. 1558)
26. a (p. 1558)
27. Primary, or congenital; secondary, or acquired (p. 1560)
28. a. Bone marrow aspiration, which demonstrates the conversion of red bone marrow to yellow, fatty bone marrow
    b. Anemia; leukopenia; low platelet counts
    c. Immunosuppressive therapy; bone marrow transplant (p. 1560)

29. d (pp. 1560-1561)
30. d, e, a, b, c, g, f (p. 1562)
31. a (p. 1562)
32. a (p. 1563)
33. b (p. 1563)
34. d (pp.1564-1565)
35. a (p. 1566)
36. Idiopathic thrombocytopenic purpura (p. 1566)
37. d (p. 1566)
38. a (p. 1568)
39. Oral ulcerations; skin infections (p. 1568)
40. Nonthrombocytopenic purpura; arthritis; nephritis; and abdominal pain (p. 1569)
41. d (p. 1573)
42. Lymphadenopathy; hepatosplenomegaly; oral candidiasis; chronic or recurrent diarrhea; failure to thrive; developmental delay; parotitis (p. 1574)
43. Slowing growth of the virus; preventing complicating infections and cancers; promoting or restoring normal growth and development; improving quality of life and prolonging survival (p. 1575)
44. T, T, F, T, F (pp.1574-1575)
45. c (p. 1575)
46. c (p. 1577)
47. b (p. 1578)
48. ELISA and Western blot will be positive because of presence of maternal antibodies derived transplacentally. Maternal antibodies may persist in the infant up to 18 months of age. (p. 1574)
49. d (p. 1579)
50. a (p. 1579)
51. Thrombocytopenia, recurrent and chronic infections, eczema, malignancy (p. 1579)
52. c (pp. 1549-1550)
53. Plan preventive schedule of medication around the clock, *not* only when needed to prevent pain; prevent resistance to administration by reassurance to child and family that analgesics, including opioids, are medically indicated, that high doses may be needed, and that children rarely become addicted. (p. 1556)
54. d (p. 1552)
55. a (p. 1556)
56. Implement and carry out standard precautions to prevent the spread of virus, including the following: wear gloves when in contact with any body fluid, wash hands carefully, wear gowns, masks and eye protection, use needle precautions and precautions with trash and linen. Instruct family in appropriate precautions. Clarify any misconceptions about communicability of virus among the family and community. Assess home situation and implement protective measures. Place restrictions on behaviors and contact for affected children who bite or who do not have control of their bodily secretions. (p. 1577)
57. Cindy will experience minimized risk for infection; will not spread disease to others; will receive optimum nourishment; will participate in family activities and peer-group activities; will exhibit minimal or no evidence of pain or irritability; and will exhibit safe, healthy expressions of sexuality. Family will receive adequate support and will be able to meet needs of the infant. (pp. 1577-1578)

CHAPTER 36

1. e (p. 1585), i (p. 1586), g (p. 1586), a (p. 1583), h (p. 1586), b (p. 1584), c (p. 1584), f (p. 1585), d (p. 1584)
2. o (p. 1594), f (p. 1586), t (p. 1594), n (p. 1594), b (p. 1586), g (p. 1587), d (p. 1586), h (p. 1592), a (p. 1588), i (p. 1592), c (p. 1586), j (p. 1592), e (p. 1586), k (p. 1592), p (p. 1594), r (p. 1594), v (p. 1594), l (p. 1592), x (p. 1594), m (p. 1592), w (p. 1594), q (p. 1594), y (p. 1595), s (p. 1594), u (p. 1594)
3. g, f, e, d, c, b, a (p. 1595)
4. c (p. 1596), f (p. 1600), e (p. 1600), a (p. 1596), d (p. 1599), b (p. 1596)

5. t (p. 1618), c (p. 1612), e (p. 1612), u (p. 1618), g (p. 1630), a (p. 1610), d (p. 1612), b (p. 1612), i (p. 1615), f (p. 1614), k (p. 1615), l (p. 1618), h (p. 1615), m (p. 1617), j (p. 1615), n (p. 1617), v (p. 1626), o (p. 1617), w (p. 1630), p (p. 1617), x (p. 1630), q (p. 1617), y (p. 1631), r (p. 1617), aa (p. 1631), s (p. 1618), z (p. 1631)

6. c (p. 1583)

7. a (p. 1584)

8. b (p. 1585)

9. d (p. 1586)

10. b (p. 1586)

11. c (p. 1587)

12. c, a, d, b, e (pp. 1587-1591; Table 36-2)

13. a (p. 1593)

14. Gastrointestinal tract—nausea and vomiting; give antiemetic around the clock
    Skin—alopecia; introduce idea of wig; stress necessity of scalp hygiene
    Head—xerostomia (dry mouth); stress oral hygiene and liquid diet
    Urinary bladder—cystitis; encourage liberal fluid intake and frequent voiding (p. 1593; Table 36-3)

15. b (p. 1594)

16. *Possible answers:* Unusual mass or swelling; unexplained paleness and loss of energy; sudden tendency to bruise; persistent, localized pain or limping; prolonged, unexplained fever or illness; frequent headaches, often with vomiting; sudden eye or vision changes; excessive, rapid weight loss (p. 1595; Box 36-1)

17. Colony-stimulating factor (p. 1596)

18. c (p. 1597)

19. a (p. 1599)

20. *Possible answers:* Liberal oral and/or parenteral fluid intake; frequent voiding immediately after feeling the urge, including immediately before bed and after arising; administration of drug early in the day to allow for sufficient fluid and frequent voiding; administration of mesna, a drug that inhibits the urotoxicity of cyclophosphamide and ifosfamide (p. 1600)

21. d (p. 1600)

22. a (p. 1601)

23. d (p. 1602)

24. d (p. 1603)

25. c (p. 1603)

26. d (p. 1612)

27. *Possible answers:* Anemia, infection, and bleeding (p. 1610)

28. b (pp. 1611-1612; Table 36-4)

29. b (p. 1613)

30. c (p. 1612; Table 36-4)

31. c (p. 1612)

32. b (p. 1614)

33. d (p. 1614)

34. a (p. 1614)

35. b (p. 1614; Box 36-3)

36. d (p. 1615)

37. c (p. 1616)

38. b (p. 1616)

39. b (p. 1617)

40. e, c, d, b, a (p. 1618; Box 36-5)

41. d (p. 1618)

42. d (p. 1619; Table 36-5)

43. *Possible answers:* Braid the hair if it is long; then cut it and save the braid. Show child how he/she looks at each stage of the process. Give the child a cap or scarf to wear. Ensure privacy during the procedure. Emphasize that the hair will begin to grow back after surgery. Introduce the idea of wearing a wig. (p. 1620)

44. d (p. 1621)

45. c (p. 1621)

46. a (p. 1623)
47. c (p. 1624)
48. d (p. 1625)
49. b (p. 1626)
50. c (p. 1628)
51. d (p. 1629)
52. d (p. 1629)
53. a (p. 1630)
54. b (p. 1632)
55. b (p. 1633)
56. c (p. 1633)
57. c (p. 1604)
58. d (p. 1606)
59. b (p. 1607)
60. a (pp. 1607, 1608)

CHAPTER 37

1. r (p. 1641), j (p. 1640), c (p. 1641), l (p. 1640), e (p. 1640), n (p. 1641), g (p. 1640), s (p. 1641), h (p. 1640), b (p. 1639), i (p. 1640), f (p. 1640), k (p. 1640), m (p. 1640), t (p. 1641), o (p. 1641), d (p. 1640), p (p. 1641), a (p. 1639), q (p. 1641)
2. b (p. 1646), d (p. 1645), a (p. 1646), f (p. 1645), l (p. 1647), e (p. 1645), h (p. 1645), c (p. 1646), n (p. 1650), i (p. 1646), r (p. 1651), j (p. 1647), t (p. 1647), m (p. 1647), o (p. 1650), k (p. 1647), p (p. 1647), g (p. 1645), q (p. 1651), s (p. 1651)
3. k (p. 1665), c (p. 1663), a (p. 1663), q (p. 1668), o (p. 1666), m (p. 1665), i (p. 1664), e (p. 1663), b (p. 1663), r (p. 1668), n (p. 1665), f (p. 1663), d (p. 1663), g (pp. 1663-1664), s (p. 1668), h (p. 1664), l (p. 1665), j (p. 1664), p (p. 1666)
4. i (p. 1676), b (p. 1674), j (p. 1681), d (p. 1675), c (p. 1681), e (p. 1675), g (p. 1675), a (p. 1674), h (p. 1676), f (p. 1675)
5. b, f, l, g, k, c, i, e, d, h, j, a (p. 1642; Table 37-1)
6. a (p. 1640)
7. b (p. 1683), i (p. 1684), a (p. 1682), k (p. 1685), s (p. 1685), p (p. 1685), m (p. 1683), f (p. 1684), h (p. 1684), dd (p. 1690), c (p. 1683), d (p. 1684), e (p. 1684), j (p. 1683), l (p. 1683), n (p. 1684), r (p. 1685), t (p. 1685), v (p. 1690), g (p. 1684), w (p. 1686), cc (p. 1690), q (p. 1685), x (p. 1686), bb (p. 1689), u (p. 1690), z (p. 1687), aa (p. 1687), o (p. 1685) , y (p. 1687)
8. d (p. 1643)
9. c (p. 1643; Table 37-1)
10. b (p. 1645)
11. Function of the cerebral cortex is permanently lost; eyes follow objects only by reflex or when attracted to the direction of loud sounds; all four limbs are spastic but can withdraw from painful stimuli; hands show reflexive grasping and groping; the face can grimace; some food may be swallowed; the child may groan or cry but utters no words (p. 1646; Box 37-4)
12. a (p. 1647)
13. d (p. 1647)
14. c (p. 1649)
15. c (p. 1650)
16. c (p. 1650)
17. a (p. 1651; Table 37-2)
18. c (p. 1651; Table 37-2)
19. b (pp. 1652, 1653)
20. d (p. 1653)
21. b (p. 1654)
22. c (p. 1656)
23. a (p. 1656)
24. d (p. 1658)
25. a (p. 1663)

26. c (p. 1663)
27. c (p. 1664)
28. a (p. 1665)
29. b (p. 1666; Table 37-4)
30. c (p. 1667)
31. a (p. 1669)
32. b (p. 1668; Box 37-6)
33. d (p. 1670)
34. d (p. 1671)
35. Inadequate supervision, the child's natural sense of indestructibility, and the child's need to explore (p. 1672)
36. a (p. 1673)
37. d (p. 1674)
38. c (p. 1675)
39. a (p. 1675)
40. b (p. 1676)
41. b (p. 1678)
42. d (p. 1679)
43. a (p. 1679)
44. a (p. 1680)
45. b (p. 1681)
46. c (p. 1681)
47. a (p. 1681)
48. b (p. 1682)
49. Birth injuries and acute infections (p. 1683)
50. a (p. 1685; Table 37-7)
51. c (p. 1687)
52. b (p. 1686)
53. a (p. 1687)
54. d (p. 1687)
55. c (p. 1688)
56. a (p. 1688)
57. a (p. 1690)
58. d (p. 1690)
59. c (p. 1693)
60. d (p. 1693)
61. b (p.1692)
62. c (pp. 1693-1694)
63. a (p. 1696)
64. d (p.1697)
65. c (p. 1698)
66. d (p. 1784)
67. b (pp. 1660-1662)
68. c (pp. 1660-1662)
69. b (pp. 1660-1662)

CHAPTER 38

1. g (p. 1702), e (p. 1702), a (p. 1701), n (p. 1703), h (p. 1702), c (p. 1701), k (p. 1703), f (p. 1702), i (p. 1702), b (p. 1701), j (p. 1703), l (p. 1703), d (p. 1703), m (p. 1703)
2. j (p. 1712), q (p. 1713), c (p. 1708), m (pp. 1714, 1715), e (p. 1710), o (p. 1713), f (p. 1715), h (p. 1712), a (p. 1707), i (p. 1712), d (p. 1710), k (p. 1713), g (p. 1711), l (p. 1712), n (p. 1713), p (p. 1713), b (p. 1707)

3. u (p. 1727), b (p. 1715), d (p. 1716), c (p. 1715), e (p. 1717), g (p. 1720), f (p. 1719), o (p. 1722), l (p. 1721), m (p. 1721), h (pp. 1722, 1723), j (p. 1721), q (p. 1723), i (p. 1721), k (p. 1721), n (p. 1721), p (p. 1722), r (p. 1723), s (p. 1727), a (p. 1715), t (p. 1727)

4. j (p. 1732), c (p. 1731), g (p. 1732), b (p. 1731), q (p. 1733), d (p. 1731), m (p. 1732), n (p. 1733), f (pp. 1730, 1732), i (p. 1732), e (p. 1731), k (p. 1732), w (p. 1734), a (p. 1731), p (p. 1733), h (p. 1732), t (p. 1733), l (p. 1732), v (p. 1734), s (p. 1733), o (p. 1733), r (p. 1733), u (p. 1734)

5. c (p. 1735), b (p. 1735), d (p. 1736), a (p. 1735), f (p. 1736), e (p. 1738), m (p. 1747), h (p. 1739), j (p. 1745), g (p. 1739), i (p. 1741), l (p. 1747), k (p. 1745)

6. Target tissues:
   a. Thyroid gland
   b. Ovaries, testes
   c. Bones
   d. Gonads
   e. Skin
   f. Adrenal cortex
   g. Renal tubules
   h. Ovaries, testes
   i. Uterus, breasts
   j. Ovaries, breasts
   Hormone's effect: g, c, f, h, a, j, e, i, d, b (pp. 1703, 1705, 1706)

7. Tropic (p. 1702)

8. h, e, j, f, b, g, c, k, d, i, a (pp. 1705-1706; Table 38-1)

9. c (p. 1707)

10. d (p. 1708)

11. c (p. 1709)

12. a (p. 1710)

13. c (p. 1712)

14. c (p. 1710)

15. Acromegaly results from hypersecretion of growth hormone that occurs after epiphyseal closure. Hyperfunction of the pituitary that occurs before the epiphyseal closure is not considered acromegaly. (p. 1711)

16. c (p. 1713)

17. b (p. 1714)

18. c (p. 1714)

19. a (p. 1716)

20. d (p. 1717)

21. c (p. 1719)

22. c (p. 1720)

23. b (p. 1720)

24. a (p. 1722)

25. b (p. 1723)

26. d (pp. 1724, 1726; Table 38-3)

27. b (p. 1727)

28. a (p. 1729)

29. c (p. 1730)

30. d (pp. 1731, 1732; Table 38-4)

31. d (p. 1731)

32. a (p. 1734)

33. c (p. 1734)

34. To maintain near-normal blood glucose values while avoiding too frequent episodes of hypoglycemia (p. 1734)

35. b (p. 1736)

36. c (p. 1737)

37. 10 to 15 g of simple carbohydrate; for example, a sugar cube, 8 ounces of milk, fruit juice, Insta-glucose, carbonated sugar drinks, sherbet, gelatin, cottage cheese, cake icing, Life Savers, Charms (p. 1738)

38. c (p. 1739)
39. c (p. 1739)
40. a (p. 1740)
41. d (p. 1741)
42. c (p. 1742)
43. d (p. 1743)
44. a (p. 1744)
45. c (p. 1745)
46. b (p. 1746)
47. d (p. 1747)
48. b (p. 1748)
49. *Possible answers:* Feelings of guilt as with any chronic disease; overprotectiveness, neglect, fear of the unknown; may block feelings that give pain; may feel threatened by independent development; may feel left out (p. 1749)
50. b (p. 1751)
51. c (p. 1751)
52. c (p. 1752)
53. d (p. 1752)

CHAPTER 39

1. Motor vehicle accidents; fires/burns; drowning; falls; bicycle injuries; firearm injuries; sports injuries; poisonings (p. 1756)
2. b (pp. 1756-1757)
3. b (p. 1758)
4. The cervical spine is immobilized by holding the head in a neutral position and not allowing movement of the head or body in any direction. (p. 1758)
5. a (p. 1760)
6. Orthostatic hypotension; increased workload of the heart; thrombus formation (p. 1761)
7. Numbness, tingling, changes in sensation, and loss of motion (p. 1764)
8. a (pp. 1766-1767)
9. Orthotics; prosthetics (p. 1771)
10. a (p. 1768)
11. c (pp. 1772-1773)
12. Financial strains decrease or eliminate family resources; focus of attention is placed on the affected child and other family member's needs may not be met; family members may have difficulty accepting child's altered body image; family members may be unable to express feelings and may have difficulty coping with crises; parents often experience guilt and have the perception of failing to protect the child. (p. 1765)
13. d (pp. 1777-1780)
14. b (p. 1779)
15. h, a, d, e, b, c, f, o, p, j, i, r, n, l, m, k, g, q (pp. 1761, 1774, 1776, 1777)
16. Pain, pallor, pulselessness, paresthesia, and paralysis (p. 1778)
17. b (p. 1779)
18. To regain alignment and length of the bony fragments by reduction; to retain alignment and length by immobilization; to restore function to the injured parts; to prevent further injury (p. 1779)
19. d (p. 1784)
20. c (p. 1785)
21. c (pp. 1784, 1791)
22. To fatigue the involved muscle and reduce muscle spasm so that bones can be realigned; to position the distal and proximal bone ends in desired realignment to promote satisfactory bone healing; to immobilize the fracture site until realignment has been achieved and sufficient healing has taken place to permit casting or splinting (p. 1786)
23. b (p. 1789)
24. a (p. 1790)

25. b (p. 1792)
26. b (p. 1793)
27. l, j, k, a, b, n, d, c, e, f, m, i, h, g (pp. 1786-1788, 1790, 1792)
28. c (p. 1793)
29. c (p. 1793)
30. a (p. 1794)
31. c, a, e, b, d (pp. 1796-1797)
32. d (p. 1797)
33. a (p. 1798)
34. Ligaments; epiphysis; growth plate (p. 1798)
35. T, T, F, T, T, F, F, T, F, T, T, T, F, T, T (pp. 1798-1803)
36. b (p. 1800)
37. a (p. 1803)
38. a (p. 1805)
39. d (p. 1805)
40. a (pp. 1806-1807)
41. Lordosis; kyphosis; spondylolisthesis (pp. 1807-1808)
42. d (p. 1808)
43. Realignment and straightening with internal fixation and instrumentation, along with bony fusion of the realigned spine (p. 1810)
44. b (p. 1809)
45. a (p. 1812)
46. a (p. 1815)
47. b (p. 1816)
48. d (p. 1816)
49. b (pp. 1816-1817)
50. d (pp. 1817-1818)
51. a (pp. 1819-1820)
52. NSAIDs: Take with food; be aware of potential for gastrointestinal, renal, hepatic, and reduced clotting side effects.
    Diet: Eat a well-balanced diet without exceeding caloric expenditure and maintain appropriate weight on corticosteroids.
    Sun exposure: Avoid excessive exposure; use sunscreen, hat, and protective clothing; schedule outdoor activities in morning and evening.
    Birth control medications: Take low-dose estrogen or progesterone only. (pp. 1826-1827)
53. To minimize disease activity with appropriate medications; to help child and family cope with the complications of the disease and treatment (p. 1826)
54. Corticosteroids (p. 1826)
55. Fostering adaptation and self-advocacy skills (p. 1827)
56. d (p. 1819)
57. c (pp. 1819-1820)
58. a (p. 1822)
59. c (p. 1823)
60. Liver enzymes and complete blood count with differential and platelet counts (p. 1820)
61. A well-balanced diet without problems of weight control often resulting from potential for more than body requirements related to decreased mobility (p. 1821)

CHAPTER 40

1. T, F, T, F, T, T, T, T (p. 1831)
2. d, e, c, b, a (p. 1832)
3. a (p. 1833)
4. b (p. 1836)
5. f, e, d, c, a, g, b, i, j, k, h (p. 1833)
6. a (p. 1834)

7. d (p. 1835)

8. d (p. 1835)

9. b (p. 1836)

10. c (p. 1841)

11. Electromyography (p. 1841)

12. a (p. 1844)

13. c (p. 1844)

14. a. Proximal muscle weakness, especially of the lower limbs and muscular atrophy

   b. Management is primarily symptomatic and supportive and related to maintaining mobility as long as possible, preventing complications, and providing child and family support. (pp. 1844-1845)

15. c (p. 1845)

16. b (p. 1845)

17. a (p. 1845)

18. Progressive stiffness and tenderness of the muscles in the neck and jaw, with difficulty opening the mouth and spasms of facial muscles (p. 1847)

19. a. Spores are found in soil, dust, and the intestinal tracts of humans and animals, especially herbivorous animals; they are most prevalent in rural areas but readily carried to urban areas by wind.

   b. Incubation period is 3 days to 3 weeks. (p. 1846)

20. b (p. 1846)

21. d (p. 1846)

22. d (pp. 1847-1848)

23. a (p. 1848)

24. b (p. 1848)

25. History, physical examination, and laboratory detection of toxin or the organism in the patient or the food (p. 1849)

26. d (p. 1848)

27. a (pp. 1849-1850)

28. c (p. 1854)

29. b (p. 1855)

30. The paraplegic patient who has function down to and including the quadriceps muscle or who has muscle function below the L3 level will have little difficulty in learning to walk with or without braces and crutches. (p. 1855)

31. a (p. 1856)

32. May enable the child to sit, stand, and walk with the aid of crutches, a walker, etc.; can be used to elicit grasp and release from the hand; helps cardiovascular conditioning; decreases pressure ulcers and increases blood flow; helps to reduce complications due to bladder and bowel incontinence, as well as assisting males in achieving penile erection (p. 1856)

33. d (p. 1858)

34. b (p. 1860)

35. b (p. 1861)

36. c, b, a, b, c, a (pp. 1861-1862)

37. Contractures, disuse atrophy, infections, obesity, and cardiopulmonary problems (p. 1836)

38. c (p. 1864)

39. c (p. 1864)

40. d (pp. 1834-1835)

41. b (p. 1842)

42. d (pp. 1842-1843)

43. Kevin will acquire mobility within personal capabilities; acquire communication skills or use appropriate assistive devices; engage in self-help activities; receive appropriate education; develop a positive self-image; receive appropriate nutrition and feeding assistance. The family members will receive appropriate education and support in their efforts to meet Kevin's needs. Kevin will receive appropriate care if hospitalized or in the community. (pp. 1842-1843)

44. c (p. 1841)

Notes

Notes

Notes

Notes

Notes

Notes

Notes